DISCOVER
YOUR
MENOPAUSE
TYPE

JOSEPH COLLINS, N.D.

Previously published as
WHAT'S YOUR MENOPAUSE TYPE?

PRIMA PUBLISHING

To the women in my family:

My wife, Ann E. Collins; my mother, Frances Collins-Eiferman; my sisters, Frances, Theresa, and Geraldine; and in memory of Ann's mother, Alphonsine Boucher.

Published by Prima Publishing, Roseville, California. Member of the Crown Publishing Group, a division of Random House, Inc. Previously published in hardcover in 2000 in slightly different form by Prima Publishing as *What's Your Menopause Type?*

PRIMA PUBLISHING and colophon are trademarks of Random House, Inc., registered with the United States Patent and Trademark Office.

Menopause Type® is a registered trademark of YourMenopauseType.com, Inc.

Disclaimer
This book is intended to provide general information about its subject. It is not intended to provide medical advice and should not be used as a guide to any treatment. As with other medical conditions, specific questions and concerns about menopause as it relates to any individual are matters that should be discussed with a doctor or other health care professional.

Library of Congress Cataloging-in-Publication Data

Collins, Joseph
    Discover your menopause type : the exciting new program that identifies the 12 unique menopause types and the best choices for you / Joseph Collins.
    p. cm.
  Includes bibliographical information and index.
  ISBN 0-7615-1815-0
  ISBN 0-7615-3749-X (pbk.)
    1. Menopause—Complications—Prevention. 2. Middle aged women—health and hygiene. I. Title.

RG186.V623 1999
618.1'75—dc21   99-15127
                                     CIP

02 03 04 05 06 HH 10 9 8 7 6 5 4 3 2 1

Printed in the United States of America

First Paperback Edition

Visit us online at www.primapublishing.com

CONTENTS

FOREWORD

As a woman and a physician, I have focused my practice and passion for many years on women's health issues. As cofounder and acting medical director of a unique, integrated clinic in Fort Collins, Colorado, I am part of a team that incorporates numerous modalities when working with patients. Because of this I have had the opportunity to assist many women through various transitions in their lives.

Menopause is a normal transition all women must experience, but it is a unique experience for each woman. Just as pregnancy or birth may be drastically different between two women, so will the menopausal journey. Menopause marks the beginning of the second half of life. I like to refer to these years as the wisdom years—when all of a woman's life experiences come together—and with the knowledge she gains, she may serve herself, as well as others, better.

One of the most disturbing things I encounter in medicine is people being treated as protocols. Menopausal women have been treated per protocol for years—as if all women are the same. There has been little consideration as to how each woman differs in terms of bone and heart risks, diet, lifestyle, need for supplements, and finally her personal hormonal levels. As each woman enters menopause, she should be individually supported, medically evaluated, and given the appropriate advice tailored to her particular needs.

In 1998, over 22 million prescriptions were written in the U.S. for Premarin alone, yet Gallop polls show only 34 percent of women are taking their hormone-replacement therapy (HRT) and 58 percent never fill their prescriptions. This is because women were either not satisfied with their evaluation and treatment, or they were leery of the side effects and/or risks from the synthetic hormones prescribed.

If practitioners really want to assist women in this transition and decrease cardiac and bone risks, as well as discomfort related to menopause, we must do a better job of individualizing treatment. In this book, Dr. Joseph Collins has written a thorough and concise reference on how to approach this unique transition. He clearly addresses the complexity and variations of menopause and discusses how to appropriately evaluate and treat menopause on an individual basis. An excellent addition to this book is the complete questionnaire Dr. Collins has created to assist in this process. This book provides a wealth of information and is a wonderful guide for both patients and practitioners. I truly hope you enjoy it.

Jacqueline C. Fields, M.D.

PREFACE

As a man, I can never truly know what it feels like to experience menopause. As a physician, I can observe how each woman experiences menopause differently, and I can be motivated to treat each woman as a unique individual. As a researcher, I can see many questions still unanswered, but am often encouraged by the growing amount of research taking place. As a writer and teacher, I can recognize the need for honest, balanced teaching and be inspired by the opportunity to provide such teaching. And, as a man, I may experience andropause (the "male menopause"), but I will never experience menopause the way women do. Yet I am still drawn to discover the most subtle truths of this passage in women's lives.

My most personal understanding of menopause has come through the experiences of my wife—my closest friend and soul mate. Though I was already working with many women encountering menopause, and had already realized the benefits of balanced and individualized care, it was when my wife shared her experiences with me that I developed a heartfelt mission to change the way menopause is treated on a larger scale. I was motivated to write this book and teach everyone about the different types of menopause.

Although I would rather focus completely on the research and the cases that describe the menopause types, a brief overview of my personal history and experiences will shed light on what else has motivated the writing of this book. It will also reveal why I am such a strong proponent of balanced and individualized care.

Before I became a naturopathic physician, I worked as a registered nurse in various hospital settings. I was often puzzled to see women who were on estrogen coming into the intensive care units because of heart disease or complications from a broken hip. The estrogen was supposed to decrease the risk of heart disease and osteoporosis. I was concerned that they were not getting the right dose, or that something else was missing. Occasionally, I was able to talk a doctor into ordering tests to check hormone levels, and was able to see dosages adjusted so that the woman's hormones were in proper range. Most often, I was informed that the patient was on "the proper dose" and that was the end of the story. Over time, as doctors became more aware of hormones, some even tested for testosterone levels. But for the most part, we were still in the dark ages of women's health care.

When I began practicing as a licensed naturopathic physician, I developed a program of testing women for levels of the three major hormones: estrogen, progesterone, and testosterone. I found that an evaluation of all three hormones gave patients tremendous insight into their unique hormonal needs.

My approach was founded on one of the most basic philosophies of naturopathic medicine: Treat the patient, not the condition. I was able to see that there was no single "menopause condition." Each woman I worked with had unique and special needs to help her regain vitality and health. There was no single protocol or medical program that was successful for every woman. I treated women with hormonal imbalances due to less-than-ideal menopause the same way I treated all patients: as new and unique. I had no preconceived ideas about what they needed. Since I had not been indoctrinated into any camp that promotes "estrogen for all women," "progesterone for all women," or "testosterone for all women," I was free to treat all my patients as individuals. The naturopathic goal of restoring balance was the guiding force.

In recent years, my work has been heavily focused on providing clinical consultation and technical support to hundreds of physicians, pharmacists, and other health-care professionals. This is because I have been given the privilege and responsibility of working at diagnostic laboratories that provide salivary testing of hormones. I have overseen the development of these tests.

While maintaining a limited private practice, the lab work has allowed me to personally review and interpret thousands of hormone tests. Under my direction, testosterone has become a routine part of female hormone testing, and an evaluation of the progesterone to estrogen ratio has become standard as well.

Over the years, I have consulted with, and been inspired by, hundreds of physicians who embraced balance as the absolute goal, and who seriously and diligently changed their practices so that women routinely receive individual-ized care.

In the course of this work, I have dedicated a significant amount of time to analysis of hormone research, with a focus on salivary hormone assessment, including my personal study and interpretation of thousands of research papers. From this research and the information from the many lab tests, I have gained a unique understanding of the salivary hormone test. Through these studies, I have also confirmed a simple truth: there are many types of menopause.

I have incorporated my personal experience and re-search in physician educational guides, lectures, treatment protocols, and computerized interpretation of hormone tests. In this book, I present this experience and research to you, the reader. It is my sincere hope that this book will bring positive changes to women's health care, and particu-larly to your own personal care and well-being.

ACKNOWLEDGMENTS

The genesis of this book reaches back to the training I received at the National College of Naturopathic Medicine in Portland, Oregon. Thank you to the faculty and to my classmates. You have each revealed to me that practicing the art and science of medicine, while still honoring the uniqueness of each individual, is the very heart of healing. Your influence permeates this book.

I would like to acknowledge my father, Charles G. Collins, RN, MS, CS, and retired assistant professor. Thank you for so much, but particularly for teaching me to look beyond diagnostic codes and into the special needs of each patient. Those lessons comprise the very essence of my practice and of this book.

I would also like to thank the scientists that I have had the privilege of knowing over the years: Lindsay Hofman, Ph.D., DABCC; Patricia Kane, Ph.D.; Dennis Freer, Ph.D.; Martin Lee, Ph.D.; and Anna MacIntosh, Ph.D., N.D. Each of your work, and the work of others like you, is molding the foundation on which the scientific practice of medicine stands.

Thank you to the M.D.s, N.D.s, D.O.s, D.C.s, pharmacists, acupuncturists, nutritionists, nurses, and other health-care professionals who have attended my lectures over the years. You have each made my work pleasant and rewarding. Thank you to all the health-care professionals I have had the privilege of working with as a partner or consultant. You are each a credit to your profession. Special thanks to Aris Andy Campbell, N.D.; Richard C. Heitsch, M.D.; and Cambor Wade, nutritional consultant.

Thank you to the many women I have worked with over the years. You have each shared your suffering with grace, dignity, and patience. When I told each of you that the word "doctor" comes from the Latin word for "teacher" you listened patiently to my teaching, and have taught me in return.

Special thanks to the editorial staff at Prima Publishing: Julia McDonald, Susan Silva, Carol Poole, and especially Michelle McCormack who has transformed my original manuscript into the book you now hold in your hands. Thank you, Patricia Henshaw and the publicity team at Prima, for your help in bringing this book to the public. Thank you, Dr. Kerry Kamer, for your scientific edits and encouragement. Extra thanks to Dr. Steven Bratman—an accomplished author of numerous health books—for your scientific edits, for first encouraging me to write the manuscript, and for your guidance. Thank you Lara Owen—another accomplished author—who has significantly guided the development of this book.

Above all, my deepest gratitude and thanks to Ann, my wife. You have patiently encouraged me, shared your passage with me, and inspired the very substance of my work.

INTRODUCTION

This book will radically change your understanding of menopause. In these pages, you will find detailed and clear information about an entirely new way of looking at this crucial passage in a woman's life. This new way will identify and explain your unique set of symptoms and feelings, and enable you to create a personalized treatment that really works for you.

You will learn about the 12 menopause types and how to determine which of these is closest to your own experience. You will learn to analyze your own symptoms by using the Menopause Type Questionnaire. You'll find out how to test your own hormone levels by using your saliva.

Once you have determined your menopause type, you will learn about the right treatment for that type, and about all the available options in both conventional and natural medicine, so that you can make your own informed choice about the treatment that is right for you. This revolutionary new method will give you control over your symptoms and help you to have a healthy menopause.

We are in the midst of a revolution in women's health care. These are tumultuous and exciting times for improving women's health. New technological advances are making it possible for us to understand the intricacies and wonders of the female hormonal system in far greater depth. We can now measure hormone levels more accurately, using the simple and inexpensive method of saliva analysis. Researchers are working with physicians and pharmacists to develop the most effective hormone supplements and natural remedies.

As a result of the postwar baby boom, more women than ever are at menopausal age, and these women tend to have higher expectations for maintaining their health and vitality than women in previous generations. Women today want more quality in their lives, and expect to stay productive and engaged with the world for decades after experiencing menopause. Menopause is no longer viewed as a change that women must endure. We can finally recognize it for what it is: simply a change. As we embrace and accept changes in science, technology, and society, we are finally able to embrace, accept, and openly discuss this change that is a natural part of life.

Without a doubt, we live in an era of profound change. Concepts and ideas we once commonly believed to be medical facts we now recognize as myths that were based on incomplete information. To say "every woman needs estrogen replacement" is as outdated as saying "the world is flat." Given the rapidity of all these changes, it is not surprising that many people, medical professionals included, are not always fully informed about current knowledge regarding the most effective management of menopause.

In recent decades, women suffered from the indiscriminate dispensing of estrogen. Their doctors rarely tested their estrogen levels, but nonetheless prescribed significant dosages of this powerful hormone because the doctors were certain that every woman needed it. Of course, some women did very well on estrogen because they had a real need for the hormone. Unfortunately, many more women have been hurt by this indiscriminate use of estrogen.

Currently, there is tremendous zeal over the use of progesterone. The similarity between the current progesterone craze and the estrogen craze of years gone by is frightening. Success stories are embellished and widely circulated, while side effects and documented problems are ignored. And the next craze looks set to be testosterone which may, in its turn, be hyped as the hormone every woman needs.

Today's truth is this: There is no magic hormone or combination of hormones that can be indiscriminately used by all women. Each woman is an individual, and hormonal balance must be the ultimate goal for all women.

All three major hormones—estrogen, progesterone, and testosterone—need to be in balance in order for menopause to be a healthy transition, rather than a debilitating struggle. With what we now know, it is possible for us to achieve this goal. I look forward to sharing this information with you throughout this book.

CHAPTER ONE

Menopause
One Size Doesn't Fit All

Ellen was a 53-year-old woman who had always enjoyed good health. Active and fit, she took an interest in her health and tended to use herbal and homeopathic remedies to treat the few mild complaints that arose over the years. Accustomed to feeling good, she wasn't prepared for what happened during menopause.

"I feel so dull and lifeless," she told me. "Almost depressed." She noted that her libido had "completely disappeared." Physically, she felt more fatigued than she had in previous years, but the emotional changes were much harder on her.

When Pamela, 49, came to see me, she was at the opposite end of the emotional spectrum from Ellen. Where Ellen had been tired and depressed, Pamela was anxious and edgy. "I'm losing my mind," she said. "I'm always angry!" Pamela's distress made it obvious she was feeling something more extreme than just a passing mood. "Even my husband is getting on my nerves," she went on. "I just feel so irritable that I wind up pushing him away. It's not because I don't want to be with him, and there's nothing wrong with my sex drive."

Pamela was 49 years old when she came to see me. For 2 years prior to her visit, Pamela's periods had been increasingly irregular and recently had stopped altogether. Along with feeling angry and agitated, Pamela was having more frequent migraine headaches. She also had some trouble with acne and oily skin.

Debra, a 57-year-old patient, had an extremely uncomfortable array of symptoms after menopause, including vaginal dryness, fatigue, thinning skin, memory problems, decreased libido, decreasing breast size, and insomnia. When she came to see me, she was 6 years into menopause—and her symptoms had been getting a little worse every year.

> Pamela was anxious and edgy. "I'm losing my mind," she said. "I'm always angry!"

Then there was Amelia. She had a hysterectomy years prior, but her ovaries were still intact. She didn't have vaginal dryness, acne, or oily skin, nor did she complain of irritability, anxiety or agitation, depression, or dull moods. Her primary concern was fatigue and tiredness which she described as "a loss of vim and vigor." She said she had been to other doctors who checked her hormones and said they were fine, but they could find no answers. Amelia was not willing to write her symptoms off as part of growing old. "I'm only 46 years old, so it's too early for menopause. Even my lab tests say that's not the problem. I don't know what it is."

Contrary to what Amelia believed, her hormones were not fine. Also, age 46 is not too early for menopause, especially with a history of surgery. The hormone test had shown Amelia to have estrogen and progesterone levels within normal range—barely. There was no test run on her testosterone level. She was fortunate to still have adequate estrogen and progesterone years after her hysterectomy (many women will experience menopause at a much earlier age after a hysterectomy). But though adequate, her levels were not ideal. A saliva test confirmed estrogen and progesterone levels on the low end of normal and revealed testosterone levels below normal range.

According to the usual way of looking at it, Ellen, Pamela, Debra, and Amelia had the same problem. All four were experiencing some discomfort related to menopause, yet their experiences couldn't have been further apart.

In the years I have been working with menopausal women, I have found that no two women have shared exactly the same experience. Menopause has a surprisingly wide range of signs and symptoms. For some women, it's easy and comfortable. For others, it doesn't go so smoothly. Indeed, menopause doesn't seem to be a single condition at all.

Over time, I realized the obvious: Every woman's menopause is unique. However, I also noticed patterns. Certain signs and symptoms tend to go together.

It dawned on me that there are different *types* of menopause.

In recent years, I have interpreted the *hormone* profiles of thousands of women. I have read thousands of pages of medical journals and abstracts, and consulted with hundreds of physicians throughout the world. Through my research, it became clear that certain variations in a woman's hormone levels—that is, her menopause type—profoundly influence her health and comfort during and after menopause.

Since the 1960s, most doctors have focused primarily on one aspect of menopause: *estrogen* deficiency. As you probably know, during menopause your body's production of this important hormone fluctuates and drops. The conventional wisdom has been that menopause is primarily an "estrogen deficiency disease." Yet my research, and my patients, tell me it's not so simple. As I'll explain in chapter 2, some of Ellen's experiences are typical of an estrogen deficiency. But what about Pamela? Her symptoms indicate that something very different is going on in her body. As you'll see in chapter 2, Pamela's difficulties suggest that, for her, estrogen is *not* the problem.

NOT JUST AN ESTROGEN DEFICIENCY

Even in the 1940s, doctors often advised menopausal women to take extra estrogen to prevent osteoporosis. In 1966, the publication of *Feminine Forever*, by Robert A. Wilson, made estrogen widely popular. This book suggested that menopause, which Wilson saw as a tragic end to a woman's sexual life, could be avoided by taking estrogen. Larger numbers of women began to take estrogen after menopause. A number of health benefits emerged from this therapy. Estrogen effectively relieved hot flashes (also referred to as hot flushes) and other uncomfortable symptoms, and also may have provided some protection against osteoporosis and heart disease.[1]

In the mid-1970s, it became clear that taking estrogen by itself could be dangerous. Women who took estrogen had a much higher risk for cancer of the uterine lining (endometrium). As it turned out, the problem was that the estrogen wasn't being balanced by another important hormone: *progesterone*. In the natural course of things, estrogen and progesterone work together to orchestrate a woman's menstrual cycle. With the addition of progesterone (or another *progestogen*, a substance with similar effects) to the estrogen therapy, the risk for endometrial cancer went back down to normal. Today, the prescription for most women who take hormones after menopause is a combination of an estrogen and a progestogen.

> In the mid-1970s, it became clear that taking estrogen by itself could be dangerous.

Oddly enough, this important discovery didn't lead to a wider appreciation of hormones other than estrogen, at least among conventional medical professionals. If you read about menopause in recent medical books and journals, the main focus is still on estrogen. Yet we now know that estrogen therapy doesn't always relieve women's symptoms. Research has discovered a number of important ways that two other hormones contribute to a woman's health and well-being throughout her life (see table 1). Progesterone is one of these hormones. The other is *testosterone*. While it is well documented that changes in either hormone can contribute to menopausal discomfort, the tendency is still to overlook these two hormones and focus on estrogen when it comes to treating menopause.

PROGESTERONE AND TESTOSTERONE

Before menopause, a woman's ovaries produce estrogen, progesterone, and testosterone. Estrogen plays many critical roles throughout the body. It has an important effect on a woman's sexual and reproductive life. It also influences brain chemistry and maintains the health of the bones, heart, and other important tissues. Progesterone, an important hormone in the menstrual cycle, allows pregnancy to occur and affects bones, the heart and brain, and other tissues. Testosterone is best known as a male sex hormone, but women's bodies need it, too, for building tissue, influencing the mood and libido, and enhancing the function of the heart. During menopause, the ovaries begin to produce less of all three hormones. Eventually, other mechanisms in the body should take over the critical job of making these hormones, but the transition doesn't always go easily. Levels of all three hormones can fluctuate and drop.

My research has confirmed what my patients' widely varying symptoms first led me to suspect: many

TABLE 1

Menopause Redefined

The definitions of menopause have changed throughout the ages. In order to figure out the best way to treat menopause, we must redefine it.

The Era	The Definition	The Treatment
1940s–1960s	"Menopause is an estrogen deficiency condition."	Treat all women with estrogens. That's all they need.
1970s–1980s	"Menopause is an estrogen deficiency condition, but we are having problems treating it with estrogen only."	Treat all women with estrogen, but give a progestogen to control side effects of estrogen.
1990–1999	*Some say:* "Menopause is an estrogen deficiency condition, we are doing fine with the addition of a progestogen."	*Depending on whom you ask:* Continue treating all women with estrogen, and continue to give a progestogen.
	Others say: "Menopause is an estrogen and testosterone deficiency condition; progestogens are still a good idea though."	*Or:* Treat all women with both estrogen and testosterone, continue giving a progestogen.
	Still others say: "Menopause is actually a progesterone deficiency condition."	*Or:* Treat all women with progesterone. That's all they need.
2000	"Menopause is a transition that may show up in many different ways. There are actually 12 different menopause types."	Treat each woman according to her own menopause type. Treatment choices must also include lifestyle, nutrition, herbs, hormone precursors, and natural hormones.

menopausal symptoms are *not* caused by an imbalance in estrogen. Imbalances in either progesterone or testosterone—or both—are important factors as well. In other words, menopause is much more complicated than a deficiency in estrogen. It can be a deficiency in both estrogen and progesterone—with a normal level of testosterone. Or it can involve an adequate level of estrogen, but too little progesterone and too much testosterone. Once I began to think of it this way, it made absolute sense to me that women had such distinctly different experiences with menopause. In chapter 2, I describe the 12 different menopause types I discovered, and why each has unique symptoms.

> Menopause is much more complicated than a deficiency in estrogen.

Balance Is Everything

Ellen, whose story I told previously, had a complaint. She had read articles about progesterone and testosterone and their roles in menopause, but the articles seemed to lack balance. "For years we've been told, 'What every woman needs is estrogen,'" she said. "Now, all we're hearing is, 'What every woman needs is progesterone.' There's even someone out there saying, 'What every woman needs is a big dose of testosterone.'" Ellen had actually tried taking progesterone, and it made her feel worse. As it turned out, it was exactly the *wrong* thing for someone with her menopause type. She also knew that taking testosterone

could be a bad idea for a woman who wasn't actually deficient in it. "What every woman needs," Ellen declared,
"is to be treated as an individual!"

Ellen is absolutely right. There are no one-size-fits-
all treatments for menopause. And whenever you consider a treatment that will change your hormonal levels,
you should be aware that balance is the key to feeling
well. Hormones are powerful substances and need to be
treated with respect. Prior to considering any type of
hormone therapy, you should receive a complete evaluation from an experienced health-care professional. As I
explain in chapters 6–9, treatment for any menopause
type should be carefully designed to maintain a delicate
balance. In most cases, you'll need to have your hormone
levels monitored to make sure the treatment is promoting balance—not upsetting it.

AN IDEAL MENOPAUSE

The reason I wrote this book is that I believe menopause
can and should be an easy, smooth transition in a woman's life. For many women, menopause brings a new capacity for work, pleasure, health, and self-esteem. Many
women say they feel freer and more active once they no
longer are expending energy on a monthly period.

Through discovery of the different types of menopause, I learned that an ideal menopause is a reasonable
goal for most women. Once you know what type of hormonal imbalance you have, you and your health-care
practitioner can take steps to restore balance.

One of the frustrating things many menopausal women find is that a treatment that worked for a friend or relative doesn't work for them. In fact, it might make things worse. Understanding your menopause type is the key to making sure you get treatments that are appropriate for you, rather than for your sister, friend, or mother.

✿ IT'S NOT ALWAYS MISERABLE

One of my earliest experiences with ideal menopause involved a patient named Emily who had come to see me because I was treating her husband. She simply wanted a checkup. At 62, she spoke and walked with confidence and strength. Her mind was sharp and clear, and she did not have the thin dry skin I frequently see in women her age. Since the average age of menopause is about 52, I asked her when she had gone through menopause. She replied, "Well, I never went through menopause like my friends did. I quit having my monthly cycle, but had none of the symptoms."

In fact, she had had an ideal menopause. It went so smoothly that she scarcely noticed it happening.

Once you know which imbalance you have to begin with, there are many treatments that can help. In this book, I describe a wide range of effective treatments from conventional and alternative medicine, including hormone therapy, herbs, and nutrition. My hope is that, with these tools, you'll arrive at your own ideal hormonal balance, and sail through menopause feeling absolutely fine.

CHAPTER TWO

The 12 Types of Menopause

As we saw in chapter 1, the conventional approach to menopause focused almost exclusively on estrogen, ignoring the importance of a balance between estrogen and the two other hormones that also affect your health and comfort during and after menopause: progesterone and testosterone.

We'll see in this chapter that menopause isn't just an "estrogen deficiency disease," as it was once famously called. In fact, there are 12 menopause types. Each type is defined by a unique pattern of estrogen, testosterone, and progesterone levels emerging in menopause.

At the onset of menopause, a number of changes occur in a woman's body. Her ovaries begin to produce less estrogen, progesterone, and testosterone. Other systems in her body prepare to compensate. In an ideal menopause, these changes happen smoothly. Many women, however, don't experience the ideal. In a less-than-ideal menopause, a woman's body may not produce enough estrogen and/or progesterone. Her testosterone levels can end up being too high or too low. The result is 12 distinct menopause types, as shown in table 2, below.

WHAT CAUSES HORMONAL IMBALANCES DURING AND AFTER MENOPAUSE?

Menopause brings a significant change in the way your body manufactures estrogen, progesterone, and testosterone. Before menopause, your ovaries produce most of these hormones. During menopause, your ovaries' pro-

TABLE 2
The 12 Menopause Types

	Normal Testosterone	Low Testosterone	High Testosterone
Adequate Amounts of Both Estrogen and Progesterone	Type 1	Type 2	Type 3
Estrogen Deficiency	Type 4	Type 5	Type 6
Progesterone Deficiency	Type 7	Type 8	Type 9
Dual Deficiency of Both Estrogen and Progesterone	Type 10	Type 11	Type 12

duction of the three hormones can decrease considerably. Your body produces less estrogen and progesterone and you no longer go through the monthly cycle of ovulating and preparing for pregnancy. But since these hormones play many other roles in your health, you continue to need a certain amount of them all your life. In fact, if menopause goes smoothly, your postmenopausal hormone levels should be close to what they were in the first half of your monthly menstrual cycle.

Ideally, as you go through menopause, your levels of all three of these hormones remain sufficient to meet your needs. As your ovaries make less, other mechanisms in your body begin to produce more estrogen, progesterone, and testosterone to keep you adequately supplied. These other mechanisms primarily involve a process I call "adrenal recruitment" in which the adrenal glands are recruited to make increased amounts of precursors for the fluctuating hormones. These precursors, or "building blocks," are transformed into estrogen and testosterone by other tissues of the body such as the liver and adipose tissue (fat cells).

But if your menopause is less than ideal, your body can have a harder time adjusting to the changes and maintaining good levels of the three hormones. This means that menopause is a complex transition. For some women, like Debra in chapter 1, menopause involves hot flashes, insomnia, and other troublesome physical symptoms. For others, like Ellen, mood changes predominate. Pamela also had mood changes, but of a very different kind than Ellen's. Each woman's experience is unique.

The key to understanding—and treating—your own particular symptoms is to know which basic menopause type you have. Some menopause symptoms, such as depression, can be caused by very different hormonal imbalances. To know how to treat your symptoms, you have to know what your imbalance is, and how to correct it. If you are *not* having an ideal menopause, take heart.

For some women, menopause involves hot flashes, insomnia, and other troublesome physical symptoms. For others, mood changes predominate.

Once you know what your menopause type is, there are many effective ways to bring you closer to this ideal balance.

THE 1 2 MENOPAUSE TYPES

To follow, I describe the most typical, or classic, symptoms and health risks of each menopause type. Keep in mind, though, that I'm describing types, not individuals. Few women have every single symptom listed for their type!

As you read about these types, you may recognize some of your own menopause symptoms. But you can't generally determine your type just by reading the descriptions that follow. Chapter 3 will guide you through a questionnaire that can more reliably help you identify what menopause type you are. Chapter 4 will explain how you can use a simple, at-home saliva test to confirm

your hormone levels and your type, and chapter 5 will reveal more about your hormones and your health. Chapters 6 through 9 will discuss the 12 different menopause
types and show you how to restore balance in each type.

Type 1: Ideal Menopause

If you are lucky enough to have a Type 1 menopause, you
might find it hard to understand why your friends complain
about their menopausal symptoms. "What's the
big deal?" you might be tempted to say, since your
menopause is almost totally free of discomfort. Over the
course of a year or so, you simply stop menstruating. You
might never experience a hot flash, vaginal dryness, or
fatigue. In general, your experience of menopause is smooth
and virtually free of symptoms. And after the changes of
menopause are complete, you feel absolutely fine.

Some women with Type 1 menopause experience
very mild symptoms related to subtle changes or variations in hormonal levels. Chapter 6 describes some natural ways to keep this menopause type smooth and
maintain optimal health.

Type 2: Low Testosterone

In this type of menopause, your body is producing
enough estrogen and progesterone to meet your needs,
though your levels of both hormones might be at the low
end of the "normal" range. But your body is not making

enough testosterone. The result can be subtle, or quite intense. You might feel basically fine, but a little lacking in drive and confidence, or "vim and vigor," as Amelia said in chapter 1. Mild depression and fatigue can be signs of low testosterone levels. You may also feel some loss of libido, though probably not a complete lack of interest in sex.

It might not occur to you that these are signs of menopause and you might say, "I don't know what's wrong with me. I don't seem to have any problems with menopause—hardly any hot flashes, anyway—but I'm a bit tired and lethargic, and I keep procrastinating about things I used to love doing."

Type 2 menopause may include physical symptoms and risks. A testosterone deficiency can cause hot flashes, even when there are adequate levels of estrogen and progesterone. Testosterone deficiency can increase your risk for disorders of the vulva, such as lichen sclerosus, a condition in which the labia and vulva become thin and fragile. Low testosterone can cause your muscle tone to weaken, and is associated with wrinkles and sagging skin. And you are at a somewhat higher risk for osteoporosis, or chest pain due to spasms of the coronary arteries. You can read more about Type 2 menopause and its treatments in chapter 6.

Type 3: High Testosterone

Type 3 menopause, like the first two types, may be relatively easy. With adequate levels of both estrogen and progesterone, things can go fairly smoothly. But too high a level of testosterone can be a problem. While testosterone boosts your confidence, strength, and libido, too much of it can leave you feeling agitated and angry. This frustration can even lead to a kind of depression—not to be confused with Type 2 depression. Facial hair, oily skin, and acne are some of the other ways excess testosterone makes itself known (and unpopular!).

High testosterone levels have been linked to insulin resistance, a condition that interferes with your body's ability to regulate your blood sugar levels.

A more serious problem is that high testosterone can increase certain major health risks. High testosterone levels have been linked to insulin resistance, a condition that interferes with your body's ability to regulate your blood sugar levels. Insulin resistance can cause adult-onset diabetes, and can increase your risk for heart disease as well as cancer of the breast and uterine lining (endometrium). High testosterone levels are known to reduce blood levels of HDL ("good") cholesterol, which is another effect that can increase your risk for heart disease. Chapter 6 will discuss treatments for this type of menopause.

Type 4: Low Estrogen

With this type of menopause, your body doesn't produce enough estrogen. It could be that, because of stress or other factors, your adrenal glands aren't able to increase their production of "building blocks" for making estrogen as well as they should.

One common sign of this menopause type is hot flashes. (Actually, hot flashes can be produced by a number of hormonal imbalances, so they appear as a symptom in most of the 12 menopause types.) You may be mentally less sharp than usual, with decreased verbal skills. Many women with low estrogen levels complain that they have trouble remembering names. These problems can be frustrating. Low estrogen can also give rise to feelings of despair or depression. (Depression is a symptom that can arise for many reasons. As we'll see in chapter 4, it's important to confirm your menopause type by testing your hormonal levels before you choose a treatment for depression, since the wrong treatment might make you feel worse.)

Physically, a shortage of estrogen can show up as thinner skin; more wrinkles; reduction in breast size; stress incontinence ("wetting your pants" when you sneeze or cough); or irregular vaginal bleeding. Without enough estrogen to balance your testosterone level, you can develop oily skin and acne. Estrogen is also needed to keep the libido healthy, so you may also suffer from some loss of sexual desire. Finally, you may have a harder time doing precise work with your hands, such as the dexterity required for embroidery and other fine-motor tasks.

You probably already know that excess estrogen has been linked to certain cancers of the breast and uterus. But too *low* a level of estrogen can also cause serious health problems. As estrogen helps regulate your bone mass, a drop in your body's estrogen levels can increase your risk for osteoporosis. Estrogen is also protective against cardiovascular disease. Premenopausal women rarely suffer heart attacks. Further, too low a level of estrogen may promote the development of insulin resistance, which can contribute to diabetes, cancer, and heart disease. See chapter 7 for more about Type 4 menopause and how to bring it into balance.

Type 5: Low Estrogen, Low Testosterone

Although this type of menopause has many of the physical discomforts of Type 4, its most painful effects may be emotional. Low estrogen and low testosterone each affect a woman's mood; together, their effects can be devastating. Many women with Type 5 menopause feel dull, listless, or depressed. A characteristic sign is a lack of interest in things—or even people—of great importance in your life. Loved ones may be hurt or puzzled, not realizing that these emotional changes are signs of a hormonal imbalance. "It's as if she doesn't love me anymore" is a typical complaint of a husband whose wife has this type of menopause.

If you have Type 5 menopause, you may have trouble with your memory, or with learning new things. The deficiency in both estrogen and testosterone leaves your libido doubly diminished, and a thinning and drying of your vaginal walls can make intercourse painful. As with Type 4, stress incontinence can be a problem. A deficiency in both estrogen and testosterone can affect your skin and muscle tone, leading to premature sagging and wrinkles. The breast tissue can also shrink and begin to sag due to a loss of collagen. And you run the same health risks that come with Types 2 and 4: osteoporosis, cardio-vascular disease, and insulin resistance. See chapter 7 for more information about this type of menopause, and how to relieve it.

Type 6: Low Estrogen, High Testosterone

Women with Type 6 menopause can suffer from an awkward combination of agitation and fatigue. High testosterone levels can make you feel irritable, while low estrogen can make it hard for you to concentrate and remember names. A woman with this menopause type may have a strong libido, but feel too irritable to enjoy sexual intimacy. This type of menopause is also associated with sleep disturbance, a troublesome condition that can rob you of needed rest and leave you feeling even more tired and irritable by day. Type 6 menopause, like Type 3, involves an imbalanced testosterone to estrogen ratio. In Type 6, however, this imbalance is even more pronounced than in Type 3. In addition to oily skin and acne, it can cause a condition called "androgenic alopecia" (hair loss or even baldness).

> Treating your menopause type is not just taking hormones! Most menopause types may not need hormone replacement.

If you have Type 6 menopause, you face the greatest risk for insulin resistance, especially if your estrogen level is extremely low compared to your progesterone level. You also face all the health risks listed under Type 4. Chapter 7 will describe treatments that may be helpful for this type of menopause.

✑ TREATING YOUR MENOPAUSE TYPE

Treating your menopause type is not just taking hormones! Most menopause types may not need hormone replacement. In all cases, it should be the last thing to consider. In addition to proper *rest* and *exercise*, try the following:

1. Balance your nutrition and diet.

2. Start using herbs and consider homeopathy, if appropriate. Some menopause types may be responsive to glandulars (see chapter 13).

3. Consider hormone precursors (see chapter 14).

4. Finally, after trying the above steps, you may consider hormones.

Pay attention to antiandrogens, antiestrogens, and antiprogestogens (Chapter 10). Though they may be appropriate in some types, they should generally be avoided in most other types. Remember, hormone replacement works much better when part of a healthy lifestyle.

Type 7: Low Progesterone

Type 7's classic sign is anxiety. In the body, progesterone has a soothing effect on the nervous system. In fact, progesterone and its by-products can affect some of the same nervous system receptors that are affected by antianxiety drugs such as Valium and Xanax. Sometimes, when your progesterone levels fall too low, it can be almost as if you are withdrawing from one of these medications, the primary symptom of which is unusual irritability. A gnawing feeling of anxiety is enough to make anyone lose perspective. Since a progesterone deficiency has been associated with poor sleep, this menopause type has the added burden of inadequate rest at night.

Women with this menopause type can also suffer from pain and inflammation. This may show up as muscle aches or joint inflammation. Either way, these discomforts only worsen an already irritated nervous system.

A progesterone deficiency isn't good for your long-term health, either. When progesterone levels fall too low to balance out your estrogen, your risk for uterine (endometrial) and breast cancer increases. Low levels of progesterone also increase your risk for osteoporosis, since progesterone plays a role in bone formation. By lowering HDL ("good") cholesterol levels, low progesterone elevates your risk for cardiovascular disease.

See chapter 8 for treatments for this type of menopause.

Type 8: Low Progesterone, Low Testosterone

The symptoms of Type 8 menopause are similar to Type 7, but involve lower spirits and a greater tendency toward depression. The lack of libido, drive, and motivation that accompany low testosterone levels don't do anything to cheer up a woman who's already feeling anxious from a progesterone deficiency. Unlike the low-estrogen menopause types, this type doesn't involve memory problems or fuzzy thinking. But clear thinking isn't much comfort when you're anxious or achy.

A typical Type 8 complaint is, "I feel like my personality has taken a real downturn. I don't enjoy sex as much as I used to, I don't have the energy to do most of the things I've always loved doing, and my muscles ache. But I have plenty of energy for worrying. My kids are getting annoyed with me, because I keep phoning to see if they're okay. Nothing much seems to be wrong physically, but I just don't feel like myself." Women with this menopause type can also have trouble getting enough restful sleep.

This menopause type faces all the health risks associated with Type 7 and Type 2, plus episodes of hypoglycemia (low blood sugar) and hypoinsulinemia (or low blood insulin) if estrogen levels are too high. The low blood insulin and low blood sugar can increase feelings of fatigue and cause poor concentration. See chapter 8 for information about restoring balance in this type of menopause.

Type 9: Low Progesterone, High Testosterone

When you combine low-progesterone anxiety with high-testosterone testiness, the result isn't fun. If your menopause is Type 9, you may feel easily alarmed. Your loved ones may see you as overreacting to everything. With nerves so frayed, women with this menopause type often sleep poorly. Also, this menopause type can include episodes of sleep apnea (interruption of breathing for brief periods during sleep), which can cause further sleep disturbances. Naturally, lack of sleep doesn't improve anyone's mood.

This menopause type involves the highest risk for endometrial cancer, since both low progesterone and high testosterone contribute to this risk. You can also suffer from abnormal uterine bleeding, which can be irregular, prolonged, and quite profuse. This abnormal bleeding may begin in *perimenopause* (the years leading up to menopause), but can continue beyond the expected end of menses. Type 9 also includes the health risks listed under Types 2 and 7. In addition, you face an increased risk for hyperinsulinemia. Treatments for this type of menopause are discussed in chapter 8.

Type 10: Low Estrogen, Low Progesterone

This menopause type involves a profound lack of two important hormones in a woman's body: estrogen and progesterone.

Women with this menopause type may feel lacking in significant ways. Physically, a Type 10 menopause can include a wide array of the symptoms described for Types 4 and 7, such as hot flashes, vaginal dryness, fatigue, or poor sleep. Emotionally, you may struggle with depression, feelings of hopelessness and futility, and memory problems. Of all the types, this one is most likely to include some trouble with stress incontinence ("wetting your pants" when you laugh or sneeze). Oily skin and acne can also be a sign of a Type 10 imbalance, since the levels of estrogen and progesterone are not adequate to control the effects of testosterone.

The health risks associated with Type 10 menopause can be serious. Low levels of estrogen and progesterone have a doubly damaging affect on bones and blood cholesterol, greatly increasing your risk for osteoporosis and heart disease. Chapter 9 will discuss treatments for this type of menopause.

Type 11: Low Estrogen, Low Progesterone, Low Testosterone

Menopause is difficult enough when it involves deficiencies in both estrogen and progesterone, but when your testosterone level is low as well, you can feel deeply uncomfortable. Physically, you may be feeling hot flashes, vaginal dryness, lack of sexual desire, fatigue, or weakness. Even if you feel any desire to attempt sexual intercourse, the thinning and drying of the vaginal walls can make it too painful. Urinary incontinence can become quite a problem; you may find it hard to hold your urine even for a very short time. Mentally and emotionally, you may struggle with anxiety, depression, dullness, memory problems, and a feeling of apathy. You may feel easily tired, even while your other symptoms are making you work harder to get things done. You may have trouble sleeping. In general, you can suffer from a number of the symptoms described under Types 2, 4, and 7.

As with Type 10, this menopause type brings especially high health risks. Women with Type 11 menopause are also at risk for becoming insulin resistant and developing hyperinsulinemia. The risk for osteoporosis is especially high with this menopause type, since all three of these hormones play a role in protecting bones.

> Menopause is difficult enough when it involves deficiencies in both estrogen and progesterone. When your testosterone level is low as well, you can feel deeply uncomfortable.

If you have this type of menopause, you have probably depended on support from your family and friends; this really is about as tough as it gets! But remember that there are a number of treatments that can help. See chapter 9 for more details about natural and medical treatments.

Type 12: Low Estrogen, Low Progesterone, High Testosterone

Like Types 10 and 11, this menopause type can bring a profoundly disturbing sense of being out of balance. With a high testosterone level, you may tend to feel more agitated or frustrated. The combination of high testosterone with deficiencies in both female sex hormones can also lead to "masculinizing" effects, such as facial hair, shrinking breasts, and deepening of the voice. All of the symptoms discussed under Types 3, 4, and 7 can come into play here.

Women with this type of menopause almost always have insulin resistance, which if untreated, can increase the risk for endometrial cancer, breast cancer, non-insulin dependent diabetes, and heart disease. Type 12 menopause also involves a high risk for heart disease, but the high testosterone levels can reduce the risk for osteoporosis that comes with a dual deficiency in estrogen and progesterone.

In chapter 9, we'll see what you can do to remedy a Type 12 imbalance.

IDENTIFY YOUR MENOPAUSE TYPE

Recognizing that there are different types of menopause is the first step to redefining what menopause means for you. The next and most important step is identifying your particular menopause type.

Determining your menopause type will help you make decisions on the course of action you want to take, and help you understand why your symptoms and needs may be completely different from those of your relatives or friends. The coming chapters will introduce you to two tools to aid you in finding an answer to the question "What's your menopause type?" These tools are the Menopause Type Questionnaire and saliva hormone tests.

The Menopause Type Questionnaire (MTQ) provides you with a way to evaluate subjective *symptoms* associated with menopause, while the saliva hormone test is a means to evaluate objective *signs*. These two types of knowledge—subjective and objective—

are what experienced physicians and other health-care professionals use to guide them toward understanding the unique features of any health condition. Since menopause is a health condition involving unique changes that may require support and monitoring, it is important to evaluate these changes by systematically looking at both signs *and* symptoms. To understand this process, let's review a working definition of signs and symptoms.

Signs are objective and can be observed by the five senses. Rashes or other visible skin changes, lumps, or masses that can be felt, and heart and lung sounds that can be heard are all objective signs. X rays, EKG readouts, and laboratory tests also provide objective signs that can be used to understand a health condition. In the case of menopause, laboratory tests provide excellent objective information to evaluate menopause types. Since saliva tests that accurately measure hormone levels are now available, this information is within any woman's grasp.

Symptoms are subjective and are experienced and reported by the individual being questioned. Aches, pains, spasms, weakness, fatigue, and feelings of irritability or anxiety are all subjective. Hot flashes, vaginal dryness, and night sweats are mainly subjective, even though they may also be observed upon examination.

In the past, a doctor would determine what symptoms were present by asking the patient a series of questions. In the last few decades, physicians have begun to rely on questionnaires to help them collect more complete information. They routinely combine the answers from such questionnaires with results from laboratory tests to aid them in diagnosis (the word *diagnosis* literally means "complete knowledge"). This diagnosis defines the health condition and gives a foundation for treatment options.

In the last few decades, physicians have begun to rely on questionnaires to help them collect more complete information.

In chapter 3, you will find the Menopause Type Questionnaire, which enables women and their health-care providers to more accurately compile and evaluate the unique symptoms they are experiencing. Chapter 4 will introduce you to saliva hormone testing and reveal why this relatively new technology is rapidly becoming the lab test of choice for measuring estrogen, progesterone, and testosterone levels. Chapter 5 discusses how each of these hormones affects your health in specific ways.

CHAPTER THREE

What's Your Menopause Type?

A Questionnaire

Discovering your menopause type will help you make crucial decisions about what treatment you need. It will also help you understand why your symptoms and needs may be completely different from those of other women you know. This chapter takes you through a detailed questionnaire about your menopausal symptoms.

You may have taken a questionnaire like this before. Questionnaires have been used for decades to compile information about menopause and evaluate menopausal symptoms. In 1953, the Blatt-Kupperman menopausal index was introduced. This index has since been used throughout the world to evaluate both the initial severity of menopausal symptoms and the progress made by the use of various therapies. In 1994, a group of German,

Austrian, and Swiss experts improved on this test by creating a questionnaire called the Menopause Rating Scale (MRS). If you've taken a menopause questionnaire before, it was probably one of these two.

The questionnaire featured in this chapter, the Menopause Type Questionnaire (MTQ), is a new one, specifically designed to help determine what *type* of menopause you are experiencing. No other questionnaire has ever been designed to accomplish this.

HOW TO USE THIS QUESTIONNAIRE

While the MTQ can help you identify your menopause type, it is *not* designed to tell you how severe your symptoms are. Nor will it tell you whether your hot flashes have gotten better or worse if you repeat the questionnaire after several months of treatment. What the MTQ will show you is what group of symptoms you have, and what type of menopause is the underlying cause. This information allows you and your health-care provider to design treatment that is tailored to your specific needs.

> The Menopause Type Questionnaire is a new questionnaire, specifically designed to help determine what *type* of menopause you are experiencing.

IMPORTANT: All questions should be answered either "yes" or "no." If the answer is "yes," place a "1" in the space provided. If the answer is "no," leave the space blank.

When Do You Answer "Yes"?

Most of the questions on the MTQ actually involve multiple questions. For example, while a few questions pose a single query—"Are your hands or feet colder than usual?"—most include more than one—"Are you more irritable? Do you have more nervous tension?" The questions are posed this way to allow for variations in how different women might describe the same symptom.

⁢⁂ HISTORY OF MENOPAUSE QUESTIONNAIRES

Year	Questionnaire	About the Questionnaire
1953	Blatt-Kupperman Menopausal Index (BKMI)	First published questionnaire to help evaluate initial severity of menopause symptoms and the progress made through therapies.
1994	Menopause Rating Scale (MRS)	Expanded questionnaire. Now includes questions on libido, vaginal symptoms, and emotional/psychiatric symptoms.
2000*	Menopause Type Questionnaire (MTQ)	First questionnaire to identify a woman's specific menopause type.

*Menopause Type Questionnaire was first published in 2000. Design and use began in 1993.

When you encounter one of these plural questions, answer "yes" if you would say "yes" to any single one of the queries included. For example, in response to "Are you more irritable? Do you have more nervous tension?" you should say "yes" if you feel more irritable, even if you wouldn't really describe it as nervous tension.

A physician once asked a patient, "Do you ever get real hot and break out in a sweat?" to which the woman answered, "No." The physician concluded that she wasn't having hot flashes, and sent her home. But she actually was having episodes when she felt hot and flushed. That was why she went to the doctor. Unfortunately, the way he posed the question didn't fit her experience. She didn't feel "real hot," in her judgment, and she didn't break out in a sweat. In this case, it would have been helpful if her doctor had taken more time to ask her about her symptoms.

Keep this patient in mind when you answer the questionnaire, and answer "yes" if you recognize your experience in *any part* of a question. It's best to answer the questions simply, without trying to talk yourself out of anything. You are answering these questions for yourself first and foremost, so answer them as honestly as possible. Share your answers with your health-care professional or your partner when you are comfortable doing so.

THE MENOPAUSE TYPE QUESTIONNAIRE

Section A

1. Are you experiencing hot flashes or night sweats, or both? ____

2. Are you feeling more depressed? Are you more withdrawn or isolated? Do you feel periods of hopelessness? Do you feel apathetic? ____

3. Do you feel a loss of energy? Do you feel more fatigued? ____

4. Do you feel less receptive to sex? Do you feel less sensual? Do you feel that your sex drive has diminished? ____

5. Are you having increased vaginal pain, dryness, or itching? ____

6. Are you experiencing insomnia, difficulty falling to sleep, or difficulty staying asleep? ____

7. Are you having trouble with your memory? Are you having more trouble remembering names? Are you more forgetful? ____

8. Is your mood low, less upbeat, less positive, or less outgoing? Are you having less "good moods" and times of joy? Do you find yourself caring less about things that used to matter to you? ____

9. Are you having trouble controlling your urine? Do you have to go more often? Do you spill urine when you cough or sneeze? _____

10. Do you feel as if your perception is weakening, that it takes you longer to notice things? Are you having trouble thinking of the right word when speaking or writing? Do you feel your mental skills are diminishing? _____

Total for Section A: _____

Section B

1. Are you having more aches and pain? Are you starting to get arthritis? _____

2. Are you having more spotting or breakthrough bleeding? Have you been told you have dysfunctional uterine bleeding? _____

3. Do you seem to be getting more inflammations and swellings? _____

4. Are your allergies or asthma getting worse, or are you developing new allergies or asthma? _____

5. Do you seem to be having more twitches and spasms? _____

6. Are you experiencing times of mental fogginess, or trouble thinking clearly? _____

7. Are you having more mood swings? _____

8. Do you feel more fatigued? Are you more tired in the morning? _____

9. Are you more irritable? Do you have more nervous tension? _____

10. Are you experiencing more anxiety? Do you feel more anxious? _____

   Total for Section B: _____

Section C

1. Do you feel less motivated in general? Do you feel less assertive? _____

2. Has your libido lessened? Are you having fewer sexual fantasies or less desire? Are you less likely to become sexually aroused? Are you less pleased with sex? _____

3. Are you feeling less composed and in control? _____

4. Are you less energetic? _____

5. Are you anemic, or do you think you are anemic? _____

6. Are you feeling more irritable? _____

7. Do you have less muscle strength? Do you feel weaker? _____

8. Are you having more trouble with mental skills requiring logic and problem solving? Are you having trouble focusing and maintaining your attention? _____

9. Is your memory weakening? Are you having more trouble remembering things and events? _____

10. Do you feel more depressed? Is your mood low, less confident? Are you feeling frightened or afraid? _____

Total for Section C: _____

Section D

1. Are you noticing more wrinkles around your mouth and eyes? Is the skin tone on your arms, legs, or hands poor? Has the skin lost its firmness or fullness? _____

2. Do you feel more depressed? _____

3. Do you feel more fatigued in general? _____

4. Are you having more headaches? _____

5. Are you over 45 years old? _____

Total for Section D: _____

Section E

1. Does it seem as though your breasts are shrinking and sagging? _____

2. Are you experiencing more confusion? _____

3. Are you experiencing more morning fatigue? _____

4. Do you cry more easily or more often? _____

5. Are your hands or feet colder than usual? _____

Total for Section E: _____

Section F

1. Is your libido less than it used to be? ____

2. Is your pubic hair thinning? ____

3. Do you feel less motivated, less assertive, less confident? Have you lost your competitive edge? ____

4. Are you gaining more body fat? Do you feel less lean? ____

5. Are you having more lower back pain or hip pain? Do you feel more joint pain? Are you having more headaches? ____

Total for Section F: ____

Section G

1. Are you developing more facial hair (hirsutism)? ____

2. Is your voice changing and becoming deeper or more masculine? ____

3. Are you having trouble tolerating sugars and carbohydrates? ____

4. Are you developing or experiencing increased acne? ____

5. Do you feel more hostile, angry, agitated, or aggressive? ____

Total for Section G: ____

To determine your menopause type, there are a series of steps to follow. These steps involve a little math.

On the score sheet below, enter the total for each of your sections in the left-hand column marked "Section Totals." Then multiply each score by the specified numbers in each column to the right. You will notice some columns require more information than others.

After you have done the math, add up the figures in each of the numbered columns. Write each column's total in the bottom row, marked "Totals."

Section Totals	Column 1	Column 2	Column 3	Column 4	Column 5
A =	A × 4 =		A × 2 =		
B =		B × 5 =	B × 2 =		
C =				C × 5 =	
D =	D × 4 =	D × 5 =	D × 6 =	D × 5 =	
E =	E × 4 =	E × 5 =	E × 6 =		
F =	F × 4 =			F × 5 =	
G =					G × 20 =
TOTALS					

You will now compare the column totals to each other as the next step in identifying what menopause type you have.

You first want to determine which group your menopause type fits into: A = Adequate, D = Dual Deficient, P = Progesterone Deficient, and E = Estrogen Deficient. You will determine this using the numbers in columns 1, 2, and 3.

If the totals of columns 1, 2, and 3 are each less than 50, then enter "A" in the Group Box on page 42 (see sample below). If not, go to the next step. If *any* of columns 1, 2, or 3 are greater than 50, do not enter "A" in the Group Box.

Column 1 Less Than 50	Column 2 Less Than 50	Column 3 Less Than 50	Column 4	Column 5	A

Now you will compare the totals of columns 1 and 2 with the total of column 3.

If columns 1 and 2 are both less than column 3, enter "D" in the Group Box on page 42 (see sample below). If not, go to the next step. If either column 1 or column 2 is greater than column 3, do not enter a "D" in the box.

Column 1 Less Than Column 3	Column 2 Less Than Column 3	Column 3	Column 4	Column 5	D

Now you will compare the totals of columns 1 and 2.

If column 2 is less than column 1, enter "E" in the Group Box on page 42 (see sample below). If not, go to the next step.

Column 1	Column 2 Less Than Column 1	Column 3	Column 4	Column 5	E

If column 1 is less than column 2, enter "P" in the Group Box on page 42 (see sample below).

Column 1 Less Than Column 2	Column 2	Column 3	Column 4	Column 5	P

You now know which group your menopause type belongs to regarding estrogen and progesterone levels (A, D, P, or E). Next, you need to find out where you fit in terms of testosterone levels (H = High, L = Low, and N = Normal). You will determine this using the totals in columns 4 and 5.

If column 5 is greater than 50, enter "H" in the T Box on page 42 (see sample below).

Column 1	Column 2	Column 3	Column 4	Column 5 Greater Than 50	Type H

If column 4 is greater than 50 and column 5 is 50 or less, enter "L" in the T Box on page 42 (see sample below).

Column 1	Column 2	Column 3	Column 4 Greater Than 50	Column 5 Less Than 50	Type L

If columns 4 and 5 are both 50 or less, enter "N" in the T Box on page 42 (see sample below).

Column 1	Column 2	Column 3	Column 4 Less Than 50	Column 5 Less Than 50	Type N

You now have two letters which show your menopause type: one of A, D, P, or E; and one of H, L, or N. Enter your two letters in the boxes to the right.

GROUP BOX	T BOX

(A, D, P, or E)   (H, L, or N)

Match your two letters with those on the Menopause Type Chart below. You now know your menopause type according to subjective symptoms.

Menopause Type Chart

AN = Type 1	Adequate amounts of both estrogen and progesterone, with Normal Testosterone	Go to page 83
AL = Type 2	Adequate amounts of both estrogen and progesterone, with Low Testosterone	Go to page 87
AH = Type 3	Adequate amounts of both estrogen and progesterone, with High Testosterone	Go to page 96
EN = Type 4	Estrogen Deficiency, with Normal Testosterone	Go to page 104
EL = Type 5	Estrogen Deficiency, with Low Testosterone	Go to page 111
EH = Type 6	Estrogen Deficiency, with High Testosterone	Go to page 119
PN = Type 7	Progesterone Deficiency, with Normal Testosterone	Go to page 127
PL = Type 8	Progesterone Deficiency, with Low Testosterone	Go to page 133
PH = Type 9	Progesterone Deficiency, with High Testosterone	Go to page 139

DN = Type 10	**D**ual Deficiency of both Estrogen and Progesterone, with **N**ormal Testosterone	Go to page 149
DL = Type 11	**D**ual Deficiency of both Estrogen and Progesterone, with **L**ow Testosterone	Go to page 155
DH = Type 12	**D**ual Deficiency of both Estrogen and Progesterone, with **H**igh Testosterone	Go to page 162

An automated version of the Menopause Type Questionnaire can be found on the Internet at www .yourmenopausetype.com. Remember, this questionnaire only examines the subjective symptoms of menopause. It is not a replacement for primary care medical screening.

CHAPTER FOUR

Using Saliva Tests to Measure Your Hormone Levels

N ow that you've taken the Menopause Type Questionnaire, you can confirm your menopause type by testing your hormone levels. This chapter will tell you how to use an easy, painless saliva test to measure your levels of estrogen, progesterone, and testosterone.

A BETTER HORMONE TEST

When you think of hormone tests, what comes to mind? For many women, the words conjure up an image of needles, discomfort, and uninformative results. Too often in the past, a woman has undergone a blood test only to be assured that the results were "within normal limits" despite her signs and symptoms. The problem is that a woman's hormone levels may fall within a "normal" range, but still be less than optimal for her well-being.

To make things worse, until recently often the only hormone measured was es-

> Saliva testing is unique in that it measures the most active part of the hormone.

trogen. If a woman's estrogen levels were anywhere within the "normal" range, her doctor informed her that she was "normal." Testing typically didn't include her levels of progesterone and testosterone.

But times are changing. Through new technology, we are now able to assess hormonal levels by measuring the hormones that are detectable in your saliva. Saliva collection is simple. You can collect the saliva yourself in the privacy of your home, and it's not as invasive as blood drawing. I have found saliva testing to be an extremely useful tool in helping women identify their menopause types.

A TEST YOU CAN DO AT HOME

In the blood, most of the measurable hormones are bound to proteins that carry the hormone throughout the body. These individual proteins have specific names like albumin and sex-hormone-binding globulin, but collectively they are referred to as carrier proteins.[1] Though much of the estrogens, progesterone, and testosterone in circulation are bound to these carrier proteins, a small amount of these hormones is unbound. Saliva testing is unique in that it measures the unbound hormones. It is the unbound or the "free" amount of the hormones that is completely available to the cells of the body, and is the most active part of the hormone.[2]

Saliva tests are available for estrogen, progesterone, and testosterone, as well as other hormones such as *cortisol* and *DHEA*. (See chapter 5 for more information on

⟡ THE RULES OF SALIVA HORMONE TESTING WHEN TAKING HORMONES OR PRECURSORS

When taking hormones* or precursors during saliva testing, you should abide by the following rules:

1. Wait at least one month after starting or changing your dosage to take the hormone or precursor. This allows the new dosage to equalize with the proteins in the blood that carry them through the body.

2. Collect saliva specimen 24 hours after last dose of hormone or precursor, in the morning. This allows the daily dose to equalize.

Since these hormones affect each other, these two rules apply to any hormone test if you're taking any of the hormones or precursors. If you do not wait a month, or do not allow 24 hours between doses, your saliva test results will be inaccurate.

*Hormones should be taken once a day in the morning to preserve their normal 24-hour rhythm.

these hormones and the roles they play in maintaining hormonal balance during and after menopause.)

The amount of hormones detectable in saliva have a consistent relationship to the levels in the blood and the rest of the body.[3-6] As research has found that salivary progesterone levels are an accurate and reliable measure of body levels, they are shown to be useful to evaluate and monitor women who have fertility problems.[7-10] Salivary *estradiol* (the most important estrogen) levels are similarly accurate and reliable, so have been useful to determine when ovulation has occurred, as a means of evaluating fertility.[11, 12] Saliva testing is also promising as a method of identifying both normal and abnormal levels of testosterone in women.[13, 14] For menopausal and postmenopausal women, saliva tests have proven to be a helpful, noninvasive, and economical way to measure hormones.[15-17]

These tests may be used for women who are taking hormone replacement, as well as for those who are not. Many practitioners regard saliva tests as scientifically and clinically valid for the routine assessment of hormones; thousands of physicians around the world employ such tests.

INTERPRETING YOUR LABORATORY TEST RESULTS

Once you receive the results of your hormone test, you will need to do some interpreting. The first thing to look at is whether your hormones fall within the normal

range. This may seem a quite simple assessment at first—
you just need to compare your levels to the levels that the
lab indicates are normal. This "normal" reading is defined by the hormone's *reference range*. Reference ranges
are created by each laboratory according to standard
guidelines, and are monitored by agencies that grant li-
censes for labs to be in business. Reference ranges for any
given test may vary slightly from one lab to another, but
are usually fairly similar.

It's important to realize that reference ranges are created based on large groups of women. The reference range
reflects the most typical hormone levels found in most
women. But it doesn't necessarily describe the ideal hormone level for you, or for any individual. Individual needs
vary widely enough that it's important to pay attention to
your signs and symptoms, as well as your test results.

A woman with estrogen levels that just barely fall
within the low end of the reference range might be quite
healthy and feel great. Another woman with the same
levels might have signs and symptoms of low estrogen,
and feel quite miserable. For many doctors, the varying
needs of individuals pose a significant problem. How can
a doctor make different recommendations to two women
with identical test results? For this reason, many doctors
simply do not routinely monitor hormone levels in
menopause-aged women.

What is needed is to evaluate lab tests in such a way
as to incorporate a consideration of a woman's symptoms,
while still working with the reference range. This is why
I interpret laboratory tests by looking at the *quartiles*.

Quartiles

A quartile is a fourth of the reference range. The first quartile is at the lowest end of the reference range, the second and third are close to the middle, and the fourth is at the high end of the reference range. I have found quartiles to be very useful in determining the unique needs of menopause-aged women, and expect the use of quartiles to be a growing trend in customized health care.

Consider the case of a woman whose saliva test revealed that her estrogen levels were at the low end of normal, within the lowest quartile of the reference range. Let's say that she is experiencing vaginal dryness and depression, and the MTQ identifies her as having an estrogen-deficient type of menopause, such as Type 5. Even though her estrogen levels register as "normal" in her lab test, they are clearly not ideal for her. In fact, I have seen many such cases in which a woman feels better when her estrogen levels are raised to the second quartile.

The same scenario can occur with progesterone (a borderline "normal" lab test may show up as low on the MTQ). It's important to look at the lab test and the results of the MTQ together. Remember, diagnosis must be based on complete knowledge. The test must be interpreted with symptoms in mind. A woman with testosterone levels in the fourth quartile may develop facial hair or other signs and symptoms of a high-testosterone menopause type, even though she is technically still normal. Her symptoms cannot be ignored, however. Lab work is only half of the diagnosis.

So, when you take the saliva test, you should always interpret its results by looking at your quartiles, along with your Menopause Type Questionnaire results. If your MTQ says you have low testosterone, but your saliva test categorizes you in the lowest quartile (the first quartile), this means you are low. You may do much better in the second quartile. While reviewing your lab results, you will also want to calculate the progesterone to estrogen ratio. The significance of this ratio and how to calculate it are discussed in detail in chapter 5.

WHEN TO USE THE SALIVA HORMONE TEST

Even if you feel great, and have not entered menopause yet, or have an "Ideal Menopause Type" (Type 1), it is a good idea to do a test to determine your hormone levels. This can be used for future reference. It helps to know what your levels are when you're feeling well, to give you an idea of what levels are best for you. This "baseline" testing is optional.

Women who are taking any form of prescribed or alternative hormone-replacement therapy should always use saliva or other hormone tests to monitor the effects of the therapy, and to make sure that the dosages are right. It is advisable to measure levels every 6 months until they are stable, and then perhaps annually after that. No woman should take hormones or hormone *precursors* without being evaluated regularly. (Hormone precursors include DHEA, *androstenedione*, and *pregnenolone*, which are discussed in chapter 14).

Unmonitored hormone replacement is never safe. Hormones are powerful substances that directly cause changes in many different areas of your body. Your health depends on keeping a balance among your hormone levels. Regular monitoring of your hormone levels can help you and your healthcare professional adjust your dosages as needed to keep you in balance.

> Even if you feel great, and have not entered menopause yet, or have an "Ideal Menopause Type," it is a good idea to do a test to determine your hormone levels.

Even if a woman is not using hormone-replacement therapy or hormone precursors, I still encourage yearly evaluation. Many women use exercise, nutrition, herbs, and/or nutritional supplements instead of supplemental hormones. With the help of the Menopause Type Questionnaire, a woman using these alternatives can monitor her health and comfort. But a yearly saliva test is still a good idea. A test result can be an early warning sign that your hormone levels are dropping. This is an important point because some women experience no symptoms, such as hot flashes, but may still have estrogen levels low enough to cause significant osteoporosis. The tests can be used also to evaluate the effects of exercise, nutrition, diet, herbs, glandular, hormone precursors, or hormones on your hormonal levels, and help you determine how to modify your lifestyle program.

WHO RUNS SALIVA HORMONE TESTS AND HOW DO I FIND A "HORMONE EDUCATED" DOCTOR?

A number of specialty laboratories throughout the world currently perform saliva hormone testing. Some of these labs are also involved in ongoing research to continue the advances made in saliva testing. Currently, there are dozens of laboratories and research facilities conducting saliva testing worldwide. Most alternative medicine physicians who use these tests belong to professional organizations that help keep physicians updated on new tests and therapies related to menopause and other important health-care issues.

To find a "hormone educated" alternative medicine doctor, refer to the list of professional organizations in the Resources section of this book. This list is also available on the Web site www.yourmenopausetype.com.

Consumer-direct hormone tests are also accessible through different Internet sites, pharmacies, health-care organizations, and even directly from some laboratories. *Consumer direct* implies that you do not need a physician's order to obtain the test. This direct-to-consumer approach is a growing part of the self-care movement.

Ordering a kit directly has its advantages. The saliva collection kit, which usually comes with easy-to-follow instructions, is sent to your home. Once you collect the saliva sample, you ship it back to the lab for processing according to the instructions the lab provides. After the hormones are evaluated, the results are usually mailed to your home. This provides a quick way to find out your hormone levels. The saliva test is an educational tool to help you understand more about your hormone levels.

Though you can do the test on your own, in reality, consumer-direct testing works best if you consult a qualified health-care professional who has taken the time to learn how to interpret these tests. That may mean ordering the kit through a physician, pharmacist, nurse, women's health teacher, nutritionist, or herbalist. In this way, you have access to someone who has studied and interpreted dozens, or even hundreds, of tests—which is probably more than you have interpreted.

At this point in time, diagnostic laboratories do not directly advise patients on individual lab results. Most saliva tests sold to the public do not provide as much information as professional tests sold to professionals. Tests sold to the public only measure hormones once, and most experienced health-care professionals do not feel confident interpreting consumer tests when they could use a more accurate test that measures each hormone a few times. It is important to realize that self-care does not mean "by myself care"—it means caring enough about yourself to gain better use of available resources.

> It is important to realize that self-care does not mean "by myself care"— it means caring enough about yourself to gain better use of available resources.

WHAT ABOUT USING BLOOD TESTS TO MEASURE HORMONES?

Measuring serum (or blood) hormone levels is still considered by many physicians to be the gold standard of hormone testing. However, measuring only estrogen for menopause assessment disregards the vital roles that progesterone and testosterone play in women's health. To properly determine your menopause type, serum tests must include all three hormones—estradiol, progesterone, and testosterone—as well as sex-hormone-binding globulin (SHBG). Recall that SHBG is a carrier protein that carries estradiol and testosterone throughout the blood (see page 45) and maintains the body's *equilibrium* by sustaining a steady state between bound and unbound levels of hormones. SHBG levels may be affected by natural estrogens, synthetic estrogens, soy isoflavones, and tamoxifen, as well as conditions such as thyroid disease.

Serum testing also allows for accurate measurement of certain estrogen metabolites that are used to assess breast cancer risk and risk of other cancers. Two of the most promising estrogen metabolites for cancer risk assessment are 2-hydroxyestrone and 16-alpha-hydroxyestrone (see pages 325 and 328). The increased awareness of the need to measure estrogen metabolites, all three hormones, as well as SHBG has led to significant advancements in serum-hormone testing for women.

CHAPTER FIVE

Your Hormones and Your Health

By the time most women reach their early forties, they have ovulated regularly for almost 30 years. At that age, the ovaries gradually begin to produce less estrogen. In the transition to menopause, ovulation happens less frequently, and some months pass without an egg being released at all. There is also a reduction in progesterone production as well. When progesterone and estrogen levels are low, the pituitary gland tries to compensate, leading to irregular periods as hormone levels fluctuate. Eventually, the ovaries stop producing eggs. Menopause usually occurs between the ages of 40 and 60, with 52 being the average age. When a woman has ceased having menstrual periods, she is considered post-menopausal.

YOUR BODY DURING MENOPAUSE

During and after menopause, the adrenal glands take over much of the body's hormone production. They do this by secreting increased amounts of the hormone *androstenedione*. Androstenedione is a precursor—a building block—for both testosterone and estrogen. Ideally, the adrenal glands continue to make adequate amounts of progesterone as well, since before menopause they made as much as 60% of the body's progesterone during the first half of the menstrual cycle.

> Understanding the steroidogenic pathway and the changes that it goes through in menopause is the key to understanding the unique needs that arise during this time.

The adrenal glands may not be able to maintain the same levels of estrogen, progesterone, and testosterone in the body as before menopause, but they should be able to supply enough to meet a woman's postmenopausal needs. All three hormones are needed for a variety of physical and mental functions long after menopause, and your body has ways of meeting these needs all your life. See table 3 on page 63 for the different effects these hormones have on the body.

This is true in an ideal menopause. Unfortunately, the transition doesn't always go so smoothly. Sometimes the adrenal glands don't step up to their new responsibilities quite as well as they should. Especially at first, the adrenal glands' production may fluctuate, causing hormone levels to spike and fall several times a month. And stress or poor diet can leave your adrenal glands fatigued.

The complex processes by which building blocks (precursors) such as androstenedione are made into steroid hormones such as estrogen and testosterone are known as the *steroidogenic pathway*. If there are weak points anywhere along this hormone-creating pathway, the body may have trouble converting androstenedione into estrogen or testosterone.

❧ NOT AN IDEAL MENOPAUSE

Sometimes, menopause happens early due to stress, chronic illness, or toxic chemical exposure, all of which can influence the production of hormones. In other cases, early menopause results from the surgical removal of the ovaries, or as a consequence of radiation or chemotherapy. Excessive exercise or weight loss can also stop the menstrual cycle, and may produce some of the problems of menopause, via an unrelated mechanism. Certain chronic diseases such as Addison's disease can also lead to premature menopause.

Women who have early menopause for one of these reasons are less likely to have a Type 1 menopause. But the imbalance patterns I describe under the 12 menopause types apply also to early menopause due to illness, surgery, or other factors.

An important thing about the steroidogenic pathway is that it shows us how and why progesterone, cortisol, DHEA, testosterone, and estrogen affect each other. For instance, the pathway shows that as DHEA travels down the path it may be changed into testosterone, or even estrogen. In fact, progesterone may travel down the steroidogenic pathway and be changed into testosterone or estradiol. Progesterone could have also been changed into *cortisol,* an important adrenal hormone that helps your body adapt to stress (see diagram in Appendix E).

Understanding this pathway and the changes that it goes through in menopause is the key to understanding the unique needs that arise during this time.

Estrogen and You

You may not recognize all its effects by name, but you're already intimately familiar with estrogen. All your life, this hormone has been quietly, profoundly affecting your health and well-being in a number of ways. From your menstrual cycle to your brain, bones, and heart, estrogen plays many important roles in the body.

As you go through menopause, your body's estrogen levels change. The effects can be quite noticeable. Below, I describe the signs and symptoms that suggest your estrogen levels may have fallen too low to meet all your needs.

Your Menstrual Cycle, Skin, and Breasts   For many women, one of the first signs of menopause is a menstrual cycle that changes in length, becoming either shorter or longer. Estrogen maintains the regular length of your cycle. If your cycle suddenly changes from 30 days to 40 (or 20), it may be a sign of low estrogen levels.

Estrogen works with progesterone to prepare your uterine lining each month to receive and nourish a fertilized egg. If no conception occurs, the uterine lining sheds in menstruation. As menopause approaches and estrogen levels fall, the amount and length of bleeding in a period may become erratic.

After menopause, your adrenal glands take over more of your body's production of estrogen. But this transition can be erratic. Further, the shifting of estrogen levels can result in changes in *neurotransmitters*, which can also initiate hot flashes.[1]

Estrogen maintains the structure of your vulva and vagina. When estrogen levels are low, both the inner and outer labia shrink, and the vulva becomes thinner. The vagina's mucous membranes shrink and become thinner and smoother. (These changes are known as vulvar atrophy and vaginal atrophy.) The vagina produces less lubrication, and the pH of the vagina changes, making it more vulnerable to harmful bacteria such as *E. coli*, which increases the risk of urinary tract infections.

Estrogen seems to have a direct effect on the libido, and not just because it makes sex more comfortable by keeping the vagina healthy and well lubricated. Estrogen makes women feel sexier; many premenopausal women notice a surge in sexual interest around ovulation, when their estrogen level is at its peak. A decline in estrogen levels can make a woman less interested in sex. Decreased estrogen levels cause shrinking of the urethra, which can lead to bladder control problems as well as urinary tract infections.[2]

During puberty, estrogen causes the growth of the breasts and the milk-producing breast ducts. Once the breasts are developed, estrogen plays a role in maintaining their size and density. When estrogen levels fall during menopause, the breasts may shrink.

As estrogen stimulates some cell growth, estrogen may play a role in the development of certain forms of breast cancer. However, new research suggests that it is actually abnormal metabolism of estrogens that results in increased cancer risk and that some metabolites of estrogen can actually decrease the risk of breast cancer. Excessive estrogen replacement can result in breast pain (mastalgia).

Estrogen contributes to the health of the skin, which is largely made of a protein called collagen. The amount of collagen in the skin is maintained by estrogen, and decreases after menopause.[3] Estrogen increases the water content of the skin, thus contributing to its thickness and softness.[4, 5] Estrogen also increases the number of blood vessels in the skin.[6] This increase in blood vessels makes the skin feel warmer and is one of the factors that cause hot flashes.

The thickness of the skin in postmenopausal women decreases with each passing year that estrogen levels are low. This thinning is due in part to decreased amounts of collagen and in part to decreased water content of the skin. In this way, a decline in estrogen levels can contribute to skin wrinkles. (Decreased testosterone, decreased growth hormone, and diminished muscle strength also contribute to wrinkling of the skin.)

Mood and Mental Functioning

Many women find that when their estrogen level goes down, they get depressed. While medical science has yet to fully understand estrogen's role in brain chemistry, we know that it affects a number of *neurotransmitters* that influence mood, memory, and motivation. As with certain types of antidepressants, estrogen increases the release of the neuro-transmitter norepinephrine in the brain, and may decrease the action of monamine oxidase. It also plays a role in the normal function of other neurotransmitters that affect mood, including seratonin, dopamine, and GABAA (gamma-amino-butyric acid type A).[7]

As well as having mood-elevating effects, estrogen improves memory and certain mental functions.[8] Studies have shown that estrogen improves verbal memory (the ability to remember words and names) and helps one learn new things.[9, 10] There is also evidence that estrogen enhances a woman's reasoning, formation of new concepts, and fine motor skills.[11, 12] Estrogen helps the brain function properly by stimulating nerve growth and maintenance.[13]

> Many women find that when their estrogen level goes down, they get depressed.

An important area of current inquiry is whether estrogen protects against Alzheimer's disease and other severe age-related mental impairment. We know that Alzheimer's disease affects women more often than men, and that postmenopausal women who take supplemental estrogen have a lower risk for Alzheimer's than women who don't.[14–16]

Your Heart and Bones

One of the most common reasons for taking estrogen is to prevent osteoporosis and heart disease. Estrogen protects your bones and heart, and when your estrogen levels drop during menopause, your risk of serious health problems increases.[17–19]

Estrogen helps maintain your bones by restraining the activity of special cells (known as osteoclasts) that break down bone tissue.[20, 21] It may also promote the formation of new bone cells.[22–25] When you enter menopause, your bones can rapidly deteriorate as your body's lower estrogen levels allow too much bone to be broken down. Research has demonstrated that estrogen-deficient women are much more vulnerable to bone loss than women with sufficient estrogen.[26]

However well you take care of yourself, there is evidence that you become more vulnerable to heart disease once your estrogen level begins to drop. Some of the reasons for this increased risk are believed to be due in part to changes in lipids (fat molecules) in the blood.

Cholesterol is the chief blood lipid. Estrogen lowers LDL ("bad") cholesterol levels and prevents it from being *oxidized*, a change that makes it more harmful to the walls of the blood vessels.[27] Estrogen also increases HDL ("good") cholesterol, and has a positive effect on other important lipids and components of the blood.[28–31]

Estrogen supplementation after menopause has also been found to help reduce high blood pressure and improve blood flow to the coronary arteries.[32, 33]

Another health risk to consider is insulin resistance, a condition I describe later in this chapter. As we'll see, insulin resistance increases the risk for heart disease and other serious health problems. Estrogen protects against insulin resistance.

TABLE 3
Effects of Estradiol, Progesterone, and Testosterone
on Various Parts of the Body

	Estradiol (the most active estrogen)	**Progesterone**	**Testosterone**
Menstrual Cycle and Endometrium	Too much increases risk of endometrial cancer.	Decreases risk of endometrial cancer. Can decrease uterine contractions, cramping, and pain. May decrease dysfunctional uterine bleeding.	Possibly increases risk of endometrial cancer.
Vagina and Urinary Tract	Prevents vaginal dryness and atrophy, decreases urinary tract infections and urinary incontinence.	Can increase urinary incontinence and counteract the beneficial effects of estrogen.	Appears to have most beneficial effect on the vulva.
Libido	Increases sexual satisfaction, libido, sexual desire, interest and responsiveness.	Can decrease libido, especially if testosterone levels are low.	The most important hormone to increase and maintain libido.

(continued)

TABLE 3 (continued)

	Estradiol	Progesterone	Testosterone
Blood Sugar (Glucose) and Insulin	Maintains normal glucose and insulin function, can prevent hyper-insulinemia.	Interferes with the action of insulin—pro-motes insulin resistance; in-creases hyper-insulinemia.	Can cause insulin resistance and hyperinsulinemia.
Brain	Stimulating to the brain—may improve learning and memory. Decreases appetite.	Calming to the brain—decreases anxiety. Can be sedating. Induces sleep. Stimulates appetite.	Decreases depression. Increases confidence.
Breast	Maintains breast fullness. Increases risk of estrogen-sensitive cancer.	Maintains breast fullness. Normal levels may prevent breast cancer. High levels may promote breast cancer.	High levels may promote breast cancer.
Skin	Maintains proper levels of collagen—may maintain skin thickness.	Increases blood flow to the skin. Increases tem-perature of skin.	May maintain skin collagen and skin thickness. Maintains function of sebaceous glands which moisturize the skin. Too much can cause acne or facial hair.

	Estradiol	Progesterone	Testosterone
Bones	Decreases the activity of the bone-clearing osteoclasts. Increases osteoblastic bone-building activity.	May increase the "building up" of bone by osteoblasts. Works best with estrogen.	Promotes bone building and bone repair by stimulating osteoblast cell growth.
Heart	Promotes cardiac health in many ways: Is thought to increase HDL (good) cholesterol and decrease LDL (bad) cholesterol. Decreases lipoprotein (a) and homocysteine, markers of increased risks of cardiac disease.	Can decrease high blood pressure. May decrease HDL (especially synthetic progestogens).	Can decrease HDL. Can cause insulin resistance. May help increase blood flow through coronary arteries.

Progesterone

Progesterone is best known for its role in pregnancy. (The name comes from the word *gestation* which means "pregnancy.") If you've had a child, you've probably felt some of progesterone's stronger effects: a faster metabolism (and bigger appetite), a tendency to feel warm or even hot, and a calmer libido. But this hormone is also important for a woman's health during and after menopause. As I'll explain in detail below, progesterone influences your mood and protects against several serious health problems.

Your Menstrual Cycle, Skin, and Breasts   Together with estrogen, progesterone regulates your menstrual cycle. Estrogen stimulates the uterine lining to grow; progesterone ensures that it sheds in monthly periods (if no conception occurs, that is). If you're familiar with hormone-replacement therapy, you know that taking estrogen can increase your risk for uterine cancer, unless you also take progesterone (or another progestogen—that is, a substance with a similar effect) to protect you against a potentially harmful buildup of tissue in the uterine lining.[34]

> Progesterone influences your mood and protects against several serious health problems.

One sign that your progesterone levels are too low during menopause is that you begin to have more painful menstrual periods, with uterine cramps. Low progesterone-to-estrogen ratios may in some cases be associated with a serious medical condition known as dysfunctional uterine bleeding (DUB), which is characterized by heavy, erratic bleeding.[35]

Progesterone doesn't actually seem to play a direct role in preventing vaginal dryness or pain, despite the claims of some health professionals. It may be that, when women take progesterone, their bodies convert some of it to estrogen, which does have a protective effect against vaginal dryness and pain.

While estrogen makes women feel sexier, progesterone is likely to have the opposite effect. It tends to moderate the effects of estrogen and testosterone.[36, 37] In fact, progesterone is given to sex offenders to decrease their sexual thoughts, desires, and satisfaction.[38–41] This loss of libido may be accompanied by depression.[42] This is why some women with low estrogen but adequate progesterone feel depressed and have decreased libido.

Progesterone increases your body's metabolic rate, and literally warms you.[43] It can enhance your tolerance of cold. The higher metabolism and body temperature are accompanied by more blood flow to the skin, and an increased ability to sweat and lose the extra heat through the skin.[44, 45] Although it is under debate, progesterone's effects on skin may be partly responsible for hot flashes. Also, this is why some women who experience low-progesterone menopause types have cool skin.

Early studies suggested that too little progesterone might play a role in the development of breast cancer, probably because the low level of progesterone created an imbalance in relationship to estrogen.[46]

Mood and Mental Functioning   Your body uses progesterone to make chemicals that soothe your nervous system.[47] These chemicals, which affect some of the same nervous system receptors as medications such as Valium and Xanax, tend to calm and sedate you.[48–52] Progesterone's effect is so strong that it has been used to decrease seizures in women with epilepsy.[53, 54]

If your progesterone levels fall too far during menopause, you can feel anxious and irritable, and your loved ones may tell you that you've become unusually critical. Or you can have trouble sleeping, or suffer from feelings of confusion, depression, or mood swings.[55] These feelings can become exhausting if the imbalance goes on too long. A drop in your progesterone level can actually cause you to go through symptoms that are similar to those experienced in withdrawal from sedatives or alcohol.[56]

Progesterone has a stimulating effect on respiration, so it may protect women from abnormal breathing patterns during sleep.[57–60] A low progesterone level can produce sleep disturbances known as sleep apnea, in which a person stops breathing for brief periods during sleep. Sleep apnea is more common in men and in overweight people, but some women are more prone to sleep apnea after menopause.[61] Estrogen appears to play an indirect role in progesterone's helpful effects on breathing.[62]

Progesterone is also involved in the regulation of appetite. Low-progesterone menopause types can have a decreased appetite.[63, 64]

Your Bones   Although its effects are not as well-known as estrogen's, progesterone protects against osteoporosis. Like estrogen, progesterone protects bone, but in a different way. Estrogen restricts the breakdown of old bone cells; progesterone stimulates the growth of new ones.[65–77]

Some animal studies suggest that high progesterone levels are able to maintain or increase bone formation even when there is low estrogen.[78, 79] However, other researchers have found that progesterone alone does *not* have a positive effect on bone mineral density and bone volume, two measures of bone strength and health.[80] There is also evidence that estrogen enhances progesterone's bone-building power.[81, 82]

Testosterone

We usually think of testosterone as a "male" sex hormone, but every woman has it, too. You need testosterone for proper function of the brain, heart, bones, and many other tissues. After menopause, your testosterone levels may remain adequate to your needs, but if the hormonal changes don't go smoothly you may end up with too much or too little. When it comes to testosterone, the adrenal glands do not appear to be equipped to make up for a total loss of ovarian testosterone—some ovarian testosterone is usually needed. But if the adrenal glands produce a lot of an-

> We usually think of testosterone as a "male" sex hormone, but every woman has it, too. You need testosterone for proper function of the brain, heart, bones, and many other tissues.

drostenedione—the building block (precursor) from which both testosterone and estrogen are made—the result may be too high a level of testosterone in the body.

Testosterone and Your Sex Life   There is growing evidence that testosterone is the most important hormone for maintaining sex drive in women, just as it is in men.[83] Before, during, and after menopause, testosterone boosts a woman's libido. Too little testosterone can leave a woman feeling uninterested in sex. Too much can make her feel edgy and aggressive, even if her level of desire is just fine.

Testosterone also has important effects on the vagina and vulva. The vaginal and vulvar atrophy that can occur with menopause are often at least partly caused by testosterone deficiency.[84] Like estrogen, testosterone directly affects the tissue of the vagina, and helps keep it healthy.[85]

Testosterone deficiency can cause a medical condition called lichen sclerosus, in which the labia and vulva become thin and fragile. This ailment creates chronic inflammation, itching, and pain, and, in severe cases, significant scarring and changes in the tissue. Testosterone ointment has been used to treat this condition.[86]

Testosterone also maintains muscle tone, and a loss of it can contribute to the aging of your skin. Low testosterone can also contribute to stress incontinence or other bladder control problems.

Mood and Mental Functioning   Low testosterone can have a negative effect on a woman's mood and sense of well-being.[87] In fact, depression is one of the major symptoms brought on by testosterone deficiency in women.[88] Testosterone is a hormone that greatly influences motivation, drive, and confidence, and perhaps even feelings of self-worth.[89]

In moderation, testosterone can be very beneficial for your skin. Proper testosterone levels work with estrogen to preserve skin collagen, and thus protect against wrinkling and aging.[90, 91] When testosterone levels are low, the skin is affected by a loss of collagen and muscle tone.

Decreased testosterone levels may be partially responsible for the increased dryness of skin that can occur during and after menopause. The sebaceous glands, which excrete lubricating oil-like substances from the pores onto the skin, often work less efficiently after menopause due to low testosterone.[92]

On the other hand, too much testosterone isn't good for your skin, either. The signs include excessive oiliness, acne, and increased hair on the face or body. High levels of testosterone in women can also result in a thinning of the scalp hair, a condition called androgenic alopecia.

It is now understood that testosterone also plays a role in women's hot flashes. In fact, new therapies for hot flashes include the use of testosterone.

Testosterone and Your Breasts   There is a significant concern that high levels of testosterone can increase the risk of breast cancer in postmenopausal women, although the evidence is mixed.[93] Though high testosterone levels have been observed to occur with breast cancer, or before, there is reason to doubt that it is actually testosterone that is stimulating cancer.[94-97] As I explain later in this chapter, one possible culprit is insulin resistance, which can result from an imbalance between testosterone and estrogen, and can contribute to the development of breast cancer. Since estrogen is associated with an increased risk for certain types of breast cancer, and testosterone is a precursor for estrogen (which means that your body can use testosterone to make estrogen), it raises the question of whether testosterone or estrogen is the problem.[98-100]

Osteoporosis   It's long been known that estrogen protects against osteoporosis. More recently, we've learned that testosterone also has a direct, beneficial effect on bone.[101] When we consider that, of all the steroid hormones, testosterone plays the greatest role in building tissue, it makes sense that it would be involved in bone-building, too.[102-109] The tissue-building effect of testosterone can accelerate the repair of damaged bone.[110] Testosterone and estrogens appear to work together to maintain and rebuild joint cartilage between bones.[111] Testosterone can effectively decrease bone deterioration associated with aging.[112] A testosterone deficiency can lead to osteoporosis.[113-115]

Testosterone and Your Heart   Too much testosterone isn't good for your heart. (This is something for you and your doctor to keep in mind if you take supplemental testosterone.) Testosterone decreases HDL ("good") cholesterol.[116, 117] In addition, as discussed below, high testosterone levels can cause insulin resistance, which results in a significant increase in heart disease.

Testosterone also has some heart-healthy effects, however. It relaxes the coronary arteries, thus allowing more blood to flow to the heart, and decreasing symptoms of angina.[118-121] Low-testosterone menopause types may have an increased risk for angina.

Blood Sugar and Insulin Problems

Blood sugar problems can arise with various menopause types, due to imbalances in all three of the steroid hormones we've been looking at: estrogen, progesterone, and testosterone. These are some of the most serious health risks of menopause.

Insulin is a hormone that enables your cells to use molecules of sugar (glucose) from your blood. Glucose is the main source of energy for most of your body's cells. To receive molecules of glucose, your cells must be sensitive to the influence of insulin.

For various reasons, your cells can become "insulin resistant," or less sensitive. Your body still provides the same amount of insulin, but your cells seem to need more. When this happens, your body tries to compensate by making more insulin. This leads to a condition called *hyperinsulinemia*, literally meaning "too much insulin in the blood."

Hyperinsulinemia with insulin resistance is responsible for a range of serious illnesses in postmenopausal women, including adult-onset diabetes, heart disease, and cancer of the breast and uterus.[122–129]

It was once thought that insulin resistance was mainly a problem of obesity, but this isn't true. Insulin resistance is a widespread but largely unrecognized threat to women's health. As many as 44% of healthy postmenopausal women may have insulin resistance.[130]

> Insulin resistance is a widespread but largely unrecognized threat to women's health.

What causes insulin resistance? Imbalances in estrogen, progesterone, and testosterone levels in women make insulin resistance more likely with each year after menopause.[131]

A deficiency in estrogen can produce insulin resistance.[132–134] Estrogen plays an important role in your body's normal insulin sensitivity, the uptake of glucose by muscle cells, the normalization of proteins that carry hormones in the blood (which help normalize testosterone levels), and the liver's ability to clear excess insulin from the blood.[135–139]

Progesterone has the opposite effect: It can *cause* insulin resistance.[140–142] The elevated progesterone seen in pregnancy has been suspected to contribute to the formation of gestational diabetes.[143–145] Supplemental progesterone used in hormone-replacement therapy has also been found to interfere with insulin and glucose metabolism.[146-151] (See chapter 14 for more information on hormone-replacement therapy.)

⚭ YEARLY EXAMINATION, EVALUATION, AND HEALTH ASSESSMENT

Whether or not you choose hormones to improve your health, your annual physical examination and evaluation will help add both years and quality to your life. Choose a special month to have this complete health assessment, perhaps each year in your birthday month, your anniversary month, or in January. This annual event should include:

A Complete Physical Exam

Complete Gynecological Exam

Pap Smear

Hormone Assessment (all three)

Manual Breast Exam

Mammogram

Colon Cancer Screen

Blood Tests

For more information regarding your yearly examination, evaluation, and health assessment, see Resources.

Later in this chapter, I explain the importance of the progesterone-to-estrogen ratio. If the level of estrogen is too low to balance progesterone, even a normal level of progesterone can promote insulin resistance. This may occur with low-estrogen and normal-progesterone menopause types.

A high testosterone level can also cause insulin resistance and hyperinsulinemia, especially when it is not balanced by estrogen.[152-157] This is true for premenopausal women, as well as women who are in or past menopause.[158]

Thus, any menopause type that includes low levels of estrogen or high levels of testosterone has an increased risk for insulin resistance—especially if there is an imbalance between estrogen and progesterone, or estrogen and testosterone. Since insulin resistance can contribute to so many serious health risks, from diabetes to heart disease and cancer, this is one of the strongest reasons for identifying your menopause type and getting appropriate treatment.

COMMON PATTERNS OF HORMONE IMBALANCE

As we've seen, it's important to determine your levels of testosterone, estrogen, and progesterone. Each of these hormones plays a number of critical roles in your health during and after menopause. But it's not enough to consider each one separately; you also need to look at the patterns of balance or imbalance of the three in relationship to each other. The relationships between the hormones are a crucial piece of the puzzle.

Though any imbalance can cause problems, the two most common imbalances are the testosterone-estrogen imbalance and the progesterone-estrogen imbalance.

Testosterone and Estrogen Imbalance

Estrogen controls testosterone, so when estrogen levels drop during and after menopause, it's possible that there will be excessive testosterone, at least until the body finds its new balance.

When testosterone is high and estrogen is low, a common manifestation is the development of excessive facial or other body hair after menopause.[159-161] This imbalance between testosterone and estrogen can be called *hyper-androgenism* (excessive "male" hormones) and has been linked to numerous other health problems, including acne, abnormal glucose metabolism, insulin resistance, and increased risk of heart disease.[162-165]

Progesterone and Estrogen Imbalance

During menopause, some women maintain adequate levels of estrogen because their adrenal glands produce more androstenedione, which is converted to estrogen. The adrenal glands may also continue to make adequate progesterone, in which case an ideal balance is maintained. If progesterone levels are not high enough to balance the actions of estrogen, however, significant health problems can result.

Since the late 1980s, this condition has been referred to as "estrogen dominance"—though a more accurate description would be "progesterone deficiency." This progesterone deficiency is most pronounced when there is still enough estrogen present, but not enough progesterone. If there is a dual deficiency of both estrogen and progesterone, the increased symptoms and health risks may not be as evident.

> If progesterone levels are not high enough to balance the actions of estrogen, significant health problems can result.

In the early 1990s, my studies into the relationship between estradiol (the most potent estrogen) and progesterone led me to recognize that the ratio between progesterone and estradiol could have a major impact on how women felt. By the mid-1990s, I was calculating the progesterone-to-estradiol ratio in women who had the saliva hormone test performed. Later, when I started my work in diagnostic laboratories, I made P:E ratio analysis a routine part of menopause testing. With P:E ratio analysis, we finally had a number to tell us if a women was "progesterone deficient." Now you can monitor your estrogen-progesterone balance by calculating your P:E ratio.

Before menopause, P:E ratios vary from about 20:1 (20 parts progesterone to 1 part estrogen) to about 170:1, depending on the time of the month.[166, 167] For pregnancy to occur, an ideal ratio of 30:1 or possibly 60:1 may be needed. For many women, the highest natural P:E ratio is about 120:1.[168] A low P:E ratio (such as 10:1) can lead to infertility in premenopausal women and abnormal uterine bleeding in women of menopausal age.[169, 170] An increased risk for breast cancer also has been attributed to a low P:E ratio.[171]

A low P:E ratio represents *unopposed estrogen*, which means there is not enough progesterone to oppose (or balance) the actions of estrogen. As estrogen stimulates the nervous system, it should always be balanced with the proper amount of progesterone, so as not to produce the anxiety seen with fluctuations of these hormones.[172] Irritability, pain, inflammation, and increased risk of breast and uterine cancer can occur with a low P:E ratio. A saliva progesterone of 100 with an estrogen of 6.0 would give a P:E ratio of less than 17:1 (not healthy).

A high P:E ratio isn't healthy, either, since it can promote insulin resistance, depression, fatigue, and a decreased libido.

Keep these ratios in mind when you have your hormones tested. Your body should have between 20 to 170 molecules of progesterone to one molecule of estrogen. To arrive at this ratio, divide the progesterone by the estrogen. For example, a progesterone of 100 divided by 2.5 gives a P:E ratio of 40:1, which is in the normal range of 20:1 to 170:1. Note: This P:E ratio must be calculated from tests which are measured in pMol or nMol, since we are concerned about molecule ratios.

Pain and Inflammation   A low P:E ratio is associated with increased levels of molecules that cause inflammation. These molecules are called *kinins*. Estrogen increases kinin levels, and giving progesterone can decrease them.[173] Kinins occur naturally in the body but promote the release of histamines. In conditions of allergic inflammation, kinins are elevated. High levels of kinins are linked to asthma, rheumatoid arthritis, psoriatic arthritis, and a number of bowel diseases.[174]

TREATING YOUR MENOPAUSE TYPE

Now that you understand how hormone deficiencies and imbalances can affect your health in annoying, uncomfortable, or even dangerous ways, you're probably ready to find out how to treat them. In the next several chapters, I'll present specific treatments designed for each menopause type. For every menopause type, there are effective treatments that can bring you back into balance and make your menopause closer to the ideal, Type 1 experience every woman deserves.

CHAPTER SIX

Adequate Menopause Types

Type 1, Type 2, and Type 3

In chapter 1, we met Emily, who didn't think she had gone through menopause. She'd had a hysterectomy several years before, so there were no menstrual cycle changes to tell her when she was in menopause. She also lacked some of the other "classic" signs of menopause— she had no hot flashes or vaginal dryness. She was fortunate enough to be spared the emotional roller coaster some women experience. She knew something was going on, but she wasn't sure what it was.

Women with adequate menopause types often doubt that they've gone through menopause at all. They sometimes have no symptoms, apart from no longer having periods. (Even though women who have had hysterectomies are less likely to have an ideal menopause, it sometimes happens, as it did for Emily.) Or they may have a vague sense that something is different. They just go on with their business as usual—managing a home, running a business, or going back to school for a graduate degree. In their bodies, changes do take place, but so smoothly that the women barely notice it. As the ovaries' manufacture of hormones slows down, the adrenal glands move right in and take over.

> Women with adequate menopause types often doubt that they've gone through menopause at all. They sometimes have no symptoms, apart from no longer having periods.

If you are having an adequate type menopause, you will probably do fine using gentle alternative methods—nutrition, lifestyle changes, or herbs—to address any symptoms you have. Your body has adapted to menopause to a significant degree. Some women need help with only one hormone, such as a 64-year-old patient of mine who had perfect estrogen and progesterone levels, but needed help with her testosterone. Others appear to have adequate levels of all three major hormones, but have a vague sense that something is less than ideal. Hormone levels may be within normal range, but not be at the optimal levels for your unique needs. To follow, I discuss treatments and tonics that are appropriate for the three adequate menopause types.

After you read about the treatments described here, turn to the later chapters in this book for more in-depth information about nutrition (chapter 11), herbal treatments (chapter 12), glandular extracts (chapter 13), and hormone-replacement therapy (chapter 14).

TYPE 1: IDEAL (ADEQUATE ESTROGEN AND PROGESTERONE, WITH NORMAL TESTOSTERONE)

Ann was 58 years old when she came to me for a hormone checkup. She was a married homemaker, with two grown children. She told me that her periods had gradually dwindled and finally stopped 6 months previously, but otherwise she'd had no menopausal symptoms at all—no hot flashes, no discomfort of any kind. She came to me because she wanted to make sure everything was all right.

Testing showed that all of Ann's hormones were within normal range and that she was in good health. Ann had experienced an ideal menopause.

What to Expect From Ideal Menopause

In an ideal menopause, hormonal changes happen so smoothly that you might not even notice them. As your ovaries' hormone production drops, your adrenal glands compensate by making more hormone precursors (building blocks). You may have a few hot flashes or a little

fatigue, but these transient signs of minor hormone fluctuations don't last. Once you stop having monthly periods, you feel completely well.

This is what menopause should be like. The changes
you feel, if any, should be subtle, and not too uncomfortable. You might be aware that you're going through a
transition, but a very graceful one.

In a truly ideal menopause, your levels of estrogen,
progesterone, and testosterone are all within the normal
reference range. Though many women with ideal
menopause are in the lower quartile for all three hormones, there seem to be just as many women with ideal
menopause who have levels in the second quartile, and
even a few in the third. If you have hormone levels in the
first quartile, you will of course have some sense of decreased hormones. But if the levels are in a higher quartile, you may have no signs or symptoms.

I have seen women in their sixties and seventies
whose hormone levels were as high as those of women in
their thirties. Even though they have stopped menstruating, these women still have the same level of estrogen,
progesterone, and testosterone that younger women have
in the first half of their menstrual cycle.

For a woman to have an ideal menopause, with sufficient amounts of all hormones, she must have very
healthy adrenal glands and ovaries. (Women whose
ovaries have been surgically removed rarely have ideal
menopause.) This healthy state depends on a number of
factors, including genetic tendencies, exercise, nutrition,
and stress. Most of these factors can be influenced to
some degree by choices a woman makes. Having a ge-

netic tendency doesn't necessarily determine the out-
come, since diet, exercise, and stress all play such important roles in staying healthy.

Even if you have Type 1 menopause, you should get
your hormone levels checked periodically to make sure
they stay in balance. And if you haven't done so already,
you might consider having your osteoporosis risk evaluated by a bone density scan. Some women with no
menopausal symptoms have *masked osteoporosis*—they feel
fine, but their bones are nonetheless weakening. If you
have this condition, you can take the appropriate action
to remedy the situation. And if everything shows up fine
in the tests, you will be fully reassured that you are indeed having an ideal menopause.

Nutrition and Diet

The adrenal glands function best when your body is well
supplied with all the trace minerals and vitamins needed
for producing hormones. A balanced diet and a high-
quality vitamin and mineral supplement will help maintain your health before, during, and after menopause.

Herbal Remedies

Herbs that help the body adjust to stress and aging will
also help you maintain an ideal menopause. These herbs
are called *adaptogens* because they help the body adapt to
stress. Herbs that have adaptogenic actions include

Siberian ginseng *(Eleutherococcus senticosus)*, Asian ginseng *(Panax ginseng)*, ashwagandha *(Withania somnifera)*, and astragalus *(Astragalus membranaceus)*. Other herbs that have some adaptogenic action include sarsaparilla *(Smilax* spp.*)*, damiana *(Turnera diffusa)*, and licorice *(Glycyrrhiza glabra)*. Dong quai *(Angelica sinensis)* is also considered to have some adaptogenic actions.

> A balanced diet and a high-quality vitamin and mineral supplement will help maintain your health before, during, and after menopause.

If you are having an ideal menopause, you can maintain the function of your adrenal glands and ovaries and keep your hormone levels healthy by adding adaptogenic herbs to your routine health care.

Glandular Extracts

If you have Type 1 menopause, but experience some fatigue, glandular extracts such as adrenal extracts may help. However, there are several cautions to consider when using these extracts. Chapter 13 tells you how to use them, and discuss the associated risks.

Ann's Treatment

Ann began taking *Panax ginseng* 2 to 3 times a week. She also started taking a high-grade vitamin and mineral supplement, with additional calcium with boron for her very mild osteoporosis, and began to exercise more frequently.

✑ TREATMENT OPTIONS FOR TYPE 1 MENOPAUSE

Nutrition and diet: vitamin and mineral supplement

Herbs: Siberian ginseng, Asian ginseng, ashwa-gandha, astragalus, sarsaparilla, damiana, licorice, dong quai

Glandulars: If experiencing fatigue, consider adrenal extract

Note: Avoid antiandrogens, antiestrogens, and antiprogestogens.

TYPE 2: LOW TESTOSTERONE

Amelia, whom we've met, was 46 when she came into my office. Married with two grown children, she'd had a hysterectomy at the age of 39. Her main complaint was fatigue and what she described as a loss of "vim and vigor." Her hormone tests showed low testosterone. Her estrogen and progesterone were within normal range, although they were at the low end, suggesting some degree of adrenal fatigue. Amelia had a classic Type 2 menopause.

It's interesting to note here that Amelia went into menopause several years earlier than her mother had, probably because of her hysterectomy. Even if the hysterectomy is partial, removing only the uterus and leaving the ovaries, the woman tends to go into menopause earlier than other family members did.

What to Expect From Type 2 Menopause

In Type 2 menopause, the estrogen and progesterone levels are adequate, but testosterone is low. This is still an adequate type menopause, but the low testosterone level can cause a loss of energy, or "vim and vigor," as Amelia put it. If you have this type of menopause, you'll feel a decrease in energy that persists after your periods have completely stopped, but you'll generally be free of the major low-estrogen and low-progesterone symptoms described in chapter 2.

Typically, a woman who has a Type 2 menopause has levels of estrogen and progesterone that are normal, but in the lowest quartile. Though the adrenal glands are helping to some degree, they are not able to produce quite enough hormone precursors to fully meet the body's needs. Since the ovaries should still make some testosterone after menopause, Type 2 menopause suggests that even remnant ovarian activity is gone. The adrenal glands are able to maintain adequate estrogen and progesterone levels, sometimes even higher than the lowest quartile, but the testosterone is low.

If you have this type of menopause, you may feel some slight changes in your energy level or mood, but not severe enough to interfere substantially with your life. You may pass off the slight changes as part of "growing old" and not even realize that you have a chance to improve them.

With this type of menopause, you may suffer when under extreme stress. Severe stress taxes your adrenal glands, and can leave them without enough reserve to continue making hormones and hormone precursors. At that time, you can temporarily show signs of estrogen and/or progesterone deficiency. It may then seem as if you've gone into menopause overnight.

> If you have Type 2 menopause, you may feel some slight changes in your energy level or mood, but not severe enough to interfere substantially with your life.

Though you can have normal vaginal lubrication with this menopause type, it may be slightly diminished, especially if your estrogen levels are at the low end of the normal range. The low testosterone increases the risk for vulvar disorders, such as lichen sclerosus. You may have some decreased libido, but not a complete loss of desire, because estrogen also helps keep your libido active.

As long as your estrogen and progesterone levels are balanced, Type 2 menopause does not increase your risk for insulin resistance or endometrial cancer. But if you remain testosterone-deficient for a long time, your muscular strength can diminish, since testosterone plays an important role in maintaining muscle tissue.

Another effect of Type 2 menopause is low-grade depression, which may be felt as a loss of motivation, drive, or confidence. These symptoms may be too mild and vague to be recognized as depression.

There is usually no dramatic change of breast tissue in this type of menopause, though there can be gradual shrinking if your estrogen and progesterone levels are lower after menopause than before. As long as your progesterone and estrogen levels remain in balance (with a ratio between 20:1 and 170:1), an adequate type menopause shouldn't increase your risk for breast cancer.

With this menopause type, you may notice the most change occurring in your skin. If your testosterone level remains too low, you can expect an increased number of fine wrinkles because you may not have enough testosterone to help maintain skin collagen. The low testosterone will also result in weakening of the fine muscles of the face until there is some sagging of the skin, which will make the wrinkles more pronounced.

You also have an increased chance of osteoporosis, even if your estrogen and progesterone levels are above the first quartile. The lack of testosterone will decrease your body's ability to build and repair bone.

One of the benefits of testosterone is that it increases coronary artery blood flow. If you have low testosterone, you may experience chest pain (angina pectoralis) or shortness of breath.

Nutrition and Diet

A high-grade multiple vitamin and mineral is also important for Type 2 menopause. In addition, consider using boron which may increase testosterone levels. Keep an eye on all your hormone levels, however, since boron can also increase estrogen.

✑ TREATMENT OPTIONS FOR TYPE 2 MENOPAUSE

Nutrition and diet: vitamin and mineral supplement, additional boron

Herbs: Siberian ginseng, sarsaparilla, damiana, licorice. *If fatigued, consider:* **Asian ginseng, rehmannia, schisandra, ashwagandha.** *For low-grade depression, consider: Ginkgo biloba*

Homeopathic remedies: damiana, *Ignatia, Sabal serrulata, Zincum metallicum*

Glandulars: adrenal and ovarian

Hormone precursors: DHEA or androstenedione

Hormones: testosterone

Note: Avoid antiandrogens and the herbs vitex and saw palmetto.

Herbal Remedies

Herbs that can aid in *increasing* testosterone include Siberian ginseng, sarsaparilla, damiana, and licorice.

If you have fatigue, the following herbs may be useful: astragalus, bupleurum, Asian ginseng, rehmannia

(*Rehmannia glutinosa*), schisandra (*Schisandra chinensis*), or ashwagandha (*Withania somnifera*).

For the low-grade depression that often accompanies Type 2 menopause, ginkgo (*Ginkgo biloba*) is particularly helpful.

Homeopathic Remedies

For low testosterone symptoms, the homeopathic damiana, *Ignatia*, lecithin, *Sabal serrulata*, or *Zincum metallicum*, can be used to restore libido and help reestablish balance during menopause. Please note that homeopathic remedies have a different effect than herbal remedies (see chapter 10).

Herbal Don'ts
There are certain herbs you definitely should *not* take if you have low testosterone. Vitex (chasteberry, *Vitex agnus-castus*), a main ingredient in many herbal formulas for menopause, could possibly reduce your testosterone level, or impair your body's ability to use available testosterone. If you're experiencing a low-testosterone menopause type, vitex may make some of your symptoms worse, and throw you further out of balance. Before you take any herbal formula designed for menopause, check the label to make sure it doesn't contain vitex.

Saw palmetto (*Sabal serrulata*) is another herb that women with low testosterone should avoid. Like vitex, saw palmetto may have an antiandrogenic effect—that is, it may lower your testosterone levels, or diminish how well the testosterone can be used by your body. See chapter 10 for a list of other substances that have antiandrogen activity.

Glandular Extracts

Studies have found that taking adrenal or ovarian tissue extracts can significantly increase a woman's testosterone levels. There are several cautions to consider when using glandular extracts. Chapter 13 contains information on how to use these extracts, and the risks involved in doing so.

Hormone Replacement and Precursors

Testosterone-replacement therapy is one option in cases of low testosterone, especially for severe deficiencies. If you do take supplemental testosterone, your hormone level should be monitored to make sure you don't get too much. Too high a level of testosterone isn't good for you, either, and can leave you with facial or body hair that remains even after your testosterone level returns to normal. Likewise, hormone therapy can cause or worsen serious medical conditions. You should consider significant hormone therapy only after a full medical evaluation, and use it only under the close and ongoing supervision of your medical doctor, to prevent serious complications.

Another approach is to use a hormone *precursor*, or a "building block" your body can convert into testosterone. DHEA and androstenedione are two important precursors for both testosterone and estrogen. After menopause, as you know, the adrenal glands take over much of the ovaries' hormone-making function. What the adrenal glands produce is actually androstenedione, which can be converted into either estrogen or testosterone. These changes are made through the *steroidogenic pathway* (see appendix E).

When you are low in testosterone, sometimes taking a precursor can bring you back into balance. There's a simple way to tell whether precursors are likely to help you: Have your levels of androstenedione or DHEA tested, either through a saliva or blood test? If they are low, chances are, taking them would help you. If they aren't low, then the problem lies elsewhere; your body already has enough precursors, but isn't effectively converting them into testosterone.

When you have Type 2 menopause, even though your estrogen levels may seem adequate (falling in the "normal" range), they may not be ideal. If your levels of DHEA or androstenedione are low, taking precursors might be an effective way to bring your estrogen up to an ideal level, along with your testosterone levels. Otherwise, you may need to consider another therapy to raise your "normal" estrogen levels to meet your needs ideally.

Similarly, if your progesterone levels are "normal" but not ideal, progesterone precursors such as *pregnenolone* can be effective. However, you should monitor the results by checking your progesterone levels 1 month after starting pregnenolone.

Antiandrogens

If you have low testosterone, you should avoid taking medications that act as antiandrogens and decrease your testosterone levels. (See chapter 10 for a list of antiandrogens). In fact, if you're already taking such a medication, make sure it is not causing your testosterone deficiency. Certain anti-ulcer and high blood pressure medications are antiandrogenic. Always read the information that comes with any prescription to see whether it affects *androgen* levels.

Amelia's Treatment

Amelia chose to try precursors, taking 10 mg of pregnenolone and 5 mg of DHEA daily, along with a high-grade vitamin and mineral supplement.

After a month, she was not satisfied with her progress, so she added adrenal and ovarian glandular supplements. A month later, she reported that her energy and libido had both improved.

After another month, she dropped the adrenal glandular extract because she was feeling too hyperactive, and reduced the DHEA to every other day. Taking precursors in this manner can decrease the chance of the body becoming dependent on steroid hormones and "forgetting" how to make them naturally.

Follow-up saliva tests showed that all of Amelia's hormones were now in the second quartile, and she felt completely better, with all her usual "vim and vigor" restored.

TYPE 3: HIGH TESTOSTERONE

Angela, 56, was a banking officer. Married, without children, she suspected that in her premenopausal years, she had been infertile. Her periods had always been irregular, and had come to an end in her early fifties. She had struggled with facial hair for years, and had electrolysis periodically.

> Since going into menopause, Angela felt she had become more agitated than before, and she was experiencing blood sugar problems, such as fatigue and sleepiness after a high-carbohydrate meal. Her facial hair was becoming even more pronounced.

Since going into menopause, Angela felt she had become more agitated than before, and she was experiencing blood sugar problems, such as fatigue and sleepiness after a high-carbohydrate meal. Her facial hair was becoming even more pronounced. She'd previously had her hormones tested and was assured they were fine. When we tested all three of Angela's major hormones, however, I was not surprised to see that, along with normal levels of estrogen and progesterone, she had high testosterone.

What to Expect From Type 3 Menopause

When your body produces more testosterone than you need, it may make you feel agitated or irritable. This is one of the classic signs of an overly high testosterone level. The increase in testosterone that occurs in this menopause type can start when the adrenal glands gear up to take over some of the ovaries' hormone-making responsibility. The adrenal glands produce androstenedione, which the body can make into either testosterone or estrogen. Ideally, the body makes appropriate amounts of both testosterone and estrogen. But sometimes too much of the androstenedione gets changed into testosterone, and the result is Type 3 menopause.

High levels of testosterone and other androgens can be dangerous for a woman's health. In younger, premenopausal women, high androgen levels are associated with ovarian diseases and menstrual irregularity, as well as symptoms that are distressing if less serious: facial hair, a deepening of the voice, oily skin, and acne. In postmenopausal women, high testosterone levels can have similar effects.

Of the risks and complications associated with high testosterone, blood sugar problems (insulin resistance) and excessive insulin (hyperinsulinemia) may be by far the most serious. Some studies have proposed a link between high testosterone levels in women with a higher risk for endometrial cancer.[1, 2]

There is a bright side to high testosterone: It can boost a woman's strength and libido, as well as her drive and confidence. Also, high testosterone levels are not known to harm the vagina or urinary tract. But the manifestations of too much testosterone can leave a woman feeling so frustrated that she actually ends up depressed.

Type 3 menopause may not be a problem for your bones. High levels of testosterone can actually benefit your bones because it's a hormone that promotes bone building and repair.

There is considerable concern, however, that a high testosterone level can make a woman more vulnerable to heart disease and other serious problems. Testosterone tends to decrease HDL ("good") cholesterol levels and increase insulin resistance that can contribute to diabetes, cancer of the breast and uterus, and heart disease.

Nutrition and Diet

A high-grade multiple vitamin and mineral is very important for Type 3 menopause, especially if the body is stressed with anxiety and agitation. However, do not use boron with Type 3 menopause since it may increase testosterone.

Herbal Remedies

One of my favorite herbs for Type 3 menopause is hops (*Humulus lupulus*), which has mild antiandrogenic activity and is also calming and sedating. Saw palmetto or vitex are also antiandrogenic and may help bring down high testosterone levels.

The classic menopause herb black cohosh (*Cimicifuga racemosa*) is excellent for this menopause type.

❧ TREATMENT OPTIONS FOR TYPE 3 MENOPAUSE

Nutrition and diet: vitamin and mineral supplement; avoid boron

Herbs: hops, saw palmetto, vitex, black cohosh.
 For agitation, consider: **passion flower, skullcap, St. John's wort, valerian, vervain**

Glandulars: not recommended do not use with this menopause type

Hormone Precursors: not recommended do not use with this menopause type

Hormones: estrogen in the oral form can help decrease testosterone (if estrogen is on the low end of normal)

Note: Consider using antiandrogens.

For the sense of agitation, try passion flower (*Passiflora incarnata*), skullcap (*Scutellaria lateriflora*), St. John's wort (*Hypericum perforatum*), valerian (*Valeriana officinalis*), or vervain (*Verbena officinalis*).

Glandular Extracts

Extracts of glandular tissue are not a good idea for this menopause type. Ovarian and adrenal extracts are likely to increase testosterone levels and thus make you feel worse.

Hormone Replacement and Precursors

Taking oral estrogen can be a useful way to lower the effect of your high testosterone levels while also boosting borderline low estrogen if it is present. If you do this and you have an intact uterus, you should also take progesterone or another progestogen. (See chapter 14 for more information about the risks of taking estrogen without progesterone.) As with all hormone therapies, only consider this option after a thorough medical evaluation, and under a doctor's supervision.

In general, DHEA and androstenedione are *not* recommended for this menopause type, because they usually work to raise testosterone levels.

Antiandrogens

Earlier in this chapter, I mentioned that some medications and herbs tend to bring down levels of testosterone and other androgens. These antiandrogenics make Type 2 menopause worse, but they can be used to relieve Type 3 symptoms (see Herbal Remedies on page 98). See chapter 10 for a list of these antiandrogens.

Angela's Treatment

Angela chose to try herbal remedies. Black cohosh and hops soothed her nervous system, and she felt considerably less agitated. After 6 months, a lab test showed that her testosterone levels had decreased. She also took saw palmetto, hoping that it would decrease her facial hair. It didn't reduce already-established hair, but she chose to stay on a low dose in the hope of preventing further hair growth.

In addition, Angela took a high-grade vitamin and mineral supplement with extra chromium, and changed her diet to one with lower carbohydrates and more protein. This diet helped manage insulin resistance.

CHAPTER SEVEN

The Low-Estrogen Menopause Types

Type 4, Type 5, and Type 6

This chapter takes a look at the menopause types that have low estrogen levels, but normal levels of progesterone.

Remember Ellen from chapter 1? Her symptoms included some classic signs of low estrogen levels. On her initial visit, she felt, in her own words, "dull and lifeless, almost depressed," which I could see very well from her manner. Her speech was monotonous and lifeless. She was going through the motions of life. She wouldn't even have come to see me, she said, without the prodding of her family. Her spark was missing. But I had a sense that she'd been a vibrant, active woman all her life until menopause.

Ellen turned out to have a Type 5 menopause—low estrogen with low testosterone. Later in this chapter, I'll tell you how Ellen's treatment worked.

Having read about Types 4, 5, and 6 in chapter 2, you have some idea how an estrogen deficiency can affect you. Estrogen normally stimulates the brain and has a powerful influence on mood, memory, and learning. It keeps the vagina and labia healthy, and enhances sexual desire. Estrogen also protects the skin and breasts against advanced aging, and helps prevent serious health problems such as osteoporosis and heart disease.

Some of the most upsetting signs of estrogen deficiency are changes in mood, memory, or even personality. The good news is that there are several effective ways you can raise your estrogen levels. In this chapter, I'll discuss a number of natural and conventional therapies for each of the low-estrogen menopause types. After you read about the treatments described here, turn to the later chapters in this book for more in-depth information about nutrition (chapter 11), herbal treatments (chapter 12), glandular extracts (chapter 13), and hormone-replacement therapy (chapter 14).

A number of medications, herbs, and other substances can reduce your levels of estrogen. If you are already estrogen deficient, these antiestrogens could make you feel worse. See chapter 10 for more information.

TYPE 4: LOW ESTROGEN

Elizabeth was 50 when she felt the need to seek treatment for her menopausal symptoms. A housewife with three grown children, Elizabeth had recently embarked on a demanding MBA program. She had no history of illness, gynecological or any other kind, but for the first time in her life she was feeling tired and unmotivated. She also felt a little depressed. She was still menstruating, but her periods had become lighter over the past year, and the last two cycles had been longer than usual. She was diagnosed as being in *perimenopause* (early menopause), with low estrogen levels.

> A number of medications, herbs, and other substances can reduce your levels of estrogen. If you are already estrogen deficient, these antiestrogens could make you feel worse.

What to Expect From Type 4 Menopause

If you have low estrogen, you may feel mentally and physically depressed and weighed down. Physically, low estrogen can lead to hot flashes, which can range from mild to severe. For some women, hot flashes come as often as several times a day.

When the body's hormone-making pathway is working properly, androgens (such as testosterone and androstenedione) move through the pathway to become estrogens. In Type 4 menopause, there is an obstacle toward the end of the pathway, where estrogen is produced. The adrenal glands appear to be doing their job of producing androstenedione, but the body is being blocked from making it into estrogen.

This type of menopause is often accompanied by some feelings of frustration. The lack of estrogen causes feelings of mental dullness, and an increased risk of depression. After all, it's depressing and frightening to find that you can't remember names or learn new things as well as you used to. But women with this menopause type have normal levels of testosterone, which can help ward off depression and maintain a certain amount of drive and motivation.

Still, testosterone can't make up for a low level of estrogen in every respect. Estrogen increases verbal skills, making speech easier and names more readily recalled. It also helps with fine motor skills, such as precision work with the hands, and with learning concepts. Even with normal testosterone levels, a woman with Type 4 menopause may find it harder to speak fluently, remember names, use a computer, or thread a needle.

These signs of low estrogen can be quite frustrating, especially for a woman whose motivation and drive are still strong. If this situation goes on long enough, despair and depression can result. While normal testosterone levels should guard against depression, estrogen deficiency can have a stronger effect here than testosterone, and the result may be at least a low-grade depression.

With Type 4 menopause, you can suffer from stress incontinence (the involuntary leaking of urine when you sneeze or cough) and vaginal dryness. Your normal testosterone levels may help maintain your libido, but without enough estrogen you're probably feeling less desire. Vaginal dryness and thinning of the vaginal walls can also make sex painful and unsatisfying. Though the presence of testosterone may decrease the incidence of hot flashes, they can still occur in this menopause type.

In Type 4 menopause, there may be some advanced aging and thinning of the skin. Having normal testosterone levels means that your muscle tone—including the small muscles of the face—will probably remain good, but without enough estrogen your skin will lose moisture and collagen, thus becoming drier and thinner. Another problem with this menopause type is that, if you have too little estrogen to balance out your testosterone, you can have some problems with oily skin and acne.

With a low estrogen level, you are at risk for bone loss and heart disease. Your normal testosterone level decreases your risk for osteoporosis somewhat; testosterone has some bone-protecting effects. But you should still take steps to protect against osteoporosis as well as the other serious health problems that can arise when you have too little estrogen.

There are a number of different approaches you can take to treat a Type 4 menopause. For some women, the best option might be hormone-replacement therapy. (See this chapter and chapter 14 for more information about hormone therapy to restore estrogen levels). Other women might prefer to use natural alternatives such as diet, herbal medicine, and nutritional supplements.

The treatments I discuss here will suit this type of menopause.

Nutrition and Diet

As well as using a high-grade multiple vitamin supplement with additional boron, foods which contain phytoestrogens can also be helpful for Type 4 menopause.

✨ TREATMENT OPTIONS FOR TYPE 4 MENOPAUSE

Nutrition and diet: vitamin and mineral supplement, phytoestrogens, boron

Herbs: alfalfa, dong quai, false unicorn root, fenugreek, hops, sage. *For fatigue, consider:* Asian ginseng, licorice, rehmannia, schisandra. *To enhance memory and mental ability, consider:* bacopa or ginkgo

Homeopathic remedies: *Cantharis, Causticum, Graphites, Juniperus communis, Apis mellifica, Lachesis, Belladonna, Natrum muriaticum*

Glandulars: ovarian extracts

Hormone precursors: DHEA or androstenedione

Hormones: estrogen (oral, creams, or gels)

Note: Avoid antiestrogens.

Soybeans and soy products are rich in a particular type of phytoestrogens that can also be good for your heart and bones. Other phytoestrogens can be found in certain vegetables. (See table 4: Foods with Phytoestrogens, on page 214.)

Herbal Remedies

There are several herbs that behave like estrogen in the body. These herbs, known as *estrogen mimetics*, include alfalfa *(Medicago sativa)*, dong quai *(Angelica sinensis)*, false unicorn root *(Chamaelirium luteum)*, fenugreek *(Trigonella foenumgraecum)*, hops *(Humulus lupulus)*, and sage *(Salvia officinalis)*. Sage can be very helpful for hot flashes. This common cooking herb has mild estrogenic actions and also has the ability to suppress perspiration.

If you have fatigue, the following herbs may be helpful: astragalus *(Astragalus membranaceus)*, bupleurum, Asian ginseng *(Panax)*, licorice *(Glycyrrhiza glabra)*, rehmannia, schisandra *(Schisandra chinensis)*, or ashwagandha *(Withania somnifera)*.

If you feel that your memory and ability to focus are not as good as they used to be, try a brain tonic herb such as bacopa *(Bacopa monniera)* or ginkgo.

Homeopathic Remedies

For urinary problems, such as stress incontinence and increased risk of urinary burning associated with low estrogen, the following homeopathic remedies can be useful: *Cantharis, Causticum, Graphites, Juniperus communis,* and *Apis mellifica*. You can treat your hot flashes with *Lachesis* or *Belladonna*. A remedy for vaginal dryness is *Natrum muriaticum*.

Glandular Extracts

Ovarian extracts can raise weak estrogen levels. They can also increase testosterone levels, however, so use these supplements with caution and stop taking them if you develop any signs of excessive testosterone, such as agitation.

Hormone Replacement and Precursors

The fact that you have adequate testosterone probably means that you have all the precursors (DHEA and androstenedione) your body needs. In this case, taking DHEA or androstenedione is less likely to help you. The problem isn't that you lack precursors; it's that your body is having trouble converting them into estrogen. Taking DHEA or androstenedione in this case can even hurt you by raising your testosterone level too high.

The best course of action might be estrogen replacement, especially if your estrogen deficiency is severe. Mild symptoms of estrogen deficiency often respond to herbal and nutritional therapies. One problem with taking estrogen is that it can cause a drop in your testosterone levels, especially if oral estrogen is used instead of estrogen creams or gels. As your body can make testosterone from precursors, it may be appropriate to take a small amount of DHEA or androstenedione when taking the estrogen to keep your testosterone levels from dropping too low. Be sure to monitor all hormone levels regularly if you are taking any hormone or hormone precursor.

In chapter 14, you can read more about the risks and benefits of estrogen-replacement therapy.

Elizabeth's Treatment

Elizabeth was just going into menopause—an ideal time to use nutritional and herbal remedies. She began taking a high-grade vitamin and mineral supplement daily, along with *Panax ginseng* to stimulate and balance her adrenal glands, and dong quai, an estrogen-mimetic herb long used by the Chinese to balance female hormones and promote gynecological health.

Six weeks later, Elizabeth felt somewhat better, but complained of increased flatulence. This side effect was most likely due to the dong quai, so she added fennel to soothe her digestion. This solved the problem.

But there was more to do. Despite the fact that Elizabeth reported feeling better, her estrogen levels had not improved, so she started taking 10 mg of DHEA daily, a dosage that gave her jitters. After 3 days of no dose, she resumed with a dose of 5 mg, which felt much better. After 6 weeks at this dosage, she showed a slight increase in testosterone, but her estrogen was still too low.

> Be sure to monitor all hormone levels regularly if you are taking any hormone or hormone precursor.

At that point, Elizabeth chose to start taking supplemental estrogen. She used a skin patch that delivered 0.05 mg of estrogen daily, a typical dose. Her older sister had experienced good results with the patch, so it made sense that Elizabeth did well with it, too. (This is more likely to be the case when sisters share the same menopause type.)

To reduce health risks associated with taking estrogen, Elizabeth also started on a cyclical program of oral-*micronized* progesterone. (See chapter 14 for a discussion of the risks involved in taking estrogen alone.) Within a couple of months, all her hormone levels were within normal range, and she felt much happier and had more energy. To make sure her hormones remained in balance, she was advised to retest her levels every 6 months.

TYPE 5: LOW ESTROGEN WITH LOW TESTOSTERONE

Let's return to Ellen's case. The first clue that her menopause might be Type 5 was her remarkable, uncharacteristic listlessness, combined with the near disappearance of her libido. A deficiency of estrogen is enough to dampen a woman's mood and sexual desire. But when testosterone levels are also low, these effects are magnified. Testosterone normally plays a major role in the libido, and also boosts a woman's energy, drive, and confidence. When both of these hormones are lacking, the result can be a profound loss of drive, energy, sexual desire, confidence, and mental clarity. I was not surprised when Ellen's lab tests confirmed my diagnosis: She had Type 5 menopause.

What to Expect From Type 5 Menopause

This type of menopause produces a pronounced effect on a woman's mood and even, apparently, her personality. She may seem indifferent to things that she normally cares about. Loved ones may even feel that she cares less about them.

A woman going through a Type 5 menopause may also feel somewhat estranged from herself, and from who she was in her life before menopause. The decreased estrogen is changing the actions of virtually every type of neurotransmitter in her brain. Norepinephrine, seratonin, dopamine, and GABAA are all affected. Her moods, her desires, her every thoughts are different due to these changes. Depression can occur as estrogen levels drop.

Unfortunately, her changes in mood may be misinterpreted as a need for an antidepressant. Taking an antidepressant will not correct an estrogen imbalance. (If feelings of depression are severe or persistent, it's a good idea to get a full medical evaluation to rule out other possible health conditions and determine whether medication might help.) It is this slowing of the mind that can be most frustrating for women who have Type 5 menopause.

Memory starts to slip, it becomes more difficult to learn new things, and your perception of the world can begin to dull. The world actually appears less interesting to you. You are not as easily pleased; and you feel less excitement and less joy. This dulling of the mind and alienation from the world just feed into your sense of depression and indifference. Your libido drops and may become nonexistent. All these changes will alter the way you interact with the world around you. Your personality can change.

These changes are evident to the people around you. They notice the spark is gone. If your significant other is going through andropause (male menopause—yes, it is real!), he may be poorly equipped to be supportive during this time. He is struggling with decreased testosterone levels, and the depression, decreased libido, and low self-esteem that go with this drop. He may not understand your change in mood, change in personality, and decreased libido. This misunderstanding can bring conflict, and further estrangement, into the relationship. On the other hand, his decreased testosterone levels may make him kinder and more patient, which can help him be understanding as you go through this passage.

If you are going through Type 5 menopause, you will experience some significant changes in your body in addition to the mental and emotional changes. Some of these changes could have a major impact on your body image—your personal image of your physical self. The changes are significant enough that you may feel estranged from your own body. This is most likely to occur if you also suffer from an underlying depression, which can result in your disliking yourself.

You may have vaginal atrophy and dryness. These conditions make sexual intercourse painful and difficult, which obviously tends to further diminish sexual desire. The low estrogen can result in a weakening of the urethra and an increased occurrence of stress incontinence.

There can also be a risk to your heart as you lose the protective effects of estrogen. Resulting changes in cholesterol can increase the chance of cardiovascular diseases.

Since both estrogen and testosterone are important for the maintenance of skin collagen, thinner skin and more wrinkles are likely. Low testosterone can cause drier skin and decreased tone of small facial muscles, which can produce premature sagging of tissues. With less breast collagen, the breast tissue can also shrink and begin to sag.

Likewise, your risk of osteoporosis increases as you lose the bone-protecting effects of both estrogen and testosterone.

Nutrition and Diet

A high-grade multiple vitamin supplement with additional boron and foods rich in phytoestrogens can be helpful for Type 5 menopause. Soybeans and soy products are rich in a particular type of phytoestrogen that can also be good for your heart and bones. (See table 4: Foods with Phytoestrogens, on page 214.)

Herbal Remedies

Herbs that act as *estrogen mimetics* behave like estrogen in the body. These include alfalfa, dong quai, false unicorn

❧ TREATMENT OPTIONS FOR TYPE 5 MENOPAUSE

Nutrition and diet: vitamin and mineral supplement, phytoestrogens, boron

Herbs: alfalfa, dong quai, false unicorn root, fenugreek, sage, Siberian ginseng, sarsaparilla, licorice. *For fatigue, consider:* astragalus, bupleurum, Asian ginseng, licorice, rehmannia, schisandra, ashwagandha. *To enhance memory and mental ability, consider:* bacopa or ginkgo

Homeopathic remedies: *Cantharis, Causticum, Graphites, Juniperus communis, Apis mellifica, Lachesis, Belladona, Natrum muriaticum, Turnera diffusa, Ignatia,* lecithin, *Sabal serrulata, Zincum metallicum*

Glandulars: ovarian extracts

Hormone precursors: DHEA or androstenedione

Hormones: estrogen (creams or gels), testosterone

Note: Avoid antiestrogens and antiandrogens.

root, fenugreek, and sage. Sage can be very helpful for hot flashes: This common cooking herb has mild estrogenic actions and also has the ability to suppress perspiration.

Saw palmetto and vitex (chasteberry) both reduce testosterone levels, so these herbs should be avoided because you already have a testosterone deficiency. As with Type 2, you should be wary of combination menopause remedies, because if they contain either of these herbs (and they commonly contain vitex) they will not be good for you. Also avoid hops, due to its antiandrogen effect.

Herbs that may help increase testosterone and other androgens include Siberian ginseng, sarsaparilla, and licorice.

If you have fatigue, the following herbs may be helpful: astragalus, bupleurum, Asian ginseng, licorice, rehmannia, schisandra, or ashwagandha.

If you feel that your concentration and memory are not as good as they used to be, try a brain tonic herb such as bacopa or ginkgo.

Homeopathic Remedies

If urinary problems such as burning or incontinence occur, consider using *Cantharis, Causticum, Graphites, Juniperus communis*, or *Apis mellifica*. Try *Lachesis* or *Belladonna* for hot flashes, and *Natrum muriaticum* for vaginal dryness.

For low testosterone, the homeopathic remedies damiana, *Ignatia*, lecithin, *Sabal serrulata*, or *Zincum metallicum*, are helpful for restoring libido and reestablishing balance during menopause.

Glandular Extracts

Ovarian extracts can effectively raise both estrogen and testosterone levels and so can be very useful for Type 5 menopause.

Hormone Replacement and Precursors

With Type 5 menopause, there is a good chance that you also have low levels of the precursors DHEA and androstenedione. Estrogen and testosterone share the same precursors and, if both hormones are low, chances are their precursors are low as well. Many women with this menopause type show low DHEA on their lab tests. In some cases, DHEA supplementation has been a successful way to raise both testosterone and estrogen levels. If you do choose to use precursors, get a hormone test every 6 months to make sure the precursors are working to raise the levels of both estrogen and testosterone.

DHEA supplementation is unlikely to be successful in women who have had a hysterectomy or who have a chronic endocrine system disease, such as diabetes. Precursors also appear not to work well when there is a current underlying disease, adrenal fatigue, or history of surgery.

If precursors don't raise your hormone levels to a healthy balance, you may consider both estrogen-replacement therapy and testosterone-replacement therapy. If you have an intact uterus, you shouldn't take estrogen without combining it with progesterone, or another progestogen. (See chapter 14 for a more detailed explanation of the risks of taking estrogen alone.)

The form of estrogen may be important to consider. Oral estrogen can actually reduce the effectiveness of your testosterone. If you take oral estrogen for Type 5 menopause, you may also need to take supplemental testosterone or implement other steps to maintain your testosterone levels.

Ellen's Treatment

Ellen chose to try DHEA at a dosage of 5 mg daily to treat her low estrogen and testosterone levels. She also took a high-grade nutritional supplement. When we retested her hormone levels after 6 weeks, her estrogen and testosterone levels were significantly higher, her hot flashes had diminished, and her mood and energy had improved. After another 6 weeks, we dropped the DHEA to 2 mg daily because she reported feeling a little agitated at times. In another 6 weeks—18 weeks after beginning the therapy—all her hormone levels were within normal range, and she felt dramatically better. Ellen's energy and vitality had returned, along with her libido. She felt mentally sharp and

> For Ellen, using DHEA as a precursor was a great success. Her energy and vitality had returned, along with her libido. She felt mentally sharp and physically fine.

physically fine. For Ellen, using DHEA as a precursor was a great success.

TYPE 6: LOW ESTROGEN WITH HIGH TESTOSTERONE

Samantha, a business consultant, single, and childless by choice, was 44 years old when she consulted me. She had always been in good health, until recently, when she had begun to experience irritability, thinning hair, oily skin, and insomnia. Her periods had been quite irregular for the past 3 years, with accompanying mood and sleep changes. When she came in to see me, she had not had a period for 6 months. In fact, she was already through menopause. She had gone through menopause somewhat early, probably because she is a smoker and of slight build, two factors associated with early menopause.

Samantha was most concerned about her hair loss, which was beginning to get quite noticeable. A hormone test revealed that she had low estrogen and high testosterone levels.

What to Expect From Type 6 Menopause

If you have this type of menopause, you will probably feel more easily irritated than usual. As with all of the high-testosterone menopause types, Type 6 menopause has significant effects on the body and mind. Though low estrogen carries its own symptoms and risks, the high testosterone levels seem to exacerbate things. Some symptoms may be more intense, certain risks are now more serious, and the nervous system may feel more on edge.

Of course, high testosterone levels affect the brain and mood. If you have Type 6 menopause, your drive and motivation are probably strong, but the high testosterone level can make you feel irritable. Thanks to the testosterone, you probably feel at least some sexual desire, but you may also feel too agitated or even hostile to want to relate sexually. Many women with this menopause type report that sex isn't satisfying, as can happen when low estrogen levels result in vaginal dryness.

If you have this menopause type, you may have more trouble sleeping, possibly to the point of developing a sleep disturbance. You may wake up feeling exhausted, which only increases irritability. So, the overall effect of high testosterone is bad for your nervous system.

If your testosterone is high for too long, you can develop oily skin or even acne. Another effect of high testosterone and low estrogen is the loss of scalp hair. This condition is called androgenic alopecia, which means hair loss due to excessive androgens.

There are some unanswered questions as to whether high testosterone levels can make up for the lack of estrogen and decrease the risk of developing osteoporosis in women with low estrogen. We do know that estrogen protects women against bone loss, but we see the same effect with testosterone in men. One study has shown that high testosterone levels decrease bone loss in young women with polycystic ovary disease, but at this time there's no research showing whether this is true for post-menopausal women.[1]

❧ TREATMENT OPTIONS FOR TYPE 6 MENOPAUSE

Nutrition and diet: vitamin and mineral supplement, phytoestrogens; avoid boron

Herbs: alfalfa, dong quai, false unicorn root, fenugreek, sage, vitex, saw palmetto, hops. *For fatigue, consider:* astragalus, bupleurum, Asian ginseng, licorice, rehmannia, schisandra, ashwagandha. *To enhance memory and mental ability, consider:* bacopa or ginkgo

Homeopathic remedies: *Lachesis, Natrum muriaticum*

Glandulars: not recommended—do not use with this type of menopause

Hormone precursors: not recommended—do not use with this type of menopause

Hormones: estrogen (orally)

Note: Consider using antiandrogens.

Nutrition and Diet

As with the other low-estrogen menopause types, foods containing phytoestrogens can be helpful for Type 6 menopause. A high-grade multiple vitamin and mineral supplement is a good idea, but avoid boron. Information on phytoestrogens can be found in table 4: Foods with Phytoestrogens, on page 214.

Herbal Remedies

As discussed, estrogen-mimetic herbs behave like estrogen in the body. These include alfalfa, dong quai, false unicorn root, fenugreek, and sage. Sage can be very helpful for hot flashes. This common cooking herb has mild estrogenic actions and also has the ability to suppress perspiration.

Vitex and saw palmetto can both be used to reduce testosterone levels. Vitex is a common ingredient in many herbal formulas for menopause. Hops is an excellent choice for this menopause type.

If you have fatigue, the following herbs may be helpful: astragalus, bupleurum, Asian ginseng, licorice, rehmannia, schisandra, or ashwagandha.

If you feel that your concentration and memory are not as good as they used to be, try a brain tonic herb such as bacopa or ginkgo.

Homeopathic Remedies

Hot flashes are not usually frequent in Type 6 menopause, but if they occur you can treat them with *Lachesis* or *Belladonna*. Try *Natrum muriaticum* for vaginal dryness.

Glandular Extracts

Glandular extracts are not suitable for Type 6 menopause. Ovarian and adrenal extracts are likely to increase testosterone, so menopause types with high testosterone do best to avoid them. Aggression and agitation can occur when women with high testosterone take ovarian extract.

Hormone Replacement and Precursors

Taking estrogen orally has the dual effect of boosting estrogen levels and lowering testosterone levels, so this is a good treatment for this menopause type, if herbal or nutritional therapies are not effective enough.[2] Topical estrogen will not be as effective as oral estrogen in lowering testosterone levels.

Estrogen precursors such as DHEA or androstenedione are not usually suitable for Type 6 menopause, because they can raise testosterone levels as well.

If you have an intact uterus and take supplemental estrogen, you should also take progesterone or another progestogen. (See chapter 14 for more information on the risks of taking estrogen alone.)

Other Treatments

Drugs such as spironolactone, ketoconazole, and other antiandrogens have been used with some success in treating androgenic alopecia.

Samantha's Treatment

Samantha wanted to use herbs to balance her hormones. She began taking high-potency vitamins and minerals, and finally stopped smoking. She took fenugreek (for its estrogenic effects and to help stabilize blood sugar), saw palmetto (for its antiandrogenic effect), and black cohosh (which stabilizes hormones and reduces irritability).

A saliva test 2 months later showed that her testosterone was still high, while estrogen was still low. Next, Samantha started on a daily dose of 2 mg of oral-micronized estradiol from a compounding pharmacist. (See chapter 14 for a discussion of compounding pharmacists.) This was the estrogen of choice because it often lowers testosterone levels. After 3 more months, a follow-up test showed that her levels of both estrogen and testosterone were normal. Samantha was happy to see that her hair was starting to grow back in.

CHAPTER EIGHT

The Low-Progesterone Menopause Types

Type 7, Type 8, and Type 9

Having low progesterone is pretty unsettling. The low-progesterone menopause types tend to be fraught with unrest and uneasiness. The body can transform progesterone down into chemicals that have a powerfully calming effect on the nervous system. These chemicals (called progesterone metabolites) act on some of the same brain cells as antianxiety drugs such as Valium (diazepam) and Xanax (alprazolam). These brain cells have GABAA (gamma-amino-butyric acid type A) receptors (see Glossary for more information).

Without progesterone's calm, there is only storm. If you have a low-progesterone menopause, you may feel nervous or jittery most of the time. Also, too little progesterone can lead to sleep disturbance. When the nervous system is chronically sleep deprived, the consequence can be a chronic stress reaction, causing anxiety and agitation with underlying fatigue and exhaustion.

Another problem with progesterone deficiencies is that they often result in a low progesterone-to-estrogen (P:E) ratio, which can lead to increased pain, inflammation, and allergies. This increased discomfort fuels the unrest of progesterone-deficient menopause types.

> Without progesterone's calm, there is only storm. If you have a low-progesterone menopause, you may feel nervous or jittery most of the time.

The good news is that women with progesterone deficiency respond well to progesterone-replacement therapy. (But it's important to make sure your dosage isn't too high, as we'll see later on, and in chapter 14). Intriguingly, the dosage of progesterone you need depends partly on the amount of stress in your life. Do you remember the "steroidogenic pathway," the body's hormone-creating system discussed in chapter 5? When you're under stress, your body secretes the hormone cortisol. As progesterone is a precursor of cortisol, your body will need more progesterone in stressful circumstances. Taking progesterone may increase your cortisol levels and help your body meet the extra hormonal needs of stress.

Although progesterone replacement will not help all postmenopausal women, it can make a world of difference for low-progesterone menopause types.

If your progesterone is low, you should be aware that certain medications can reduce your progesterone levels even further. (See chapter 10 for more information.)

After you read about the treatments described here, turn to the later chapters in this book for more in-depth information about nutrition (chapter 11), herbal treatments (chapter 12), glandular extracts (chapter 13), and hormone-replacement therapy (chapter 14).

TYPE 7: LOW PROGESTERONE

Pauline, a 52-year-old college professor, was a healthy, strong, sensible woman who was amazed to find herself having so much trouble during menopause. "I'm irritable all the time," she complained, "and I can't sleep. I'm exhausted during the day."

Pauline had a history of PMS (premenstrual syndrome) and had recently stopped having periods altogether after 2 years of irregular cycles. She experienced some hot flashes, which decreased after she quit drinking coffee. Her hormone test showed her to be deficient in progesterone, with normal levels of estrogen and testosterone. I diagnosed her as being in early postmenopause.

What to Expect From Type 7 Menopause

The classic progesterone-deficient woman feels anxious and irritable a lot of the time. It is hard for her to relax. If the deficiency is severe, a feeling of gnawing anxiety may leave a woman uncharacteristically humorless and critical. If you have Type 7 menopause, you may feel frustrated with your loved ones more often than usual. They may complain that you're "moody" or "pouty," unlike your usual self. You may even say harsh things you normally would never say. In fact, your brain chemistry is feeling the effects of a shortage of progesterone and its metabolites. When GABAA receptors are deprived of input from progesterone and its metabolites, a woman can actually experience symptoms similar to those seen in withdrawal from drugs such as Valium, Librium (chlordiazepoxide), and Xanax, though rarely as extreme, and without the more serious medical complications associated with those drugs.

Such drugs are sometimes used to treat postmenopausal woman. When women are placed on estrogen-replacement therapy, but no progesterone, they are often put on antianxiety drugs as well. I recall one woman who became so sharp-tongued on estrogen that her family thought she'd had a stroke! Taking estrogen without progesterone is enough to throw some women into a Type 7 anxiety state, which can be mistaken for an "anxiety disorder" and treated not with progesterone but with antianxiety drugs. (If feelings of anxiety are intense or persistent, I strongly recommend a full medical evaluation to rule out other health conditions, and to determine whether treatment is needed.)

✎ TREATMENT OPTIONS FOR TYPE 7 MENOPAUSE

Nutrition and diet: vitamin and mineral supplement, extra antioxidants

Herbs: vitex, passion flower, skullcap, valerian, vervain, St. John's wort, black cohosh, wild yam. *For fatigue, consider:* astragalus, bupleurum, Asian ginseng, licorice, rehmannia, schisandra, ashwagandha

Homeopathic remedies: *Lachesis, Belladonna, Natrum muriaticum*

Glandulars: Try ovarian but watch hormone levels

Hormone precursors: pregnenolone

Hormones: progesterone

Note: Avoid antiprogestogens.

The problem is that the low progesterone level has other harmful health effects if left untreated. The low progesterone level increases your risk for endometrial cancer.

If you have Type 7 menopause, your normal levels of estrogen and testosterone should do a great deal to protect you against wrinkles, as well as vaginal and urinary problems. Your libido will likely be strong, but if you're having trouble relaxing, your sex life may suffer.

If your P:E ratio is too low, you can experience uterine bleeding (spotting).

Nutrition and Diet

A high-grade multiple vitamin and mineral is very important for Type 7 menopause, with special attention given to antioxidants needed for progesterone production. These antioxidants include vitamins C, A, and E as well as beta-carotene and selenium. Avoid boron until after the progesterone deficiency is corrected.

Herbal Remedies

Vitex reportedly increases progesterone levels, and so it is considered the herb of choice for this menopause type.

Mild nervine herbs such as passion flower, skullcap, valerian, vervain, or St. John's wort can help calm the nervous system.

The classic menopause herb black cohosh is also good for this type. The anti-inflammatory and anti-spasmodic actions of wild yam *(Dioscorea villosa)* may ease symptoms due to low progesterone levels. If the P:E ratio is low enough to cause uterine bleeding, paeonia *(Paeonia lactiflora)* will be quite useful.

If you have fatigue, the following herbs may be helpful: astragalus, bupleurum, Asian *(Panax)* ginseng, licorice, rehmannia, schisandra, or ashwagandha.

Homeopathic Remedies

Homeopathic vitex *(Vitex agnus-castus)* may improve low-progesterone symptoms. Use *Lachesis* or *Belladonna* to treat hot flashes, and *Natrum muriaticum* for vaginal dryness.

Glandular Extracts

As ovarian extracts can increase estrogen levels, menopause types that do not have enough progesterone should use ovarian extracts with caution, and keep an eye on the P:E ratio so that it is at least 20:1.

Hormone Replacement and Precursors

Progesterone-replacement therapy can be very effective for Type 7 menopause, although it may take a little time to adjust to the progesterone replacement. You may feel sleepy for the first few days on progesterone. If you can get some extra rest, the calming and balancing effects of progesterone can take effect sooner. You may need to take a few naps the first day or two on progesterone, after which you will feel refreshed, well rested, and free from anxiety—even if worry has been plaguing you for a long time.

The amount of progesterone each woman needs will depend on how much her adrenal glands are still able to contribute. The required dosage for progesterone replacement can be from 25 to 200 mg of oral-micronized progesterone daily.

Progesterone precursors, such as pregnenolone, can be effective. However, check your progesterone levels 1 month after starting pregnenolone to evaluate the results.

If your estrogen levels are adequate, but not ideal, consider estrogen precursors such as DHEA or androstenedione. They can effectively raise estrogen if levels of these precursors are low. If DHEA and androstenedione levels are adequate, and estrogen levels are not ideal, then estrogen replacement may be required.

The P:E ratio must be evaluated. If the P:E ratio is not at least 20:1, it is important to restore the proper ratio, and keep it there.

If you take progesterone, you should be aware that this may reduce your testosterone levels to below ideal. Progesterone has an antiandrogenic effect, so if you take it, you may need to take testosterone replacement as well. Taking DHEA or androstenedione can increase your testosterone levels, especially if your levels of these precursor hormones are low. However, this is not guaranteed because sometimes the DHEA and androstenedione convert into estrogen instead. If this happens, you will need to take testosterone directly. As with any hormone therapy, I advise a full medical evaluation, and the supervision of a doctor.

Pauline's Treatment

Pauline's history suggested that a chronic progesterone deficiency may have contributed to her PMS symptoms in the past. She chose to go on progesterone replacement, taking 100 mg of oral-micronized progesterone each morning. She began taking a high-grade vitamin and mineral supplement. She also chose to augment the hormone replacement with herbs, taking passion flower each evening to help her sleep, and *Panax ginseng* during the day to help with fatigue.

> Pauline's history suggested that a chronic progesterone deficiency may have contributed to her PMS symptoms in the past.

After 2 months, she felt improvements in mood and energy, and all her hormones were within normal range. She still takes passion flower and ginseng as needed, usually 2 or 3 times a week, on more stressful days, usually Mondays and Fridays. She continues to take progesterone and will retest once a year unless her symptoms change.

TYPE 8: LOW PROGESTERONE WITH LOW TESTOSTERONE

Patricia, a 68-year-old widow who owned five gift shops, was suffering from depression and restlessness. She also complained of low libido and stress incontinence. Several years earlier, she had been in a bad motor vehicle accident, which may have contributed to her menopausal symptoms because it appeared to have compromised the health of her adrenal glands. Patricia had always had normal periods and had stopped menstruating in her early fifties. Tests revealed that she had moderate osteoporosis.

What to Expect From Type 8 Menopause

Patricia's depression was typical of this menopause type. A Type 8 menopause is burdened with worry and sad thoughts. Spirits are low and you feel anxious and gloomy. You may feel melancholic and even quite deeply depressed.

Although you have a "normal" amount of estrogen in your body, in Type 8 menopause, the estrogen level is usually in the lowest quartile. A low-progesterone menopause, especially when testosterone is also low, often happens when the adrenal glands aren't producing quite enough androstenedione, the precursor hormone for both estrogen and testosterone. In other words, you're still able to make a certain amount of estrogen, but it may not be ideal. DHEA and cortisol levels are usually low in Type 8 menopause, too.

With low progesterone levels, there may be increased risk of endometrial cancer. This risk will be even higher if your estrogen levels are high, in the third or fourth quartile. The lower the P:E ratio, the greater the risk.

As with Type 7, your estrogen levels are protecting your skin against drying and thinning, as well as vaginal dryness. But in Type 8, you don't have the benefit of testosterone. Your muscle tone can suffer, along with your libido, and, of course, your general outlook on life. Low testosterone types often suffer a loss of motivation

✣ TREATMENT OPTIONS FOR TYPE 8 MENOPAUSE

Nutrition and diet: vitamin and mineral supplement, extra antioxidants; use boron cautiously

Herbs: passion flower, skullcap, valerian, vervain, St. John's wort, black cohosh, wild yam, Siberian ginseng, sarsaparilla, licorice. *For fatigue, consider:* **astragalus, bupleurum, Asian ginseng, licorice, rehmannia, schisandra, ashwagandha.** *To enhance memory and mental ability, consider:* **bacopa or ginkgo.** *Avoid:* **vitex and saw palmetto**

Homeopathic remedies: damiana, *Ignatia,* **lecithin,** *Sabal serrulata, Zincum metallicum,* **vitex** *(Vitex agnus-castus), Lachesis, Belladonna, Natrum muriaticum*

Glandulars: consider ovarian extracts

Hormone precursors: pregnenolone, DHEA, androstenedione

Hormones: progesterone, testosterone

Note: Avoid antiprogestogens and antiandrogens.

and confidence. When coupled with the nerve-wracking effects of low progesterone, the combined effect of Type 8 menopause can be deeply unsettling.

If your P:E ratio is low, you may have a higher risk for breast cancer. In Type 8 menopause, the risk for osteoporosis could be significantly increased, since both progesterone and testosterone may have a role in protecting against bone loss.

With adequate estrogen levels, you may have adequate HDL ("good") cholesterol and decreased LDL ("bad") cholesterol. These factors can add up to a decreased risk of atherosclerosis (thickening and hardening of the arteries).

Nutrition and Diet

A high-grade multiple vitamin and mineral is very important for Type 8 menopause, with special attention given to antioxidants needed for progesterone production. These antioxidants include vitamins C, A, and E as well as beta-carotene and selenium. Boron will help restore low testosterone, but it must be avoided until after the progesterone deficiency is corrected.

Herbal Remedies

Mild nervine herbs such as passion flower, skullcap, valerian, vervain, or St. John's wort can help calm the nervous system. Due to its antidepressant quality, St. John's wort is especially suited for Type 8 menopause.

The classic menopause herb black cohosh is good as well. The anti-inflammatory and antispasmodic actions of wild yam is also useful for symptoms due to low prog-esterone. If the P:E ratio is low enough to cause uterine bleeding, paeonia will be quite helpful.

Avoid herbal saw palmetto and herbal vitex because they tend to reduce testosterone levels. Herbs that can be useful in *increasing* testosterone include Siberian ginseng, sarsaparilla, and licorice.

If you have fatigue, the following herbs may be helpful: astragalus, bupleurum, Asian *(Panax)* ginseng, licorice, rehmannia, schisandra, or ashwagandha.

Brain tonic herbs such as bacopa and ginkgo can be helpful if low testosterone is leading to depression and poor concentration.

Homeopathic Remedies

When testosterone is low, the homeopathic remedies damiana, *Ignatia*, lecithin, *Sabal serrulata*, or *Zincum metallicum* can help restore libido and reestablish balance during menopause. Homeopathic vitex *(Vitex agnus-castus)* may improve low progesterone symptoms. Use *Lachesis* or *Belladonna* for hot flashes, and *Natrum muri-aticum* for vaginal dryness.

Glandular Extracts

As adrenal or ovarian tissue glandular extracts can signifi-cantly increase testosterone levels, you might want to consider taking them for this menopause type. Ovarian extracts can increase estrogen, however, so when your progesterone is low, you need to use these extracts with caution. Monitor your P:E ratio, so that it is at least 20:1.

Hormone Replacement and Precursors

Type 8 menopause often requires progesterone-replacement therapy. Supplementation with low doses of progesterone (10 to 20 mg in a cream, or 25 to 200 mg of oral micronized progesterone daily) is usually adequate to restore balance.

Testosterone replacement is often required as well. If estrogen levels are in the first quartile, then precursors (DHEA or androstenedione) may be a good way to boost both your testosterone and estrogen levels. But if your estrogen levels are in the second quartile or higher, then your body probably has enough precursors already, and taking more won't help.

Your P:E ratio must be evaluated. If it is not at least 20:1, it is important to restore the proper ratio.

Patricia's Treatment

Patricia chose to start on 2.5 mg of testosterone skin cream every morning and 10 mg of progesterone skin cream every morning. She also took a homeopathic combination remedy made from damiana, zinc, passion flower, and vitex, along with a high-grade multiple vitamin and mineral supplement.

To support her general health, she joined a swimming class to get regular exercise. Walking would have been a better exercise for preventing osteoporosis, but Patricia felt healthier and calmer as a result. After 3 months, she reported improved mood and libido. Her hormones were all in normal range, and she no longer felt depressed.

TYPE 9: LOW PROGESTERONE WITH HIGH TESTOSTERONE

Pamela, a 49-year-old executive, was having a hard time with menopause. She had panic attacks, migraines, breakthrough bleeding, and acne. When she came to see me, she rushed into my office, speaking a mile a minute.

"I feel like I'm losing my mind, Doctor. I panic over the smallest things. A traffic light turned yellow while I was just about to go under it and I almost jumped out of my skin! I feel like I'm overreacting to everything lately."

Pamela had always had irregular cycles, with frequent spotting and cramping. Significantly, she suspected she'd never been fertile. She had a history of acne and oily skin. When she came into my office, she had not had a period for 3 months. She was

> Pamela had panic attacks, migraines, breakthrough bleeding, and acne. "I feel like I'm losing my mind, Doctor. I panic over the smallest things."

in early menopause, and had had quite an uncomfortable perimenopause, with migraines and skin problems.

The Menopause Type Questionnaire revealed that Pamela had a progesterone-deficient type of menopause, with high testosterone. A subsequent saliva hormone test revealed below-normal progesterone, as expected. It also revealed quite adequate levels of both estrogen and testosterone. Though her testosterone levels were just still barely in the fourth quartile, the absence of adequate progesterone to balance the actions of testosterone and estrogen gave her high-testosterone symptoms.

What to Expect From Type 9 Menopause

A woman experiencing this type of menopause feels panicky and overcome by fright. With Type 9, you are easily alarmed, and feel apprehensive and anxious without any clear explanation. You are probably sleeping very poorly. This menopause type poses the greatest risk for developing sleep disturbance. Low progesterone and high testosterone is a bad combination for a restful night's sleep. Sleep disturbance will result in a long-term, low-grade sleep deprivation, which keeps your nerves on edge. Even if you are sleeping well, with no sleep disorder, your nervous system is still under the stimulating influences of testosterone and estrogen, without the calming and soothing effects of progesterone.

Type 9 women are at a higher than normal risk for ovarian cysts, facial hair, and obesity. You may have heard of "polycystic ovary disease" (PCO), a condition in which premenopausal women have altered hormone levels leading to ovarian cysts and infertility. Type 9 menopause includes some similar symptoms. Furthermore, a woman who has had untreated PCO is more likely to undergo Type 9 menopause.

With Type 9 menopause, you have an adequate estrogen level, which is often in the second or third quartile, occasionally in the fourth quartile, or even above reference range. Although it's good to have adequate estrogen, it's not good if your progesterone-to-estrogen ratio is too low.

The risk for endometrial cancer is greatest with this menopause type. Also likely is abnormal uterine bleeding which is irregular, unusually long, and can be quite profuse. The P:E ratio is low enough that the unopposed estrogen could cause abnormal growth of the endometrium. This growth results in excessive thickening of the endometrium, which is called *endometrial hyperplasia*. Endometrial hyperplasia causes abnormal, profuse bleeding. If endometrial hyperplasia is not properly treated with progesterone, endometrial cancer can develop.

If you have this type of menopause, your estrogen levels will maintain vaginal lubrication and the health of your urethra. Your testosterone will maintain the health of the vulva and your libido (estrogen also plays a helpful role here). However, the excessive anxiety commonly experienced by this menopause type can interfere with sexual desire.

The high testosterone levels in this type of menopause are likely to contribute to the development of insulin resistance and hyperinsulinemia, even when you have adequate estrogen levels. The progesterone deficiency may increase your risk for breast cancer.

As with the other low-progesterone types discussed in this chapter, one problem is that some women receive antianxiety drugs instead of progesterone therapy. Benzodiazepene drugs such as Valium, Librium, and Xanax affect some of the same receptor cells in your brain, as do progesterone and its metabolites. The problem is compounded when the anxiety and restlessness of a low-progesterone menopause lead to depression. Of all the menopause types, Type 9 is most likely to be mistaken for an emotional or even a psychiatric disorder, because of the intensity of anxiety you can experience when you lack the soothing effects of progesterone, but feel the full stimulating force of estrogen and testosterone. As with any question of a serious mood disorder, I strongly recommend a full medical evaluation and a doctor's supervision.

As with Types 7 and 8, there may be some increased risk for osteoporosis with this menopause type, because progesterone helps keep bones strong and healthy. But the high levels of estrogen and testosterone give significant protection to the bones.

If estrogen levels are in a good range, there will be increased HDL ("good") cholesterol and decreased LDL ("bad") cholesterol. If estrogen levels are in the lowest quartile, however, their beneficial effects can be canceled out by the high testosterone, so there may be higher risk for cardiovascular disease.

Nutrition and Diet

Like other progesterone-deficient menopause types, Type 9 benefits from a high-grade multiple vitamin and

ℰ✿ TREATMENT OPTIONS FOR TYPE 9 MENOPAUSE

Nutrition and diet: vitamin and mineral supplement, extra antioxidants; avoid boron

Herbs: vitex, passion flower, skullcap, valerian, vervain, St. John's wort, black cohosh, wild yam. *For fatigue, consider:* astragalus, bupleurum, licorice, rehmannia, schisandra, ashwagandha

Homeopathic remedies: *Vitex agnus-castus, Lachesis, Belladonna, Cimicifuga racemosa*

Glandulars: not recommended—avoid with this type of menopause

Hormone precursors: not recommended—avoid with this type of menopause

Hormones: progesterone

Note: Avoid antiprogestogens.

mineral with additional antioxidants such as vitamins C, A, and E as well as beta-carotene and selenium. Boron supplementation should not be considered since it can also raise testosterone levels.

Herbal Remedies

Vitex has the dual action of increasing progesterone levels and decreasing testosterone levels, making it the ideal herbal remedy for Type 9 menopause.

If testosterone symptoms are intense, consider using saw palmetto or hops in addition to vitex. When nervous symptoms are significant, nervines such as valerian, vervain, passion flower, skullcap, or St. John's wort can help.

The classic menopause herb black cohosh is also good for this menopause type. The anti-inflammatory and antispasmodic actions of wild yam may be helpful for the symptoms of low progesterone levels. If the P:E ratio is low enough to cause uterine bleeding, paeonia will be quite useful.

For fatigue, try adaptogenic herbs such as astragalus, bupleurum, rehmannia, schisandra, or ashwaghanda. But avoid stronger adaptogens such as Asian *(Panax)* or Siberian ginsengs, which can increase restlessness and insomnia in this menopause type.

Homeopathic Remedies

Homeopathic vitex *(Vitex agnus-castus)* may improve low progesterone symptoms. *Lachesis* or *Belladonna* can work well for hot flashes. Try homeopathic cimicifuga to help restore hormonal balance.

Glandular Extracts

It is best to avoid glandular extracts if you have Type 9 menopause. If you use them at all, do so with great caution, because both ovarian and adrenal extracts are likely to raise your testosterone levels.

✿ HOW MUCH IS TOO MUCH?
Monitoring Your Progesterone Levels

If you take any form of supplemental progesterone—whether a cream, gel, or pill—you and your health-care provider need to be careful that you don't get too much progesterone. An excessively high progesterone level can cause health problems and uncomfortable symptoms. Excessive progesterone may counteract some of estrogen's helpful effects in your body.

Progesterone creams and gels are convenient, but it's harder to determine the right dosage with these forms of progesterone. Women vary widely in how well their skin absorbs topical progesterone. Not all creams and gels contain the same amounts of progesterone. If you use topical progesterone, you and your health-care professional should monitor your hormone levels, and you should pay close attention to any signs such as fatigue, weight gain, or disorientation. (For more information about the problems that can develop if your progesterone levels are too high, see chapter 14.)

Hormone Replacement and Precursors

Most women with Type 9 menopause do well with progesterone-replacement therapy. True progesterone—

either in oral-micronized form, or in a skin cream or gel—is especially helpful for this menopause type because it tends to lower testosterone levels while raising progesterone levels. ("True" progesterone is chemically identical to the hormone your body produces naturally. Many doctors instead prescribe *progestins*, chemicals that are similar, but not identical to true progesterone.) Taking progestins can reduce your testosterone levels just as true progesterone can.

The required dosage for progesterone replacement ranges from 25 to 200 mg daily of oral-micronized progesterone. You can try the precursor pregnenolone, but the goal is to restore progesterone levels as soon as possible and, though pregnenolone can become progesterone, there is a chance that it may not. As always, the goal is to bring the P:E ratio into a healthy range.

The precursors DHEA and androstenedione are not good for this menopause type, since they tend to raise your testosterone levels.

Pamela's Treatment

Pamela chose to take saw palmetto and black cohosh, to which she responded well. She also used 20 mg daily of progesterone gel, obtained from a compounding pharmacist, applying the topical gel on her abdomen or thighs once a day. The antiandrogen effect of natural progesterone made it an ideal choice.

After 3 months, tests showed that Pamela's testosterone level had dropped, while her progesterone had increased to the third quartile. She felt much calmer, and all of her symptoms had diminished considerably. I advised her to come for a follow-up visit in 6 months, and told her that if her hormone levels were stable at that point, annual visits would be sufficient unless her symptoms changed.

CHAPTER NINE

The Dual-Deficiency Menopause Types
Type 10, Type 11, and Type 12

After a normal menstruating life, Debra, 57, had stopped having periods 6 years earlier. But ever since entering menopause, she'd been feeling worse and worse. She had signs of low estrogen: vaginal dryness, thinning skin, memory problems, and a loss of sexual de-

148

sire. She also had signs of low progesterone: insomnia, anxiety, and fatigue. Her breast size had decreased, and she felt "less feminine." She was depressed, and having trouble with incontinence. As her long list of symptoms suggests, Debra was having one of the hardest types of menopause—a dual-deficiency type, with deficiencies in both progesterone and estrogen.

Of the 12 menopause types, the ones with the most pronounced hormone deficiency fall within this group. All three of these menopause types are affected in very significant ways, both physically and mentally. Type 10 struggles with hopelessness and despair, while Type 11 feels the emptiness most acutely. Type 12 has an irritable response to the emptiness she feels inside her and is enormously frustrated by her symptoms.

When a woman with one of these menopause types talks about how she feels, she may cover the entire list of estrogen- and progesterone-deficient symptoms. This type of menopause can feel quite overwhelming, often bringing a sense of premature aging and debility. But there are many ways to restore balance to the dual-deficiency menopause types, as we'll see in this chapter.

TYPE 10: LOW ESTROGEN AND LOW PROGESTERONE WITH NORMAL TESTOSTERONE

When Diana came to see me for help with her menopausal symptoms, she was 68 years old. When she'd first entered menopause in her late fifties, she'd had a few hot flashes, but no major symptoms. Her menopause had seemed to go easily enough. But in the years that followed, her health had progressively weakened. Now she was suffering from osteoporosis, depression, vaginal dryness, decreased libido, fatigue, and an ever-increasing sense of being unable to cope.

Saliva tests showed her to be deficient in estrogen and progesterone, while her testosterone was in the normal range.

What to Expect From Type 10 Menopause

In Type 10 menopause, the adrenal glands have been unable to take over from the ovaries in making progesterone and estrogen. The ovaries may be managing to produce enough testosterone, but they can't compensate for the lack of help from the adrenal glands when it comes to the other two major hormones. Usually, women with this menopause type will have DHEA levels that are low or in the first quartile, confirming that the adrenal function is not very strong.

If you have this type of menopause, your testosterone levels are likely to be in the lower two quartiles. If they are higher, you are at risk for having multiple ovarian cysts, and you may have the symptoms of excess androgens (such as facial hair), even though your testosterone levels are still within the normal range. (If your testosterone level is within the reference range, but it's too high for your ideal health, you may actually have Type 12 menopause.)

If you have any of the dual-deficiency menopause types, you may experience many or most of the symptoms that come with low estrogen (see Type 4 menopause in chapter 7) and low progesterone (see Type 7 menopause in chapter 8). In Type 10 menopause, your normal testosterone level may give you some protection against the emotional and mental effects of an estrogen deficiency. You may still experience some degree of depression, but it probably won't be severe. You may notice that your memory isn't as sharp as usual.

> In Type 10 menopause, your normal testosterone level may give you some protection against the emotional and mental effects of an estrogen deficiency.

Your normal level of testosterone should provide some protection against lichen sclerosis, but without enough estrogen, you may experience vaginal dryness and urinary incontinence. And your sexual desire and satisfaction may be somewhat diminished.

The presence of testosterone delays the loss of skin collagen, so thinning of the skin is not as pronounced in this menopause type. Testosterone also maintains sebaceous gland activity, so dry skin is less likely to be a problem. In fact, without enough estrogen to balance the effects of testosterone, you can have trouble with oily skin. Though this is more likely to occur when testosterone levels are in the third and fourth quartiles, it may occur even if testosterone levels are not that high.

⚜ TREATMENT OPTIONS FOR TYPE 10 MENOPAUSE

Nutrition and diet: vitamin and mineral supplement, extra antioxidants, boron

Herbs: damiana, St. John's wort, alfalfa, dong quai, false unicorn root, fenugreek, sage. *For fatigue, consider:* astragalus, bupleurum, Asian ginseng, licorice, rehmannia, schisandra, ashwagandha. *To enhance memory and mental ability, consider:* bacopa or ginkgo

Homeopathic remedies: *Vitex agnus-castus, Cantharis, Causticum, Graphites, Juniperus communis, Apis mellifica, Lachesis, Belladonna, Natrum muriaticum*

Glandulars: consider ovarian and adrenal extracts

Hormone precursors: DHEA, androstenedione, pregnenolone

Hormones: estrogen, progesterone

Note: Avoid antiestrogens and antiprogestogens.

Nutrition and Diet

A high-grade multiple vitamin supplement with additional boron, and foods that contain phytoestrogens can be helpful for Type 10 menopause. Phytoestrogens are substances in plants that have a weak estrogen like action. Information on phytoestrogens can be found in table 4: Foods with Phytoestrogens, on page 214.

Herbal Remedies

Damiana and St. John's wort are antidepressant herbs that can lift the low spirits associated with this menopause type.

You can also use estrogen mimetics such as alfalfa, dong quai, false unicorn root, fenugreek, and sage.

The anti-inflammatory and antispasmodic actions of wild yam may be helpful for symptoms due to low progesterone. If the progesterone-to-estrogen ratio is low enough to cause uterine bleeding, paeonia may help.

If you are having trouble thinking due to the low level of estrogen, try brain tonic herbs such as bacopa and ginkgo.

For fatigue and to boost depleted adrenals, try adaptogenic herbs such as astragalus, bupleurum, Asian *(Panax)* ginseng, licorice, rehmannia, schisandra, Siberian ginseng, or ashwagandha.

Homeopathic Remedies

Homeopathic vitex *(Vitex agnus-castus)* may improve low progesterone symptoms. For symptoms of low estrogen, such as urinary problems, *Cantharis, Causticum, Graphites,* juniper *(Juniperus communis)*, and *Apis mellifica.* For hot

flashes, use *Lachesis* or *Belladonna*. For vaginal dryness, try
Natrum muriaticum.

Glandular Extracts

As ovarian extracts can increase estrogen, use them with
caution so your P:E ratio does not become imbalanced.
As adrenal or ovarian tissue glandular extracts also can
increase testosterone levels, it is important to check for
signs of excessive testosterone.

Hormone Replacement and Precursors

Estrogen precursors such as DHEA or androstenedione
can be effective if your levels of these precursors are low.
If your DHEA and androstenedione levels are adequate,
and your estrogen is still low, you may require estrogen
replacement.

You can bring your progesterone levels into normal range with progesterone-replacement therapy. Progesterone precursors such as pregnenolone may be effective.
You can determine the results by checking your progesterone levels 1 month after starting pregnenolone.

The P:E ratio must be evaluated also. If the P:E
ratio is not at least 20:1 and less than 170:1, it is important to restore the proper ratio.

Taking oral estrogen can cause your testosterone
levels to drop. If your testosterone levels are on the high

end of the normal range anyway, this may make oral estrogen a good choice for you.

Diana's Treatment

Diana chose oral hormone-replacement therapy and began taking 1 mg of oral-micronized estradiol, 100 mg of oral-micronized progesterone, and 1 mg of oral-micronized testosterone every morning (see chapter 14 for information about these types of hormone therapy). She also began taking a calcium supplement and a high-grade multiple vitamin and mineral supplement. She took ashwagandha, an herb to help with her fatigue. After 6 months of this therapy, she had normal estrogen, progesterone, and testosterone levels, and felt enormously better.

TYPE 11: LOW ESTROGEN AND LOW PROGESTERONE WITH LOW TESTOSTERONE

Debra, who you met earlier, was a classic example of menopause Type 11. Upon further questioning, she disclosed feelings of emptiness and depression and she had become very withdrawn. Additionally, she was having trouble holding her urine. She was only in her fifties, but she looked much older than her years and said, "I feel like I'm 80 years old." Her skin was sallow and her eyes were dull and lifeless.

Debra had no history of gynecological problems. She had experienced normal periods until 6 years before, when they gradually ceased. Nothing in her medical history suggested that she would be a candidate for such an extreme version of menopause.

Saliva tests showed that her estrogen, progesterone, and testosterone were all below the reference range. She was also low in cortisol and DHEA, two hormones that reveal adrenal gland function.

> Debra disclosed feelings of emptiness and depression and she had become very withdrawn. Additionally, she was having trouble holding her urine.

The DHEA and cortisol levels showed that her adrenal glands were fatigued. Not only couldn't they handle the extra job of taking over some of the ovaries' hormone-making function, they were having a hard time dealing with ordinary stress. Her adrenal glands were still working—she was almost able to make a normal amount of cortisol at one point in her daily cycle.

What to Expect From Type 11 Menopause

Women with this devastating type of menopause often feel alone. Life feels devoid of comfort, warmth, or hope. Even the cells of the body feel abandoned and neglected. They are not getting enough estrogen, progesterone, or testosterone. Most women with this menopause type will also have low levels of other adrenal hormones such as DHEA and cortisol.

If you have Type 11 menopause, you are probably experiencing quite severe vaginal dryness, often to the point of discomfort and pain, even bleeding. Urinary incontinence is a significant problem, and you may find it difficult to hold urine for even a very short time. You

✑ TREATMENT OPTIONS FOR TYPE 11 MENOPAUSE

Nutrition and diet: vitamin and mineral supplement, extra antioxidants, boron

Herbs: alfalfa, dong quai, false unicorn root, fenugreek, sage, wild yam, Siberian ginseng, sarsaparilla, damiana, licorice, St. John's wort, black cohosh. *For fatigue, consider:* Asian ginseng, astragalus, bupleurum, licorice, rehmannia, schisandra, ashwagandha. *Brain tonic herbs:* bacopa or ginkgo. *Avoid:* vitex and saw palmetto

Homeopathic remedies: *Vitex agnus castus, Cantharis, Causticum, Graphites, Juniperus communis, Apis mellifica, Lachesis, Belladonna, Natrum muriaticum,* damiana, *Ignatia,* lecithin, *Sabal serrulata, Zinc metallicum*

Glandulars: consider both ovarian and adrenal extracts

Hormone precursors: DHEA, androstenedione, pregnenolone

Hormones: estrogen, progesterone, testosterone

Note: Avoid antiestrogens, antiprogestogens, and antiandrogens.

might have little desire for sex, even if vaginal symptoms don't make it too painful. It may be helpful for you to review the low-estrogen symptoms described under Type 4 menopause (see chapter 7), and the low-progesterone symptoms under Type 7 (see chapter 8). Added to this dual-deficiency picture are the effects of low testosterone.

With Type 11 menopause, you are especially at risk for depression. As bad as the physical symptoms can be, the mental and emotional impacts of this menopause type are often the most troubling. You are likely experiencing memory and learning difficulties. This struggle to learn can cause considerable stress. You also may be having sleep problems, which doesn't help your mental state.

Breast shrinking and skin thinning can painfully reinforce the feeling of aging rapidly. The combination of inadequate estrogen or testosterone to maintain collagen and the decreased circulation to the skin due to progesterone deficiency results in accelerated aging of the skin.

Nutrition and Diet

A high-grade multiple vitamin supplement with additional boron, and foods that contain phytoestrogens can be helpful for Type 11 menopause. See table 4: Foods with Phytoestrogens, on page 214 for more information on phytoestrogens.

Herbal Remedies

Estrogen mimetics such as alfalfa, dong quai, false unicorn root, fenugreek, and sage may be useful.

For fatigue and to boost depleted adrenals, try adaptogenic herbs such as astragalus, bupleurum, Asian *(Panax)* ginseng, licorice, rehmannia, schisandra, Siberian ginseng, or ashwagandha.

The anti-inflammatory and antispasmodic actions of wild yam may ease symptoms due to low progesterone. If the progesterone-to-estrogen ratio is low enough to cause uterine bleeding, paeonia may help.

If you are having trouble thinking, due to the low level of estrogen, try brain tonic herbs such as bacopa and ginkgo.

Avoid the antiandrogenic herbs saw palmetto and vitex because you already have a testosterone deficiency. Herbs that may help increase androgens include Siberian ginseng, sarsaparilla, damiana, and licorice.

Damiana is also a nervine, as is St. John's wort, which means they are appropriate for Type 11 menopause because of their antidepressant qualities. The classic menopause herb black cohosh is good as well.

Homeopathic Remedies

Homeopathic vitex *(Vitex agnus-castus)* can improve progesterone deficiency.

For symptoms of low estrogen, such as urinary problems, try *Cantharis, Causticum, Graphites, Juniperus Communis,* and *Apis mellifica.* For hot flashes, use *Lachesis* or *Belladonna.* For vaginal dryness, try *Natrum muriaticum.*

For low testosterone, use homeopathic damiana, *Ignatia* (St. Ignatius bean), lecithin, *Sabal serrulata,* or

Zincum metallicum, to help restore libido and reestablish balance during menopause.

Glandular Extracts

Glandular extracts can be very useful for Type 11 menopause. Adrenal or ovarian tissue glandular extracts can raise estrogen and testosterone levels. Use ovarian extracts with caution, and consider progesterone supplementation, so your P:E ratio doesn't get out of balance.

Hormone Replacement and Precursors

Some women with Type 11 menopause need estrogen-, progesterone-, and testosterone-replacement therapy to restore hormone levels to normal, if their imbalances are too severe to correct in other ways. Precursors are worth trying, but may not work in women with significant adrenal fatigue.

In other women, estrogen precursors such as DHEA or androstenedione can be effective if levels of these precursors are low. If your DHEA and androstenedione levels are adequate, and your estrogen is still low, then you may need estrogen replacement.

Progesterone-replacement therapy can bring progesterone levels into normal range. For some women, progesterone precursors such as pregnenolone are effective. To monitor the results, check your progesterone levels 1 month after starting pregnenolone.

The P:E ratio must be evaluated also. If the P:E ratio is not at least 20:1 and less than 170:1, it is important to restore the proper ratio, and keep it there.

You can raise your testosterone with DHEA or androstenedione, especially if your levels of these precursors are low.

Debra's Treatment

Debra wanted to try taking DHEA, since she had heard that it could be made into the hormones she needed. Actually, as I explained to her, DHEA could raise her testosterone and estrogen levels, but not her progesterone. She agreed to add progesterone to her treatment plan. She started on 25 mg of DHEA (a large dose) and 50 mg of oral-micronized progesterone each morning.

After a month, Debra showed signs of increasing androgens and estrogen, suggesting she could now handle a larger dose of progesterone. I raised her dosage to 100 mg daily. She showed further signs of improvement over the following months.

> In Debra's case, taking precursors was a successful strategy. Her hormone tests after 3 months showed estrogen, testosterone, and progesterone all within reference range.

In Debra's case, taking precursors was a successful strategy. Her hormone tests after 3 months showed estrogen, testosterone, and progesterone all within reference range. Her cortisol levels had returned to normal, and her DHEA levels were at the high end of normal. She reported having much more energy, an increased libido, and improved mood and memory.

Her skin had lost its sallow look and its tone had improved considerably. (While it usually takes 6 months or so of restored estrogen levels to have any noticeable effect on skin, progesterone helps much more quickly by increasing the circulation of blood in the skin.) Debra was overjoyed to be feeling alive again.

TYPE 12: LOW ESTROGEN AND LOW PROGESTERONE WITH HIGH TESTOSTERONE

Danielle, an executive assistant at a law firm and married with two grown children, was 57 years old when she came into my office for help with her menopausal symptoms. She was suffering from irritability, feelings of agitation, facial hair, deepening of the voice, and hair loss (androgenic alopecia). She was also struggling with vaginal dryness.

What to Expect From Type 12 Menopause

Women with this type of menopause may develop masculine features such as facial hair and deepening of the voice. The high testosterone level puts a more aggressive edge on the personality, and this aggressiveness can partially disguise the underlying dual deficiency in estrogen and progesterone. There is often a strong feeling of drive and ambition, but working hard can further deplete the body.

If you have this menopause type, your libido may still be strong because of the increased testosterone, but you may experience vaginal dryness due to the low level of estrogen.

Even though some forms of memory are stimulated by the testosterone, you might have difficulty remembering names and word-related things, such as what you read, and new learning can be a struggle. The high levels of testosterone will help preserve bone, skin, and breast collagen. Without either estrogen or progesterone to enhance breast growth, however, your breast size can decrease, in spite of adequate collagen levels.

With Type 12 menopause, you will likely have more oily skin, acne, and facial hair, and androgenic alopecia (hair loss) is not uncommon.

Nutrition and Diet

A high-grade multiple vitamin supplement and foods which contain phytoestrogens can be helpful for Type 12 menopause. See table 4, Foods with Phytoestrogens, on page 214 for more information on phytoestrogens. Avoid boron in this menopause type, since boron can increase testosterone levels.

Herbal Remedies

Vitex is a good herb for this menopause type as it both increases progesterone levels and reduces testosterone levels.

Nervines such as valerian, vervain, passion flower, skullcap, and St. John's wort are appropriate for Type 12 menopause.

❧ TREATMENT OPTIONS FOR TYPE 12 MENOPAUSE

Nutrition and diet: vitamin and mineral supplement, extra antioxidants; avoid boron

Herbs: vitex, valerian, vervain, passion flower, skullcap, St. John's wort, alfalfa, dong quai, false unicorn root, fenugreek, sage, wild yam, saw palmetto. *For fatigue, consider:* Asian ginseng, astragalus, bupleurum, licorice, rehmannia, schisandra, ashwagandha. *Brain tonic herbs:* bacopa or ginkgo

Homeopathic remedies: *Cantharis, Causticum, Graphites, Juniperus communis, Apis mellifica, Lachesis, Belladonna, Natrum muriaticum*

Glandulars: not recommended—do not use with this type of menopause

Hormone precursors: pregnenolone

Hormones: estrogen (oral), progesterone

Note: Avoid antiestrogens and antiprogestogens; consider antiandrogens.

Estrogen mimetics such as alfalfa, dong quai, false unicorn root, fenugreek, and sage may be used.

For fatigue and to boost depleted adrenals, try adaptogenic herbs such as astragalus, bupleurum, Asian *(Panax)* ginseng, licorice, rehmannia, schisandra, Siberian ginseng, or ashwagandha.

The anti-inflammatory and antispasmodic actions of wild yam may be helpful for symptoms due to low progesterone. If the progesterone to estrogen ratio is low enough to cause uterine bleeding, try paeonia.

If you are having trouble thinking due to the low level of estrogen, try brain tonic herbs such as bacopa and ginkgo.

Homeopathic Remedies

Treat symptoms of low estrogen, such as urinary problems, with *Cantharis, Causticum, Graphites,* juniper *(Juniperus communis),* or *Apis mellifica.* For hot flashes, use *Lachesis* or *Belladonna.* For vaginal dryness, try *Natrum muriaticum.*

Glandular Extracts

Glandular extracts are usually not recommended for Type 12 menopause. Ovarian and adrenal extracts are likely to increase testosterone, and yours is already too high. You may experience agitation and feelings of aggression if you take ovarian extract when your testosterone is high.

Hormone Replacement and Precursors

Oral estrogen is a good choice for Type 12 menopause due to its ability to lower testosterone levels as well as restore estrogen levels. You obviously will also need progesterone supplementation, to restore progesterone levels and maintain a healthy P:E ratio.

Estrogen precursors such as DHEA or androstenedione are not a good idea because they also raise testosterone levels.

Progesterone precursors such as pregnenolone can be effective. Monitor the results of the treatment by checking progesterone levels 1 month after starting pregnenolone. If it is not working to raise your progesterone levels, you will need progesterone-replacement therapy.

The P:E ratio must be evaluated also. If the P:E ratio is not at least 20:1 and less than 170:1, it is important to restore the proper ratio, and keep it there.

As testosterone levels can be brought down to normal levels with oral estrogen, you may have no need to use antiandrogens if you are supplementing with estrogen.

Danielle's Treatment

Danielle began taking 2 mg of oral-micronized estrogen and 200 mg of oral micronized progesterone every day. We chose oral estradiol because it reduces testosterone levels. Additionally, Danielle added soy to her diet and took a high-grade multiple vitamin and mineral supplement daily.

She also took the herbs saw palmetto (to reduce her testosterone level), fenugreek (an estrogenlike herb), and a combination remedy containing hops, valerian, and other calming herbs.

Within 3 months, all three of Danielle's hormones were within normal reference range, and she felt much better.

CHAPTER TEN

Self-Care During Menopause

Each menopause type requires different care and management. Recognizing that there is more than one type of menopause helps create an effective individualized program. We know that every woman does not necessarily need estrogen or progesterone. There is no such thing as one program for all women.

But does this mean there are now 12 programs? Have we only stretched our options from one program to one dozen programs? I sure hope not!

I have included a lot of detailed information in this book so that you can create your own personalized health-care program, with the help of your health-care provider when necessary. You can eliminate menopausal symptoms once you understand how hormones work, which ones are out of balance in your body, and what treatments are available.

An increasing number of health-care professionals are surrendering some of the power and control they traditionally had over health care and giving it back to women. As radical as that sounds, it is not a new thought. There are thousands of physicians who support the concept of self-care during menopause.

> Give a woman health care, and she is well for a day; teach a woman self-care, and she is well for a lifetime.

Self-care is a rapidly emerging component of health care throughout the world. Individuals who want to have greater control of their personal health and well-being are learning more about health-related issues specific to their own personal needs. To modernize an old proverb: Give a woman health care, and she is well for a day; teach a woman self-care, and she is well for a lifetime. Self-care does not mean avoiding hospitals and medical doctors. It means a more responsible utilization of those resources.

Self-care may prove to be a solution to medical costs that are out of control. Health-care resources need to continue to grow away from the "physician as center of focus" to the "consumer as center of focus." This shift in focus encourages consumers to recognize and utilize other health-care professionals such as nutritionists, herbalists, and pharmacists.

In natural hormone-replacement therapy, a type of practitioner called a compounding pharmacist has made some of the most significant advances over the past decade.

COMPOUNDING PHARMACISTS: ANOTHER RESOURCE FOR WOMEN

Compounding pharmacists are specially trained pharmacists who prepare customized medications such as natural hormones that are designed to the unique needs of each woman. The compounding pharmacist works as a member of the health-care team, with the physician and the patient. The physician first prescribes the specific hormones a woman needs. The pharmacist then takes the necessary ingredients, compounds (or mixes) them, and dispenses the medicine to the woman after a one-on-one consultation with her. In this way, women receive the personalized care they deserve, and physicians and local community pharmacists have the opportunity to provide true patient-oriented services. You can locate a compounding pharmacist in your area by contacting one of the organizations of compounding pharmacists listed in the Resources section of this book.

SELF-CARE DURING MENOPAUSE

Self-care during menopause involves several steps. The first is self-diagnosis. You can do this by completing the Menopause Type Questionnaire (see chapter 3) and by getting laboratory testing of your hormone levels (see chapter 4). The next step involves customizing your care to fit your unique needs. It may take a month or more to design an effective treatment program for yourself.

Once you have tried and tested various treatments and found a system that you like and that seems to be balancing your body, check your hormone levels again, waiting at least one month—ideally three.

What Influences Menopausal Health?

The main factors that influence your health during menopause are your nutrition, your stress level, and whether you have any long-standing health problems. Poor nutrition, stress, and chronic disease can result in an earlier and more debilitating menopause. Lifestyle habits are also crucial, as they are with any health issue. Smoking tobacco and drinking excessive amounts of alcohol lower hormone levels and make it more likely that you will have a difficult menopause. Regular exercise helps your bones to stay strong and has a host of other benefits.

> Smoking tobacco and drinking excessive amounts of alcohol lower hormone levels and make it more likely that you will have a difficult menopause.

You can help ensure that your adrenal glands and ovaries are functioning at their optimal level by taking adequate amounts of vitamins and minerals. During times of severe stress, your body requires increased nutrition, which you can take care of by increasing your intake of vitamins and minerals.

Antiestrogens, Antiprogestogens, and Antiandrogens

An important part of self-care during menopause is knowing how your lifestyle and any medications you are taking will affect your levels of estrogen, progesterone, and testosterone. There are several medications, foods, and other substances that may decrease the level or actions of estrogens. These are called antiestrogens. (Similarly, antiprogestogens are substances that decrease the level or actions of progestogens, and antiandrogens have the same effect on testosterone. *Androgen* comes from the

✑ SUBSTANCES WITH ANTIANDROGENIC ACTIVITY[1-8]

Chasteberry *(Vitex agnus castus):* an herb commonly used in women's health

Cimetidine (Tagamet): an anti-ulcer medicine

Finasteride (Pro-Cure, Proscar, Proscar 5): an antiandrogen

Fluconazole (Diflucan): an antifungal

Flutamide (Eluexin): an antiandrogen

Fluvastatin (Locol): a cholesterol-lowering drug

Ketoconazole (Nizoral): an antifungal drug

Greek word for "male," and refers to male sex hormones including testosterone.) Collectively, we could say these medications and substances all have "antihormone" actions.

Depending on your menopause type, these *antihormones* might help you, or make things worse for you. If you have a deficiency in estrogen, you should avoid anti-estrogens. But if you have too high a level of testosterone, an antiandrogen might help bring it back into balance. See the sidebars on pages 172, 173, 174, and 175 for commonly used medications, herbs, and other substances that have notable antihormone activities.

Leuprolide (Lupron): an anti-hormone

Lovastatin (Mevacor): a cholesterol-lowering drug

Medroxyprogesterone Acetate (Depo-Provera, Provera, Cycrin): a progestin, or synthetic progestogen

Pravastatin (Pravachol): a cholesterol-lowering drug

Risperidone (Risperdal): an antipsychotic

Saw Palmetto *(Sabal serrulata)*: an herb commonly used in men's health

Simvastatin (Zocor): a cholesterol-lowering drug

Spironolactone (many brand names): a diuretic

Willow herb *(Epilobium* spp.)*: an herb commonly used in men's health

General Recommendations for the Care of All Menopause Types

The first step is nutrition. During menopause, you should treat your nutrition as seriously as you would if you were pregnant. The changes taking place in your body require a lot of nutrients to smooth the transition from being a menstruating woman to a postmenopausal

❧ SUBSTANCES WITH ANTIESTROGEN ACTIVITY[9-18]

Clomiphene Citrate (generic): an antiestrogenic drug

Gossypol (found in cottonseed oil): a component of cottonseed

Ketoconazole (Nizoral): an antifungal

Fluconazole (Diflucan): an antifungal

Leuprolide (Lupron): an antihormone

Medroxyprogesterone Acetate (Depo-Provera, Provera, Cycrin): a progestin, or synthetic progestogen

Nicotine tobacco products

Quercetin (found in onions and black tea [*Camellia sinensis*]): a flavonoid (plant pigment)

Saw Palmetto *(Sabal serrulata):* an herb commonly used in men's health

Tamoxifen (Nolvadex): an antiestrogenic drug

Willow herb *(Epilobium* spp.): an herb commonly used in men's health woman. Your adrenal glands and your organs in general need to be well nourished so they can function at their optimum levels.

Proper nutrition is the foundation for all other treatments. In order to make hormones, the adrenal glands and ovaries need a healthy supply of vitamins and minerals. So, eat right! If possible, eat the best quality, preferably organic food. Make sure to eat lots of fresh fruits and vegetables, and have sufficient protein every day. Avoid sugary snacks, sodas, and foods high in fats, salt, caffeine, additives, and preservatives.

It is a good idea for all menopausal women to take a high-grade multiple vitamin and mineral supplement. Increased intake of foods high in phytoestrogens is also recommended. For a list of these foods, see table 4 on page 214.

The next step is to investigate herbal and homeopathic remedies based on your menopause type. These remedies are generally less disturbing to the body and have fewer side effects than taking hormone

❧ SUBSTANCES WITH ANTIPROGESTOGEN ACTIVITY [19-25]

Medroxyprogesterone Acetate (Depo-Provera, Provera, Cycrin): a progestin, or synthetic progestogen

Mifepristone (RU 486): an antiprogestogen

Gossypol (found in cottonseed oil): a component of cottonseed replacements, and there are definitely benefits to creating the most "natural" treatment program that you can. See chapter 12 for more information on herbal treatments for menopause.

You may wish to consult a qualified Western or Chinese herbalist to design an herbal prescription for your unique needs. Likewise, a consultation with a homeopathic physician is a wise course, if you are interested in pursuing this treatment option. Choose a practitioner who is properly accredited. For details about the professional organizations you can contact for a referral to a practitioner in your area, see the Resources section at the back of the book.

If herbs and homeopathy are not completely effective, try glandular treatments. You must use glandular extracts cautiously if you already have symptoms of agitation or anxiety. See chapter 13 for more information.

From an optimal therapy point of view, conventional hormone-replacement therapy (HRT) is among the last options in the decision chain. While it may prove safe in many cases, conventional HRT does not always relieve menopausal symptoms. You should certainly consider this therapy when nutrition, homeopathy, herbs, and glandular extracts alone do not relieve your menopausal symptoms. For some women, hormone replacement may be the first option to try, such as when there is real risk of severe disease (for example, osteoporosis). See chapter 14 for more information on hormone-replacement therapy.

Some women do best with herbs, some with homeopathy, some with glandular extracts, and some with a mixture of therapies. How you will react to nutrition, herbs, and homeopathy is affected by a number of factors including your age, body weight, history of birth control or other hormone use, existing health problems, history of surgery, family history, and nutritional history. Because each woman is unique, no one remedy is perfect for all women.

The guidelines given for each menopause type in the previous chapters are based on treatments found to be effective for each type. As helpful as they are, don't let them become a rigid recipe for you. Study the other herbs and

> Some women do best with herbs, some with homeopathy, some with glandular extracts, and some with a mixture of therapies.

supplements in this book and allow yourself a chance to create a program unique to your needs.

EILEEN'S STORY

Eileen is a woman who has made self-care a routine part of her life. When she first assessed her hormone levels, her saliva test showed deficiencies in all three hormones: estrogen, progesterone, and testosterone. Her symptoms included hot flashes, vaginal dryness, fatigue, and decreased motivation. Eileen was having a dual-deficiency menopause—one of the hardest types there is. But Eileen had an important advantage: She understood that she needed to do more than just take a couple of pills if she wanted optimal health.

She started with a high-grade multiple vitamin, with extra calcium. In the herbal category, she took ashwagandha and *Panax* ginseng, which are both excellent female adaptogens (helping the body to deal with stress; see chapter 12). She also took 25 mg of oral-micronized progesterone and 5 mg of DHEA every day. Regular exercise, relaxation, play, and quiet time all became an important part of her health and stress reduction program.

On this regimen, Eileen feels great. Her mind is sharp, her mood positive, and her energy good. A follow-up saliva test 3 months into her program showed that she was on the right track: All hormones were within normal range. With the help of this program, her body was able to resume production of estrogen and testosterone.

Subsequent tests and Menopause Type Questionnaire results showed she was still doing well after 6 and then 12 months. She had a little problem with vaginal dryness again, but it was relieved when she started taking the estrogen-mimetic herb dong quai.

Eileen continues to visit health-care professionals for regular Pap smears and pelvic exams, and to review her hormone levels once a year. Otherwise, she manages her health on her own. To Eileen, doctors are resources for education and special services, but she is the one responsible for her health and happiness.

CHAPTER ELEVEN

Nutrition and Menopause

Including Minerals, Vitamins, and Phytoestrogens

Nutrition has a big impact on the healthy functioning of hormones throughout a woman's life, and is particularly important during menopause. The body needs nutrients to create the needed hormones.

In this chapter, we take a look at some of the specific effects that the key vitamins and minerals have on hormone production. As the body uses a wide variety of minerals and vitamins to create the steroid hormones, you may want to take a balanced combination supplement in addition to eating well. We will also take a look at phytoestrogens, plant substances that have estrogenlike activity.

MINERALS

Your body uses enzymes to make hormones. In addition to the other factors we've looked at, your body can't make hormones without certain nutrients, including essential minerals and trace minerals. Copper and iron are particularly important, but minerals from boron to zinc are required for the proper function of most endocrine tissues, including the thyroid, the ovaries, the adrenal glands, and the pancreas.[1] Specific minerals are required for every enzyme in the steroidogenic pathway.

Taking minerals is a good way to make sure that you're getting the minerals you need for making hormones. Without boron, copper, manganese, and zinc, your adrenal glands can't rise to their increased hormone-making duties after menopause. But balance and moderation are important in nutrition, as in everything else. An excess of any mineral can potentially be dangerous, so avoid extreme dosages. Give your body what it needs, but not more than it can handle.

Nutritional minerals are essential to life and are involved in many important metabolic functions. Some nutritional minerals in the body—such as calcium, magnesium, and zinc—are present in large amounts, while others—such as chromium, cobalt, and selenium—occur in trace amounts. These minerals cover such a wide range of functions in the body that an entire chapter could be written on each one.

Unfortunately, conventional medicine has paid little attention to the role that these minerals play in the production of steroid hormones, which is so important for women during menopause. This section focuses on how these minerals affect adrenal and ovarian function, as well as other functions relevant to menopause. Even though each mineral is discussed individually, minerals function best when working together (see sidebar, Using Minerals for Balance, on page 185).

Boron

Boron is a trace element that improves the body's absorption of calcium, magnesium, and phosphorus. It also helps to significantly increase estrogen production, which is good if you need more estrogen. However, a precaution is worth noting. If more estrogen might make your condition worse (as in the case of an estrogen-sensitive tumor), boron supplementation is ill-advised. I therefore recommend that you seek a full medical evaluation prior to using this supplement, just to be on the safe side.

> Nutritional minerals are essential to life and are involved in many important metabolic functions.

When postmenopausal women take a daily boron supplementation of 3 mg, it causes an increase in serum concentrations of estrogen and testosterone and a decreased loss of calcium from the bones.[2-4] A deficiency of boron will actually result in decreased levels of estrogen and testosterone.[5] Boron also works with vitamin D to decrease osteoporosis and increase mineral content in bone, and enhances cartilage formation.[6, 7]

Boron supplementation is appropriate for all menopause types, but you should use it cautiously when you have a progesterone deficiency or an excess of testosterone. The increase in estrogen without enough progesterone to balance it could upset your P:E (progesterone-to-estrogen) ratio. Likewise, since boron may increase testosterone, use it cautiously if you have a high-testosterone menopause type. Consider 3 mg a day if appropriate.

Calcium

Calcium is important for proper bone formation and preventing osteoporosis. Additionally, calcium plays a vital role in cardiovascular health, blood clotting, muscle function, and nerve function. To be most effective, calcium supplementation must include vitamin D. When calcium is taken with vitamin D, the benefit is so significant that all women should use it as their primary defense against osteoporosis. Long-term supplementation with 1 to 2 g of calcium and 500 IU of vitamin D (or 14 micrograms [mcg] of vitamin D_3) increases intestinal absorption of calcium and increases bone mineral density no matter what a woman's age, nutritional status, or hormonal status.[8] So even a woman on a healthful diet with adequate exercise and healthy hormone levels will still benefit from such supplementation.

Calcium also acts as an important messenger inside the cells of the body, particularly in making cholesterol available to enter the steroidogenic pathway.[9, 10] It's important to note that the heavy metal cadmium may interfere with calcium's ability to increase steroid production, which could result in a decreased ability to convert cholesterol to pregnenolone.[11] This is one of many ways in which cadmium can be toxic. Certain blood pressure and heart medications known as calcium–channel blockers (verapamil, diltiazem, and prenylamine) may also inhibit the making of steroid hormones, by interfering with calcium at the level of the cell.[12, 13]

The body has a mechanism to maintain healthy and stable levels of calcium in the blood, including using calcium from the bones if needed. Common dogma is that this stable calcium level will shield the cells from effects of low calcium. The fact that widely prescribed medications and cadmium can affect calcium metabolism enough to inhibit steroidogenesis reveals just how delicate the balance can be. Some data suggest that blood calcium levels (extracellular levels) can affect steroidogenesis.[14] One study in particular showed that the movement of calcium across the cell membrane is an important and common step in the stimulation of progesterone production.[15] Therefore, even a very mild calcium deficiency cannot be dismissed as insignificant.

As calcium plays such an important role in steroidogenesis, you may want to consider supplementation. Certainly, if you are taking calcium–channel blockers, you should monitor your hormone levels.

Women of all menopause types should consider calcium supplementation. An ideal daily dose is at least 1 g of elemental calcium. Calcium is best balanced with magnesium. For 1 g of calcium, 500 mg of magnesium should be sufficient.[16]

Chromium

Chromium's ability to help with glucose metabolism by improving the effectiveness of insulin is well proven. It may also aid in maintaining proper metabolism of proteins and carbohydrates and controlling cholesterol and triglyceride levels. For women during menopause, chromium can do all this and more. It can reduce bone loss by slowing down bone clearing (resorption) and also may raise levels of DHEA.[17] This ability to raise DHEA is important for postmenopausal women who are more dependent on adrenal hormones such as DHEA, which can act as a precursor to androstenedione and other androgens. Chromium is a trace mineral taken in microgram (mcg) not milligram (mg) doses. Chromium supplementation is appropriate for all menopause types. Consider taking 200 to 400 mcg of elemental chromium daily.

Cobalt

Cobalt is the most important element that makes up the core of the vitamin B_{12} molecule; therefore, a cobalt deficiency is synonymous with a vitamin B_{12} deficiency. The role of vitamin B_{12} in women of menopausal age is discussed in detail later in this chapter.

Cobalt supplementation is appropriate for all menopause types. Cobalt may be taken in the form of vitamin B_{12} supplementation at a rate of 1 mg (1,000 mcg) daily for 1 to 2 weeks, then once a week, then once a month.

Copper

Copper is one of the important minerals required for the production of adrenal and ovarian hormones, and the protection of these tissues from free-radical damage.[18-21]

☙ USING MINERALS FOR BALANCE

Mineral	Daily Recommendations for Menopause
Boron	3 mg*
Calcium	1 gm (1,000 mg)*
Chromium	200–400 mcg
Cobalt	See vitamin B_{12} in Vitamins section
Copper	2 mg
Iodine	100–150 mcg
Iron	18 mg*
Magnesium	250–500 mg*
Manganese	10–20 mg
Selenium	100–200 mcg
Vanadium	10–30 mcg*
Zinc	30 mg*

*Please see additional information in text.

Without adequate copper, hormone production may eventually cause decreased progesterone production.[22] Copper has been associated with reproductive failure, osteoporosis, and abnormal neurotransmitters with increased risk of depression and mental deficiencies.[23] Adrenal function is impaired significantly when there is a copper deficiency, which may cause decreased cortisol levels.[24–27] Thus, a copper deficiency may lead to a diminished tolerance to stress.[28] Copper is also required for production of hemoglobin and for proper fat and protein metabolism. It promotes healthy nerve function and, together with vitamin C and zinc, is essential for skin collagen production and wound healing. Copper supplementation is appropriate for all menopause types at a daily dose of 2 mg a day. Copper should especially be taken if a zinc supplement is used, since zinc supplements will lower copper levels.

Iodine

Iodine is an essential nutrient required for the production of thyroid hormone. As the key element of the thyroid hormone, iodine is involved in proper fat metabolism, ideal energy levels, and normal cholesterol levels. Iodine also plays a part in the conversion of carotene to vitamin A.

After the addition of iodized salt to the American diet, common belief held that iodine deficiency was a thing of the past. In actuality, it is of increasing concern today. In some countries, as many as one in three women are deficient in iodine. In the United States, the average person's iodine levels have dropped over 50% between 1974 and 1994—enough to pose a public health concern.[29]

Numerous studies have found an association between thyroid enlargement and breast cancer.[30]

However, there is no conclusive evidence of a direct cause between breast cancer and a goiter due to iodine deficiency.[31]

Inadequate iodine/thyroid function affects other endocrine tissues beyond the thyroid. Animal studies suggest that a chronic iodine deficiency could result in decreased adrenal gland activity.[32]

Too much iodine can be toxic to the thyroid gland, so you shouldn't take iodine supplements beyond the safe nutritional range. Likewise, if you have known disease of the thyroid gland or suspect that you do, seek a medical consultation prior to trying iodine supplements. Iodine supplementation is appropriate for all menopause types, at a daily dose of 100 to 150 mcg.

Iron

Iron is best known as the mineral required for the production of hemoglobin, the oxygen-carrying molecule in red blood cells. A deficiency of iron may result in significant anemia with fatigue, dizziness, and many complications. Iron also is involved in immune system health and is a key element in many enzymes throughout the body, which makes iron important in the proper maintenance of hormone levels.[33–36]

Since anemia has other causes, such as vitamin B_{12}, vitamin B_6, or folate deficiency, an experienced health-care provider should evaluate a suspected iron deficiency. This evaluation is important because it can be dangerous to take too much iron. You shouldn't take an iron supplement unless you've got a medically proven iron deficiency.

Iron supplementation is appropriate for all menopause types if blood tests prove that you need it. If true iron deficiency is found, continue iron replacement for about 6 months to replenish body stores. Iron supplements can interfere with the absorption of a number of different medications, including antibiotics, blood pressure medications, and blood thinners, among others. Given possible effects on medication and the necessity of a blood test to determine the appropriateness of iron supplementation, seek the advice of a medical physician before using this supplement.

> A deficiency of iron may result in significant anemia with fatigue, dizziness, and many complications.

Magnesium

Magnesium is an important mineral required for proper function of the heart muscle and of smooth muscles found in blood vessels and airways. A deficiency may increase risk of heart disease and high blood pressure. It is also needed for proper nerve and skeletal muscle function. Additionally, magnesium plays an important role in steroid hormone production.

Magnesium is one of many key nutrients that work in the initial steps of the steroidogenic pathway.[37] If early steps are not functioning, then all steroids—adrenal and ovarian—will be affected.[38] A low-grade magnesium deficiency also may play a role in insulin resistance.[39] All menopause types should use magnesium supplementation. Consider taking 250 to 500 mg of magnesium daily. As stated earlier, 1 g of calcium should be taken with 500 mg of magnesium.[40]

Manganese

Manganese is required for proper bone health and the prevention of osteoporosis.[41] It is also essential for a healthy nervous system and brain, healthy immune system, and blood formation, among many other functions. Manganese is necessary for optimal adrenal and ovarian function.[42, 43] Adequate concentrations of manganese are needed for maximum enzyme activity of the adrenal glands.[44] Manganese also is required for the production of both estrogen and progesterone in the steroidogenic process.[45] Abnormally low manganese levels may contribute to abnormal glucose metabolism, with insulin resistance and obesity. Though insulin resistance is a complex condition with many factors involved, manganese deficiency and abnormal adrenal gland function appear to play some role in its development.[46] Manganese supplementation is appropriate for all menopause types. Consider taking 5 to 10 mg of elemental manganese daily.

Selenium

Selenium is a strong *antioxidant*, a substance that prevents or counteracts the damaging effects of *oxidation* (oxygen reactions), that works closely with vitamin E and is considered to have cancer-preventive, anti-aging, and heart and liver protective properties. Although its role in endocrine health is not yet fully understood, researchers have identified selenium as an important mineral for the health of the ovary. In recent years, studies have revealed that the level of important enzymes in the ovary can fall dramatically when there is selenium deficiency.[47] Other research has shown that patients with unexplained infertility had significantly decreased selenium levels in the follicles of their ovaries.[48]

The steroidogenic pathway appears to be dependent in some way on proper selenium levels. Research has shown that when selenium concentrations increase, there is a significant elevation of progesterone concentration in steroid-producing cells.[49] Like most other minerals, selenium has functions beyond its commonly known ones. More than an antioxidant, selenium is proving an important mineral in a number of enzyme pathways.

Note that selenium is a trace mineral taken in microgram (mcg) not milligram (mg) doses. It can be dangerous to take too much selenium. It's best to stick with the recommended dose, unless you are under the care of an experienced physician. Selenium supplementation is appropriate for all menopause types. Consider taking 100 to 200 mcg of elemental selenium daily.

Vanadium

Supplementation with vanadium can produce long-term improvement in glucose metabolism because of this trace mineral's insulinlike activity.[50] Clinical trials using vanadium compounds in patients have been promising so far and suggest that vanadium may even be useful in severe blood sugar imbalances, such as diabetes.[51]

Low doses of vanadium can raise progesterone levels, while higher doses can actually lower levels.[52] It's important to have enough vanadium—but too much can interfere with hormone production.[53-56]

When you suffer from insulin resistance or weight gain due to high cortisol levels, taking vanadium may help. As long-term vanadium supplementation can lead to adrenal insufficiency, use it only to correct a proven deficiency, and only on a short-term basis, with frequent monitoring of steroid levels. Like other trace minerals, vanadium supplements are measured in micrograms. Dosages range from 10 to 30 mcg per day. It is important not to exceed dosages known to be safe.

Zinc

Zinc is required for the production of the sex steroid hormones, growth hormones, and more than 70 other reactions in the body, including the production of energy and glucose tolerance.[57] Zinc also is essential for the health of breast tissue.[58] It is needed for tissue repair, wound healing, bone repair, and bone growth. One group of researchers found that zinc may enhance estrogen's bone-building effect.[59] It is required for the formation of insulin, helps the body to synthesize proteins, and stimulates hair growth. Decreased zinc levels will result in a decreased sense of taste and smell and difficulty seeing at night.

Zinc is a critically important mineral in the steroidogenic pathway. It is required for the proper function of both adrenal and ovarian tissues.[60] In fact, a severe zinc deficiency can significantly decrease your body's production of steroid hormones.[61] A therapeutic dose is 30 mg daily. When taking zinc, take 2 mg of copper daily to prevent copper deficiency.

VITAMINS

Like minerals, vitamins cover such a wide range of functions in the body that I could write an entire chapter on each one. And also like minerals, conventional medicine hasn't paid enough attention to the role vitamins play in the production of steroid hormones. Below, I explain how vitamins affect adrenal and ovarian function and other issues of concern for women during menopause. Like minerals, vitamins work together to achieve optimal results (see sidebar, Using Vitamins for Balance, on page 197).

Thiamine (Vitamin B$_1$)

Thiamine (B$_1$) acts as a coenzyme that is critical for a number of metabolic processes in the body, including proper metabolism of thyroid hormones.[62] Required for proper nerve function, it is commonly used for nerve pains. It is needed for the activation of enzymes in the adrenal glands as part of the steroidogenic pathway.[63–65] It allows the adrenal glands to help the body adapt to stress and avoid exhaustion and burnout of the adrenal glands. Thiamine supplementation can be an effective remedy to protect the adrenal glands from functional exhaustion due to major psychological and trauma stresses such as surgery. When administered before and during surgery, 120 mg of thiamine reduced the corticosteroid stress response from the adrenal glands.[66] In a vitamin replacement study, supplementation with vitamins B_6, B_1, and C, normalized cortisol production and the 24-hour rhythm of the adrenal glands.[67]

> Like minerals, vitamins work together to achieve optimal results.

Thiamine is important for proper function of other adrenal hormones in addition to cortisol. Thiamine deficiency results in increased *cortisol* (a steroid hormone secreted by the adrenal cortex) levels and a lowered ability to increase *aldosterone* (mineralocorticoid hormone produced by the adrenal gland that regulates the balance of water and electrolytes such as potassium and sodium) levels, showing that thiamine is necessary for the steroidogenesis of aldosterone.[68] Given the steroidogenic pathway, while thiamine is helping the body maintain proper cortisol, aldosterone, and thyroid function, it is ultimately influencing androgen and estrogen activity in the body. As thiamine is an essential nutrient, women of all menopause types should take it, especially if you have thyroid or nerve problems. A daily dose of 30 to 100 mg is appropriate.

Riboflavin (Vitamin B₂)

Riboflavin is a component of two compounds called co-factors, used by many enzyme reactions in virtually every cell of the body. The body needs these two cofactors, termed FAD and FMN (see the glossary if you want to know their long technical names!), to convert vitamin B_6 into its active form. FAD and FMN also are required to produce the active form of other nutrients, including folic acid, vitamin A, and niacin. Proper thyroid function depends on adequate riboflavin levels.[69] A deficiency can result in decreased formation of aldosterone by the adrenal glands.[70]

As this is an essential nutrient, women of all menopause types should take riboflavin. A daily dose of 10 to 100 mg is appropriate.

Niacin (Vitamin B₃)

Niacin (B_3) is actually a generic term for nicotinic acid and nicotinamide (also called niacinamide). Niacin is an element in two important enzyme cofactors, NADH and NADPH. Like most B vitamins, niacin is required for proper function of the adrenal glands at specific places within the steroidogenic pathway. The first step of steroidogenesis involves a group of enzymes collectively called the *cholesterol side chain cleavage system.* These enzymes are so named because they cleave off the side chain part of cholesterol, as illustrated in the steroidogenic pathway. This cholesterol side chain cleavage system is dependent on the niacin-based cofactor NADPH for the energy required to start the steroidogenic pathway and convert cholesterol to pregnenolone.[71-73]

The cofactors NADH and NADPH are also essential for enzymes involved in the production of energy for the body, and in the metabolism of carbohydrates, proteins, and fats.[74] Research has shown that a daily dose of 1,500 to 3,000 mg of nicotinic acid can successfully decrease LDL ("bad") cholesterol and increase HDL ("good") cholesterol. Studies suggest that hormonal influence from the adrenal glands—the corticosteroids in particular—may play a significant part in the ability of nicotinic acid to decrease cholesterol levels.[75, 76] This may explain why nicotinic acid is not always effective in lowering cholesterol levels. Decreased adrenal function, due to chronic stress or medications, may diminish the availability of corticosteroids required for this process.

Women of all menopause types should take niacin because it is an important essential nutrient. You should only take high doses of nicotinic acid (for the reduction of LDL cholesterol, for example) under medical supervision because liver damage, peptic ulcer, or decreased glucose tolerance can result. I recommend taking a high-grade multiple vitamin containing all B vitamins, with additional niacin as needed to increase the daily dose to 100 mg.

Pantothenic Acid (Vitamin B_5)

Pantothenic acid (B_5) is known as the "antistress" vitamin and is required for the production of adrenal gland hormones. Chronic deficiency results in decreased function of the steroidogenic pathway.[77, 78] B_5 deficiency also has been associated with the development of high blood pressure.[79] The active form of pantothenic acid is coenzyme A (CoA), which is a coenzyme involved in energy production from fats, proteins, and carbohydrates. The deficiency that leads to adrenal weakness can result in general feelings of fatigue and a decreased ability to tolerate stress. Animal studies reveal that 1.5 mg of pantothenic acid for each pound of body weight is required to prevent symptoms of adrenal weakness due to B_5 deficiency.[80]

As healthy adrenal function is one of the factors in ideal menopause, women of all menopause types should use B_5 supplementation. Take at least 250 mg per day in a high-grade multiple vitamin. Some clinicians use daily doses as high as 1,000 mg.

Pyridoxine (Vitamin B_6)

Women are vulnerable to vitamin B_6 deficiency because high levels of estrogen interfere with B_6 metabolism. Pyridoxine (B_6) is required for a number of metabolic pathways, including the metabolism of tryptophan to serotonin. The most active form of B_6 is pyridoxal-5-phosphate, which is a cofactor for many enzyme reactions. B_6 function and tryptophan metabolism can be significantly inhibited in women taking estrogen-replacement therapy if estrogen levels get too high. As the inhibition is due to a decreased availability of vitamin B_6, this effect is best described as a relative B_6 deficiency—levels are deficient relative to the amount required.

USING VITAMINS FOR BALANCE

Vitamin	Daily Recommendation for Menopause
Thiamine (B_1)	30–100 mg
Riboflavin (B_2)	10–100 mg
Niacin (B_3)	100 mg a day
Pantothenic Acid (B_5)	250 mg*
Pyridoxine (B_6)*	250 mg*
Cobalamin (B_{12})	100 mcg*
Folic Acid	1 mg (400–1,000 mcg)
Vitamin C	1,000 mg (1 gram)*
Vitamin A	2,000–10,000 IU
Beta Carotene	2,000–50,000 IU
Vitamin D*	400 IU
Vitamin E	400–800 IU*
Vitamin K_1	100 mcg–1,000 mcg*

*Please see additional information in text.

Impaired metabolism of tryptophan can be responsible for symptoms such as depression, anxiety, decrease of libido, and glucose intolerance in estrogen users.[81] Though this problem with B_6 is widely recognized in young women who take estrogen/progestogen-based birth control pills, women of menopausal age are also at risk.

In postmenopausal women, estrogen from either the ovaries or the adrenal cortex may interfere with tryptophan metabolism if high levels are produced.[82] Estrogen-replacement therapy during postmenopause can result in the same problem. In one small study, a relative pyridoxine deficiency was found in all 12 women who were using estrogen without taking any progestogens.[83] The pyridoxine deficiency was not as bad when a progestogen was used at the same time.

Synthetic estrogens such as ethinyl estradiol have been shown to lead to a disturbance of tryptophan metabolism and to a deficiency of vitamin B_6. Natural estrogens such as estradiol and estriol caused abnormal tryptophan metabolism similar to that caused by synthetic estrogens.[84] Of course, we would expect this since even estrogens produced in the body by the ovaries or adrenal glands can cause problems with B_6 and tryptophan. The naturally increased hormone activity of pregnancy also causes a relative B_6 deficiency with an increased need for B_6 supplementation.[85]

Classic signs of an estrogen-induced relative B_6 deficiency include depression, irritability, insomnia, fatigue, and glucose intolerance. B_6 deficiency also causes abnormal adrenal growth with increased craving for salt, suggesting problems with aldosterone activity.[86] As noted earlier in this chapter, a study found that supplementation with vitamins B_6, B_1, and C, normalized cortisol production and the 24-hour rhythm of the adrenal glands.[87] Also as noted earlier, the ovary is more susceptible to damage from high homocysteine levels when there is a deficiency of vitamin B_6, vitamin B_{12}, or folate.[88]

As little as 40 mg of vitamin B_6 daily restores normal function and relieves the symptoms of B_6 deficiency in women taking estrogens or in women whose ovaries or adrenal glands are producing relatively high amounts of estrogen.[89, 90] Women of all menopause types should take this essential nutrient. You should definitely take vitamin B_6 if you exhibit signs of relative B_6 deficiency while using any form of estrogen. I recommend a high-grade multiple vitamin containing all B vitamins, with additional B_6 taken to increase the daily dose to 100 mg. You should only take a dose higher than that under the supervision of a physician, due to a potential risk of nerve injury.

Cobalamin (B_{12})

As noted earlier, cobalt is the most important element in the vitamin B_{12} molecule, and a vitamin B_{12} deficiency is synonymous with a cobalt deficiency. Vitamin B_{12} is required for red blood cell production and nerve function. This requirement is so well-known that vitamin B_{12} is commonly considered when there are signs of anemia or nerve pain or numbness. But the effects of vitamin B_{12} extend beyond blood and nerve function. A vitamin B_{12} deficiency may result in decreased progesterone and estrogen levels, and increased cortisol levels.[91, 92] This effect is due to the apparent shifting of the steroidogenic pathway—the body may respond to the specific stress of vitamin B_{12} deficiency by increasing cortisol at the expense of other hormones. The body increases cortisol output to ensure the survival of the body under conditions of stress.

In addition to this apparent shift in steroid production, a vitamin B_{12} deficiency also can result in increased levels of homocysteine, a compound that has been linked to heart disease, heart attacks, depression, Alzheimer's disease, rheumatoid arthritis, osteoporosis, insulin resistance, and an increased risk of atherosclerosis.[93-95]

> The body increases cortisol output to ensure the survival of the body under conditions of stress.

The ovaries are also susceptible to the effects of elevated homocysteine due to vitamin B_{12} (and/or B_6 and folate) deficiency.[96] Observations of decreased ovarian hormones in the presence of B_{12} deficiency clearly demonstrate the degree to which ovarian degeneration and loss of function can occur due to elevated homocysteine levels.

In addition to abnormal ovarian function, a vitamin B_{12} deficiency may affect sleep.[97-101] Because vitamin B_{12} helps normalize the 24-hour sleep-wake pattern, vitamin B_{12} supplementation may help restore normal function and effectively treat certain forms of sleep-wake disturbances.[102-104]

Vitamin B_{12} supplementation is appropriate for all menopause types. My daily recommendation for menopause treatment is 100 mcg. Since vitamin B_{12} is relatively hard to absorb, I usually advise 1 mg (1,000 mcg) once a day for 1 to 2 weeks, then once a week, then once a month. Always take vitamin B_{12} in the morning.

Folic Acid

Folic acid is a tremendously important vitamin for women. A member of the B vitamin family, it is usually included in B-complex supplements. Folic acid is required for the production of red blood cells. It is essential for proper health of all tissues, especially mucous membrane tissues, such as those lining the digestive tract, vagina, and cervix. An increased risk of cervical cancer has been associated with folic acid deficiency.[105] In fact, many practitioners use folic acid supplementation as part of their program to treat mild cervical dysplasia.

Folic acid deficiency greatly increases risk of heart disease by resulting in elevated homocysteine levels in the blood. As noted earlier, the ovary is also more susceptible to damage from high homocysteine levels when there is a deficiency of vitamin B_6, vitamin B_{12}, or folate.[106] Animal studies have shown that folic acid deficiency results in an increased number of ovarian cysts and an impaired synthesis of estrogen and progesterone by the ovaries.[107] The adrenal glands also experience problems when folic acid levels are low. Vitamin C levels may drop due to folic acid deficiency, which reveals the interdependence of these nutrients.

As folic acid protects the heart and cervical tissue and supports ovarian and adrenal health, women of all menopause types should take this supplement. I advise a high-grade multiple vitamin containing all B vitamins, with additional folic acid taken to increase the daily dose to 400 mcg.

Vitamin C

Vitamin C (ascorbic acid) is most popular for its role as an antioxidant. This vitamin, and vitamin E, are most important in decreasing the free-radical damage that results from steroidogenesis.[108] As noted throughout this chapter, the steroidogenic process involves a number of enzyme reactions with various minerals and vitamins. These enzyme reactions are actually biologically controlled chemical reactions that take place within the cells of the body at a molecular level. Free radicals are small fractions of "leftover pieces" of molecules, which are very reactive. They can react to other parts of the cell, the cell membrane, or even DNA and cause significant damage. Antioxidants such as vitamin C "quench" these free radicals by neutralizing them.

A significant deficiency of antioxidants such as vitamin C can result in decreased production of important adrenal gland hormones.[109] This point is vital because the body needs to be able to increase the production of adrenal hormones, such as cortisol, rather quickly when exposed to severe stress. Even chronic stress (menopause can be considered a kind of chronic stress in its effect on the adrenal glands) puts increased demands on the adrenal gland production of hormones such as cortisol. The adrenal glands will use an increased amount of vitamin C when stimulated to make cortisol.[110] As the body does not store vitamin C, it must be supplied daily. The ability of the adrenal glands to regulate steroidogenesis depends on blood levels of vitamin C.[111]

In addition to requirements by the adrenal glands, vitamin C is required by the ovaries for steroidogenesis.[112] This appears to be especially true for the production of progesterone. Animal studies have demonstrated that vitamin C supplementation can increase the ability to produce progesterone.[113]

Vitamin C has many other functions, including decreasing the risk of heart disease and playing a role in collagen production for skin and bones. Women of all menopause types should supplement with vitamin C. Many practitioners suggest a minimum of 1,000 mg (1 g) a day. Doses of 3 or more grams a day are not uncommon.

Vitamin A and Beta-Carotene

Vitamin A and its precursor beta-carotene are both important antioxidants required for the ongoing health of the adrenal glands and the ovaries. There is considerable evidence that vitamin A may not be directly involved in the steroidogenic pathway per se, but plays an important role in supporting the work of other antioxidant nutrients, such as vitamin C and vitamin E.[114, 115] In fact, the antioxidant capability of vitamin A directly correlates to ovary health and the ability of the ovary to make hormones.[116–117] The beneficial effects of beta-carotene are most likely limited to its ability to protect steroid-producing tissues from damage due to free radicals generated during progesterone synthesis.[118] Beta-carotene exerts its protective effect early in the steroidogenic pathway, at the cholesterol side chain cleavage system which, as noted earlier, is the first step of steroidogenesis.[119] This being the case, it is evident that beta-carotene is required for healthy production of all steroid hormones.

Research on cattle has found that lower beta-carotene levels result in cycle irregularities and depressed steroid hormone production.[120] Other researchers have demonstrated that vitamin A and beta-carotene actually stimulate progesterone secretion in pigs' luteal cells, the cells that produce progesterone.[121] The same progesterone-stimulating effect was noted by other researchers in bovine luteal cells.[122] Further research found that progesterone production was positively related to blood levels of beta-carotene and vitamin A.[123] Some researchers have stated that beta-carotene has no effect on progesterone and reproductive capability.[124–127] However, one of those primary research groups changed their position four years later and reported that heat stress and excessive protein will lower progesterone levels, and that beta-carotene will in fact increase fertility.[128]

There is enough evidence that vitamin A and beta-carotene are required for proper steroidogenesis that women of all menopause types should take these supplements. Vitamin A may be taken at 2,000 to 10,000 IU a day, with 2,000 to 50,000 IU of beta-carotene a day.

✧ IU VS. MILLIGRAM

Most fat-soluble vitamins may be labeled as either IU (International Units) or as mg (milligrams). The following list can be used to compare different products that use different numbering systems.

> Vitamin A: 1 mg = 3,333 IU
>
> Beta-Carotene: 1 mg = 1,667 IU
>
> Vitamin E: 1 mg = 1.49 IU
>
> Vitamin D: 1 mg = 40,000 IU

Vitamin D

Vitamin D plays an important role in increasing calcium absorption in the intestines and stimulating mineralization of bones. A deficiency of vitamin D (or vitamin K) will result in incomplete synthesis of osteocalcin, a protein that is synthesized by osteoblasts. Osteocalcin is required for depositing minerals into bones. A buildup of *undercarboxylated osteocalcin*, the inactive form of osteocalcin, leads to decreased mineralization, fragile bones, and increased osteoporosis.[129] Vitamin D is especially important for women of menopausal age.

The steroid hormones—estrogens, progesterone, and testosterone—all contribute to bone building and repair. The combination of hormone-replacement therapy and vitamin D supplementation increases bone mineral density much more effectively than hormones alone.[130, 131] Vitamin D supplementation can actually increase bone density even without estrogen, though not as well as estrogen.[132] Supplementation with vitamin D is beneficial to all women, including women who are already on a healthful diet that includes adequate amounts of calcium and vitamin D.[133] Even with the advent of new drugs designed to prevent and reverse osteoporosis, vitamin D still has its place and should remain an important component in the prevention and treatment of postmenopausal osteoporosis.[134, 135]

The active form of vitamin D is 1,25 dihydroxycholecalciferol—or $1,25(OH)_2D_3$. This active form has a number of different precursors. Vitamin D_3 comes from fish and animal sources, while vitamin D_2 is derived from plants. Vitamin D_3 requires half as much energy as vitamin D_2 to be converted into the most active form of vitamin D.[136] The active form is most important for the prevention and reversal of osteoporosis.

But the actions of vitamin D go beyond the control of osteoporosis. The ability of the pancreas to release insulin appears to depend on the active form of vitamin D_3.[137] Insulin release is impaired by a vitamin D_3 deficiency, but it can be restored by giving $1,25(OH)_2D_3$.[138]

Animal studies have revealed that vitamin D_3 deficiency results in a generally decreased production of insulin as well as a decreased response to a glucose challenge.[139] Supplementation with $1,25(OH)_2D_3$ significantly improved this decreased ability to tolerate glucose. Of interest is the fact that the improvement in pancreatic response required a waiting period of at least 6 hours after the administration of $1,25(OH)_2D_3$.[140] This suggests that the improvement wasn't caused directly by the action of the vitamin D_3, but was a result of changes in the tissue.

As healthy kidneys are required to convert $25(OH)D$ into $1,25(OH)_2D_3$, one study tested people with kidney failure to evaluate their insulin response to glucose. Compared to healthy people, it took them longer to lower their glucose levels, and they created less insulin and had more insulin resistance.[141]

When research compared healthy humans given $1,25(OH)_2D_3$ to healthy humans not given the supplement, there was slight evidence of increased glucose tolerance. Those taking $1,25(OH)_2D_3$ had a slight increase in the glucose uptake by cells as well as a slightly higher level of C-peptide, a substance which reveals increased insulin activity.[142] As vitamin D metabolism also is impaired by phenytoin (Dilantin), abnormal insulin function has been found in epileptic patients taking that drug.[143] This impairment was only partially improved by $1,25(OH)_2D_3$ supplementation.

> As research continues, we are sure to discover further that vitamin D is much more than a vitamin that builds healthy bones.

Vitamin D receptors are located not only in the bones and pancreas, but also in the intestines, kidney, brain, spinal cord, male and female reproductive organs, thymus, and pituitary, thyroid, and adrenal glands.[144] As research continues, we are sure to discover further that vitamin D is much more than a vitamin that builds healthy bones.

Since vitamin D supplementation is so important for the prevention of osteoporosis, it is best for women of all menopause types to take this vitamin. Vitamin D dosage should be 10 mcg (400 IU) daily, or 0.5 to 1.0 mcg per day of the active form, calcitriol. When taking vitamin D, it is also important to take 1,000 mg of elemental calcium daily.

Vitamin E

Vitamin E is another important antioxidant that protects adrenal and ovarian tissues from damage by the free radicals produced during the steroidogenic process. This vitamin is required so early in the pathway that a deficiency will result in decreased hormone production by both the ovaries and the adrenal glands.[145] There is no evidence yet that vitamin E is actually involved in any of the enzyme processes that make up the steroidogenic pathway. However, there is convincing evidence that the ovaries depend on vitamin E to function properly and efficiently.[146] Recent research confirms that the condition of the steroidogenic pathway relies on adequate levels of vitamin E and other antioxidants.[147] Though vitamin E will not actually cause hormone levels to increase, it will allow normal production to take place.

Some health practitioners recommend vitamin E supplementation as a treatment for low estrogen levels, with the belief that it will significantly raise those levels. This belief is based on reports that some women taking vitamin E have fewer hot flashes. This has led to misinformation that vitamin E raises estrogen levels and increases the risk of breast cancer. In truth, vitamin E will not increase estrogen levels. Though it may allow normal steroidogenesis to take place, vitamin E will not force estrogen levels to become elevated.

Women taking vitamin E have been found to have no significant changes in blood levels of estrogen, testosterone, or DHEA.[148] One study found that women supplementing with the vitamin showed a slight increase in progesterone concentrations, which resulted in an increase in the progesterone-to-estrogen (P:E) ratio and a reduced risk of breast cancer.[149] Other research has shown that vitamin E supplementation can inhibit growth of both estrogen receptor-negative and estrogen receptor-positive breast cancer cell cultures.[150]

Vitamin E is actually made of a number of related molecules, which include both tocopherols and tocotrienols. Recent research reveals that the tocotrienols, which are the major vitamin E components in palm oil, are the forms of vitamin E that suppress the growth of both estrogen-responsive and estrogen-unresponsive human breast cancer cell cultures.[151] The ability of vitamin E to shift P:E ratio as well as to inhibit cancer cell growth, whether estrogen receptor-positive or -negative, are good reasons for all women to consider taking this vitamin.

Studies demonstrate that vitamin E also exerts a protective effect on certain nerves in the hypothalamus that are very sensitive to the effects of estrogen.[152, 153] Animal studies show that estrogen actually can be toxic to these specific nerves (beta-endorphin neurons within the hypothalamus), and promote the aging and degeneration of the reproductive system.[154, 155] These changes are thought to be linked to anovulation (failure to ovulate), vaginal dryness, and polycystic ovary disease, as well as reproductive aging and the onset of menopause.[156–159] The capacity of vitamin E to protect beta-endorphin neurons from the potentially toxic actions of estrogen is another reason to consider taking this nutrient.

The ability of vitamin E to impede the development of atherosclerosis is due to many factors, one of the most important being its inhibition of platelet adhesion and aggregation.[160–162] Adhesion and aggregation—stickiness and clumping together—increases the risk of blood clots and heart disease. The effect of estrogen on platelet function is still controversial; science has long associated the hormone with increased risk of blood clots, even though some recent research suggests it may decrease platelet aggregation.[163] Despite this study, the predominant thought remains to use estrogens cautiously if there is a history of blood clots in the family. Research has also noted the risk for increased blood vessel disease due to increased estrogen levels in some pregnant women, so the risk is not limited to women on birth control pills or hormone replacement.[164] Fortunately, studies have shown that vitamin E is able to neutralize most of the adverse effects of estrogen on blood platelets.[165–167]

Due to the many benefits vitamin E supplementation offers, it is best for women of all menopause types to take this vitamin. The typical dosage is 400 to 800 IU daily. Some clinicians prefer a dose of 10 IU for each pound of body weight—one 400-IU capsule for each 40 pounds of body weight.

Vitamin K

Vitamin K is best known for its role in helping blood to clot properly. A deficiency of vitamin K is a contributing cause of many disorders involving excessive bleeding.[168] Though much of the research on vitamin K has focused on its role in blood clotting, this vitamin also has other important functions. Vitamin K is required for the proper synthesis of osteocalcin, a protein that is synthesized by osteoblasts.[169] As noted earlier, osteocalcin is required for depositing minerals into bones. A deficiency of vitamin K (or vitamin D) will re-

> Vitamin K is best known for its role in helping blood to clot properly. A deficiency of vitamin K is a contributing cause of many disorders involving excessive bleeding.

sult in incomplete synthesis of osteocalcin, and a buildup—"undercarboxylated osteocalcin"—leads to decreased mineralization, fragile bones, and increased osteoporosis.[170, 171]

Additionally, animal studies have demonstrated that a vitamin K deficiency can cause increased breakdown of skin collagen and a decrease in the total amount of collagen in the skin.[172] This decreased collagen will mean thinner skin. Vitamin K supplementation may prevent the loss of skin collagen and preserve skin health. Though the relationship is not fully understood, animal studies have shown that a deficiency of vitamin K is associated with a drop in vitamin C levels in the adrenal glands, liver, and other tissues.[173] At the very least, this finding supports the widely held belief that all nutrients are in some way dependent on each other. It also reminds us that we still do not know every function of every nutrient.

Of course, if you are taking blood-thinning medication (anticoagulants), you should talk to your doctor before taking any vitamin K. Otherwise, vitamin K supplementation is appropriate for women of all menopause types. The natural form of vitamin K is called vitamin K_1 or phylloquinone, and is preferable to synthetic forms. A dosage of 100 mcg to 1,000 mcg (1 mg) daily is acceptable.

PHYTOESTROGENS

There is growing evidence that eating foods rich in phytoestrogens (plant substances that have an estrogenlike activity) can be of significant help in easing the symptoms of menopause. Soybeans are high in phytoestrogens. Women in cultures that traditionally eat a lot of soy products, such as the Japanese culture, have a much lower incidence of difficult menopausal symptoms. This appears to be, at least in part, because foods rich in phytoestrogens mimic estrogen activity in the body.

Phytoestrogens don't behave exactly like estrogen, or estrogen replacement, but that can actually be an advantage when you are going through menopause. At that time, your body is adapting to having less estrogen in the system, and there may be a protective effect when you get estrogenlike activity from eating phytoestrogen-rich food, rather than taking full-strength estrogen in hormone replacement.

Phytoestrogens bind to the estrogen receptors of cells, but they do not stimulate the cells as much or as strongly as estrogen steroid hormones. But, by binding to the receptor, they accomplish two important tasks. First, they "satisfy" the receptor by binding to it. This allows the receptor site to respond by initiating changes within the cell. These changes could include helping to decrease osteoporosis, in the case of bone cells, or decreasing hot flash symptoms, in the case of blood vessels. The effect is not nearly as strong as that of a steroid hormone like estradiol, but sometimes that is better.

Second, phytoestrogens decrease cancer stimulation by steroid hormones such as estrogens by taking up the receptor space and competing with steroid hormones that would normally bind to the hormone receptors.[174]

When phytoestrogens block steroid estrogens from binding to the receptor, they are said to be *antagonists*, meaning they work against the steroid hormones. This effect could prevent strong stimulation of cancer cells in the breast or uterus. With less stimulation from steroid estrogens, cancer cells will grow much slower and may be more susceptible to control by the immune system. Additionally, research reports that some phytoestrogens, such as genistein from soybeans, actually suppress tumor growth even in tumors that are not influenced by hormonal activity.[175, 176] Research is discovering that phytoestrogens are inhibitors of breast, uterine, bowel, and prostate cancers.

TABLE 4
Foods with Phytoestrogens[177–186]

Fruits and Vegetables:	Apples, cherries, olives, plums, broccoli, cauliflower, brussels sprouts, cabbage, eggplant, tomatoes, garlic, onions, potatoes, alfalfa sprouts, peppers, chilies, carrots, yams
Herbs and Seasonings:	Alfalfa, aniseed, coconut, fennel, licorice, licorice root, parsley, red raspberry, sage, oregano, red clover, thyme, turmeric, hops, verbena, brewer's yeast, flaxseed
Beans, Grains, and Seeds:	Peanuts, soy products, peas, garbanzo beans, barley, brown rice, bulgur, oats, wheat, wheat germ, rye

Phytoestrogens found in soy foods may decrease the rate of bone loss because of their estrogenlike activity.[187, 188] They can be protective to the cardiovascular system by decreasing high cholesterol levels.[189, 190] They also help allay osteoporosis, and are also able to help control some symptoms of menopause.[191] See table 4 for a list of foods that can help add phytoestrogens to your diet.

Soy

Soy is the most well studied of foods containing phyto-estrogens, and is the source of several very important substances such as the isoflavones, genistein, and daidzein. As well as decreasing cancer risks, soy has the ability to help prevent osteoporosis and, possibly, autoimmune diseases.[192] Since phytoestrogens have an antagonist effect, the decreased risk of autoimmune disease should come as no surprise. It is well-known that women have a higher incidence of autoimmune diseases than men, and that estrogens are believed to play a role in these conditions.

The isoflavones, genistein, and daidzein could prevent postmenopausal bone loss and osteoporosis. In animal studies, genistein is as effective as steroid estrogens in preserving bone. Even synthetic isoflavones, such as ipriflavone, are able to reduce bone loss in animals with osteoporosis and show great promise for the prevention and treatment of postmenopausal osteoporosis.[193]

Animal research demonstrates that soybean phytoestrogens do not have any estrogenic activity in the uterus and vagina, and exert antagonist activity by reducing uterine cell stimulation by supplemented steroid hormones.[194] The implications are that women on hormone replacement would benefit from taking soy-based phytoestrogens. A healthful diet that includes regular intake of legumes, especially soybeans, may result in a decreased risk of endometrial cancer.[195]

In addition to decreasing risks of breast cancer, uterine cancer, heart disease, and osteoporosis, soy can relieve some of the more immediate discomforts of menopause. In a study involving 28 postmenopausal women, each having at least 14 hot flashes per week, soy reduced hot flashes by as much as 40%.[196] These same women reported an overall improvement in menopausal symptoms.

Legumes

In addition to soybeans, other legumes (members of the bean family) have phytoestrogens. These include peanuts, peas, and garbanzo beans.

Grains and Seeds

Whole grains and seeds such as barley, brown rice, bulgur, oats, wheat, wheat germ, and rye are an additional source of phytoestrogens.

Fruits and Vegetables

Common fruit and vegetable sources of phytoestrogens include apples, cherries, olives, plums, broccoli, cauliflower, brussels sprouts, cabbage, eggplant, tomatoes, garlic, onions, potatoes, peppers, chilies, alfalfa sprouts, carrots, and yams.

Herbs and Seasonings

In addition to herbs with estrogenic action, which are discussed in chapter 12, a number of culinary herbs and seasonings also contain phytoestrogens. Herbs and seasonings with phytoestrogens include alfalfa, aniseed, fennel, coconut, licorice, licorice root, parsley, red raspberry, sage, oregano, red clover, thyme, turmeric, hops, verbena, brewer's yeast, and flaxseed.

❧ DECREASING GAS CAUSED BY PHYTOESTROGEN FOODS

It is not uncommon for women who are suddenly consuming more legumes and other vegetables to have increased gas and bloating, due to the gas-producing nature of these foods. For the best remedy for these gastrointestinal problems, look to your spice rack. Many spices and culinary herbs are carminatives. These carminatives, rich in aromatic oils, help the digestive system work properly. They are soothing, help ease gripping discomfort, and help remove gas from the digestive tract. It is no surprise that many of these spices and herbs are traditionally used when preparing these gas-producing foods.

Anise*	Cardamom
Chili and Cayenne*	Celery Seed
Cinnamon	Cloves
Dill Seed	Fennel*
Ginger	Horseradish
Oregano*	Parsley*
Peppermint	Rosemary
Sage*	Spearmint
Thyme*	Turmeric*

*Carminatives that are also a good source of phytoestrogens.

THE IDEAL MENOPAUSE DIET

Menopause is a time to really look after yourself and give yourself foods that are high in the nutrients you need. Choose very fresh food that still has a high vitamin and mineral level, not vegetables that have been sitting in the fridge for a week. Organic food is preferable, when possible.

The ideal diet to follow for menopause emphasizes legumes (beans, peas, and especially soy), along with ample amounts of vegetables and whole grains, with generous use of herbs and spices. Using soymilk instead of cow's milk fulfills two nutritional functions. It is a simple way to augment the soy in your diet, while at the same time cutting out the often allergy-producing effects of dairy products.

SUMMARY

All women experience great demands upon their bodies from all the hormonal changes that occur during menopause. You can significantly improve your menopausal symptoms by eating well and by supplementing your diet with good-quality vitamins and minerals.

The steroidogenic activity that is taking place in the adrenal glands and ovaries can be supported by enhanced intake of the nutrients that are used in this process.

Additionally, other important nutrients can offer significant protection from osteoporosis, heart disease, and other menopause-related conditions.

A diet rich in phytoestrogens also will decrease some of the symptoms and many of the risks associated with menopause. The best choice for vitamin and mineral supplements is a high-grade multivitamin mineral. Since most nutrients work together, especially the B vitamins, the multivitamins will help keep your nutrition balanced.

CHAPTER TWELVE

Herbal Remedies for Menopause

Herbal remedies have been used to treat the symptoms of menopause throughout history in many cultures. The ancient Egyptians, Native Americans, and Chinese all used herbs to nourish and balance women's bodies. Today we have the benefit of modern research to enhance our understanding of how herbs work, and we also have access to herbs from all over the world, thus expanding our repertory of menopausal remedies.

Herbal remedies can be extremely useful during menopause to relieve symptoms and increase overall health. Some women find that they can resolve their menopausal symptoms by the use of herbs alone. You may want to find a qualified herbalist to help you choose the right combination of herbs for your particular menopause type.

The herbs described in this section are the most commonly used during menopause, but this is not an exhaustive list. Your herbalist may recommend other herbs not included here that are specific to your unique physical needs.

The use of herbal preparations in menopause goes far beyond relieving hot flashes. Herbs also are able to maintain the health and tone of the uterus, increase adrenal gland and ovarian function, and increase the capability of the body to adapt to the changes of aging and menopause. Several herbs are well proven to be beneficial in relieving symptoms of anxiety or depression and in preserving memory and other mental functions.

The type of herbs taken during menopause work by restoring function to tissues that have been damaged by illness, stress, hormone changes, and aging. It takes time for them to have an effect because the tissues have to be healed first, and then normal function begins to operate again.

You may not notice the beneficial effects of your herbal remedy for a couple of weeks, or even a month. Some herbs need to be taken for several months before the effect takes hold. For instance, the well-known abilities of black cohosh to relieve menopause symptoms, of ginkgo to improve memory and learning, and of St. John's wort to relieve depression all require use of the herbs for months. So, you have to be a little patient and give the herbs time to do their job.

HOW TO TAKE HERBS

Herbs are sold in different forms: unprocessed (the raw herb), in capsules or tablets, standardized (meaning that the herb has been processed to some degree to ensure that each capsule has exactly the same strength), in freeze-dried granular form, in liquid alcohol (called a tincture), or in glycerin extracts.

> Raw herbs may be hard to digest, so if you have digestive problems such as an ulcer, you should avoid taking your herbs in this form.

Raw herbs may be hard to digest, so if you have digestive problems such as an ulcer, you should avoid taking your herbs in this form. If you normally have good digestion but find that a particular herb irritates your stomach, try taking fennel or another carminative (see sidebar, Decreasing Gas Caused by Phytoestrogen Foods, on page 217), which soothe digestion. Or you can try the herb in another form.

Some people prefer herbs in tincture form (in alcohol), while others want to avoid alcohol or find that it irritates the stomach. Herbs in glycerin are very easy on the system, but are usually much weaker than alcohol extracts.

Chinese herbs are traditionally cooked for specific periods of time and in specific ways. You should consult a Chinese medical herbal specialist to learn how to prepare Chinese herbal formulas. Chinese herbs are also available in tablet form and in freeze-dried granular form. There are specific combinations of Chinese herbs designed for women with different menopausal symptoms that have been tried and tested over centuries.

In Europe, many herbs are traditionally taken as teas. The herbs are steeped in water that has just boiled, for ten to twenty minutes, then strained for drinking. This is a good method for taking some of the more aromatic herbs recommended for menopause, such as sage, vervain, and damiana. You can buy loose herbs for making teas from your local health-food store or from mail-order catalogs specializing in herbs for women. Health-food and other stores now sell herbal teas containing combinations of herbs specifically for menopause. Just make sure they don't contain any herbs which might not be suitable for your menopause type.

Menopausal herbs can be used individually or in various combinations. There are traditional ways of combining herbs which have been used for centuries, such as the Chinese tradition of using licorice with other herbs because licorice helps the other herbs in the combination be absorbed by the body. If you buy a combination of herbs designed for menopause, once again, make sure it does not contain any herbs that are not good for your menopause type, such as vitex if you have low testosterone.

Dosages

Some dosages in this book reflect higher doses than are usually given today. These higher doses were used in early herbal traditions and are currently used by many herbal practitioners in Australia and Europe. I find these doses to be most effective, especially when you are working to heal an imbalance. Once a state of harmony has been reached, you can reduce the dose to a management level.

You need to build up to these higher doses gradually, so start at the lower dose to give the body time to adjust to the tonic effect of the herb. If tolerated well, the herbs can be increased to a higher dose and taken at that dose until the benefits of the particular herb are achieved.

After the benefits are attained for a few weeks, it is often possible to lower the amount of herb and still maintain the benefit. For instance, you can start ashwagandha or Siberian ginseng at 500 mg each morning, work up to 1,000 mg in the morning and 1,000 mg at noon, and then wean back down to 500 mg each morning.

With some herbs, it is quite important *not* to exceed the recommended dosage, as those herbs have the potential to produce toxic effects. Likewise, there can be potential interaction between herbal remedies and prescription medications. If you are currently taking a prescribed medication on a daily or regular basis, it is always safest to consult your medical physician and pharmacist before trying an herbal remedy.

TYPES OF HERBS TO USE DURING MENOPAUSE

Before using any herb, it is important to know what is expected from the herb. Some of the main types of herbs used during menopause are uterine tonics, adaptogens, and nervines. The meaning of this terminology is explained in the following sections. Keep in mind that some herbs listed in this chapter are not only uterine tonics, adaptogens, or nervines. All herbs have more than one action. For example, cramp bark is an important antispasmodic, fenugreek is great for controlling blood sugar problems, and hops is included for its antiandrogen properties. Though ashwagandha is primarily thought of as an adaptogen, it also has anti-inflammatory, anti-tumor, and liver-protecting properties. Because it is useful for women with anxiety and nervousness, it may also be considered to have a nervine quality.

Uterine Tonics

Uterine tonics are herbs that strengthen the uterus and increase its tone. They work by increasing blood flow and circulation to the tissue, or by decreasing spasms and preventing congestion. Many of these herbs have an estrogenlike activity. As you learned in previous chapters, a phytoestrogen is a substance in an herb that exerts this estrogenlike activity. A phytoestrogen has very weak estrogen activity compared to the steroid estrogens that occur naturally in the body.

Phytoestrogens are beneficial in relieving the symptoms of menopause, without apparently increasing the risk of estrogen-related cancers. As these substances mimic the activity of estrogen somewhat, they are also called estrogen mimetics.

Some of the most popular uterine tonics used for menopause include black cohosh (*Cimicifuga racemosa*), paeonia (*Paeonia lactiflora*), blue cohosh (*Caulophyllum thalictroides*), wild yam (*Dioscorea villosa*), dong quai (*Angelica sinensis*), false unicorn root (*Chamaelirium luteum*), shepherd's purse (*Capsella bursa-pastoris*), and cramp bark (*Viburnum opulus*).

❧ WHAT UTERINE TONICS CAN DO FOR YOU

Uterine tonic herbs strengthen the uterus and increase its tone. They may increase blood flow and circulation to the tissue, or decrease spasms and prevent congestion. Many of these herbs have phytoestrogen activity. Uterine tonics include:

Black Cohosh *(Cimicifuga racemosa)*

Paeonia *(Paeonia lactiflora)*

Blue Cohosh *(Caulophyllum thalictroides)*

Wild Yam *(Dioscorea villosa)*

Dong Quai *(Angelica sinensis)*

False Unicorn Root *(Chamaelirium luteum)*

Shepherd's Purse *(Capsella bursa-pastoris)*

Cramp Bark *(Viburnum opulus)*

Fenugreek (*Trigonella foenumgraecum*), licorice (*Glycyrrhiza glabra*), and some of the adaptogenic herbs also have estrogen-mimetic properties, but they are not classically considered uterine tonics.

Adaptogens

An herbal adaptogen is an herb that has the ability to help the body adapt to stress. The various kinds of ginseng are the most popular herbs in this group. Though adaptogens can enhance the function of every tissue in the body, most adaptogens appear to have their most specific ef-

✿ WHAT ADAPTOGENS CAN DO FOR YOU

Adaptogens help the body adapt to stress. They may enhance the function of every tissue in the body, but most adaptogens increase the tone or strength of the adrenal glands, nervous system, and immune system. Adaptogens may slow the aging process by revitalizing and regenerating the body. They are best taken with food in the morning, with a second dose during a noontime meal if needed. Adaptogens include:

Asian Ginseng	Siberian Ginseng
Ashwagandha	Astragalus
Bupleurum	Rehmannia
Schisandra	Licorice

fects on the adrenal glands, nervous system, and immune system. They have the ability to increase the tone and strength of these tissues. In most cases, other tissues such as the liver, heart, and kidneys are strengthened as well. These herbs will decrease deterioration, and possibly slow aging, of the tissues that they affect. They have been described as having an ability to revitalize and regenerate the body.

Since decreased function and deterioration of tissues can result from decreased hormone activity, adaptogens are very helpful for menopause, especially in easing the stress created by hormonal changes. These herbs all enhance adrenal function at some level. Additionally, they can enhance the function of other systems of tissues, such as the nervous system, the immune system, or the liver.

It is best to avoid taking adaptogenic herbs after midday, so that the increased adrenal activity doesn't give you insomnia. They are best taken with food in the morning, with a second dose at the noon meal if needed.

Each adaptogen has its own unique benefits. By far the most popular adaptogens are the "ginsengs"—chiefly Asian ginseng (*Panax ginseng*) and Siberian ginseng (*Eleutherococcus senticosus*). Ashwagandha (*Withania somnifera*), the "Ginseng of India," seems to be less agitating than Asian or Siberian ginsengs for women. Astragalus (*Astragalus membranaceus*) is an adaptogen that can stimulate a weak immune system, while bupleurum (*Bupleurum falcatum*) is one that will calm an agitated immune system. Rehmannia (*Rehmannia glutinosa*) is an adaptogen used when the immune system is so imbalanced that there is autoimmune disease. Schisandra (*Schisandra chinensis*) is a great adaptogen to improve mental and nerve function, and goes well with bacopa (*Bacopa monniera*), ginkgo (*Ginkgo biloba*), or nervines. Licorice (*Glycyrrhiza glabra*) is a widely used herb that also has adaptogenic properties.

Nervines

Nervines are relaxing and calming to the nervous system. They are more sedative than stimulating, and replenish nerve energy more than they deplete it or use it up. Though they are not strong stimulants, they can increase mental function by balancing an overstimulated nervous system. Nervines are often described as "tonics" to the nervous system—they restore tone and function. This restorative ability of nervines makes them useful and popular for menopausal symptoms. Skullcap, valerian, vervain, St. John's wort, passion flower, and damiana are all examples of nervines. Some adaptogens also have nervine actions, such as dong quai, and ashwagandha.

๏ WHAT NERVINES CAN DO FOR YOU

Nervines are soothing, relaxing, and calming to the nervous system. They replenish nerve energy, but are not stimulants. They increase mental function by balancing the nervous system. Nervines include:

Skullcap	Valerian
St. John's Wort	Vervain
Passion Flower	Damiana

CHOOSING AN HERB

In truth, it is difficult and in some ways incorrect to classify herbs according to a single action. Many of the uterine tonics have mild adaptogenic properties, while quite a few adaptogens enhance uterine tone and health. Additionally, most of these herbs have antioxidant, anti-inflammatory, and digestion-balancing properties as well. Nonetheless, in keeping with traditional models of using herbs, the following herbs are described according to their most dominant properties.

Uterine tonics can be used as a general "female tonic" to enhance and fortify tissues that are feeling the effects of decreased hormones. You can select adaptogens as an alternative to, or in addition to, the uterine tonics and as the most useful herbs to help overcome fatigue. The nervine herbs can be used with adaptogens and uterine tonics when there is a need to decrease anxiety or enhance nerve function.

Alfalfa

Alfalfa (*Medicago sativa*) is an herb with estrogen-mimetic properties.[1, 2] It is also considered mildly diuretic, increasing the flow of urine.[3] Alfalfa sprouts are a popular form of this herb. Women of any menopause type can use this herb as a food (sprouts), an herbal extract, or in tablet form, at a dosage of 500 to 1,000 mg, 1 to 3 times a day.

Ashwagandha

Ashwagandha (*Withania somnifera*), an herb from India, has a very wide range of adaptogenic properties. This adaptogen helps preserve adrenal size and function, enables the body to adapt to stress, and increases muscle mass, endurance, and strength.[4] Ashwagandha also can be used to treat anemia, lower cholesterol, and increase libido and sexual performance.[5] Additionally, this herb has antibacterial, anti-inflammatory, antitumor, and liver-protecting properties.[6]

Ashwagandha may be less stimulating than other adaptogens and is ideal for women who have underlying anxiety or nervousness. This herb is suitable for any menopause type. You can take 500 to 1,000 mg in the morning, with a second dose of the same size at noon if needed.

Astragalus

Astragalus (*Astragalus membranaceus*) is an adaptogenic herb that also can strengthen the immune system. It is best for women who have a weak immune system with frequent infections. This herb aids women with a history of fatigue that came on after a virus or other infection. It is traditionally used to strengthen weakened organs, treat a prolapsed uterus and uterine bleeding, control excessive sweating, and promote urination to get rid of edema.[7] This adaptogen is also a heart and lung tonic.

The possible immune-enhancing actions of astragalus include antiviral activity and the ability to increase immune system function, which is important for fighting infection and cancer. Astragalus also warms the system and increases metabolism. Women of all menopause types can use astragalus, especially in the case of a weak immune system. Take 1,000 mg (1 g) in the morning, with a second dose of the same size at noon if needed.

Bacopa

Bacopa *(Bacopa monniera)* is an herb traditionally used in India as a brain tonic.[8] It is used to enhance memory and learning capability and to treat insomnia.[9, 10] Considered of great value for the aging brain, it is also used to promote longevity and recovery from nervous deficits due to injury or stroke.[11] Researchers have studied its potential application in treating epilepsy, nervous breakdowns, and exhaustion.[12, 13] While enhancing brain function, it also has a mild sedative and tranquilizing effect.[14, 15] Bacopa is useful for all menopause types, but especially for those with low estrogen or testosterone levels. Take 1,000 mg, 1 to 3 times a day.

Black Cohosh

Black cohosh *(Cimicifuga racemosa)* is a very popular herb for the treatment of menopausal symptoms. Herbal traditions have long recognized its hormonelike activity.[16] It does have an ability to decrease hot flashes and other symptoms of menopausal discomfort. Its estrogenlike activity makes it ideal for treating estrogen-deficient types of menopause. Its action does not stimulate uterine tissues the way estrogen does, so in that sense it lacks the complete properties of estrogen.[17] Nonetheless, it is effective in increasing blood flow to the pelvic area, and relieves spasms, cramps, and inflammation.[18] It also has a mild euphoric effect, resulting in mood elevation and control of menopause-related depression.[19, 20]

Perhaps this ability to relieve symptoms, without having a complete hormone effect, is why black cohosh is considered a safe, effective alternative to estrogen-replacement therapy for women who wish, or need, to avoid estrogen.[21] Black cohosh can be used for any menopause type, especially when there are symptoms of decreased estrogen. Take 500 mg, 1 to 3 times a day. This herb often takes 1 to 2 months to be effective.

Blue Cohosh

Blue cohosh *(Caulophyllum thalictroides)* is reported to have antispasmodic and tonic effects on the female reproductive system,[22, 23, 24] and has been used in some menopause formulas for these reasons. The ability of blue cohosh to cause abdominal irritation[22] has received more attention recently. There is renewed concern about a potential risk of high blood pressure or heart disease from use of this herb.[25] The unmonitored use of blue cohosh is now being discouraged.

Bupleurum

Bupleurum *(Bupleurum falcatum)* is a reputed adaptogen thought to enhance function of the adrenal glands and liver, while calming the immune system. This herb may increase the size of the adrenal glands and promotes ACTH secretion by the pituitary gland, which enhances adrenal gland function.[26, 27] This effect can be very helpful in encouraging the adrenal glands to help make menopause a smooth transition.

Bupleurum can significantly improve liver function, as demonstrated by improved liver enzyme levels in studies of blood tests.[28] Bupleurum also has anti-inflammatory, mildly sedative, cholesterol-lowering, and very mild laxative actions as well.[29] Bupleurum is useful for any menopause type. Take 1,000 mg (1 g) in the morning, with a second dose of the same size at noon if needed.

Cramp Bark

Cramp bark *(Viburnum opulus)* is an antispasmodic herb that can be used to decrease uterine spasms and cramps.[30, 31] It is a muscle relaxant that is helpful for any cramps in smooth muscles (found in organs and blood vessels) or skeletal muscles, especially uterine cramps and cramps in the calf of the leg.[32, 33] It is also useful in relieving spasms in asthma and spasms of the urinary bladder.[34, 35] Cramp bark also has sedative properties, which obviously contribute to its action as a muscle relaxant.[36, 37] The sedative and smooth-muscle-relaxant abilities also can help reduce elevated blood pressure.[38] This herb can be used in any type of menopause. Take 500 to 800 mg, 1 to 3 times a day.

Damiana

Damiana *(Turnera diffusa)* is an herb that acts as a tonic to the nervous system. It is considered a nervine with restorative properties.[39] Damiana is useful for the treatment of depression with anxiety.[40] Traditionally, it has been used to restore sex drive and was widely considered to be an aphrodisiac—a substance that increases sex drive.[41] In fact, the scientific name for damiana used to be

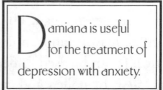

Damiana is useful for the treatment of depression with anxiety.

Turnera aphrodisiaca. It is apparently a nervine that has a direct effect on the reproductive organs. This herb is useful for conditions involving anxiety, depression, and fatigue in which sexual dysfunction is present due to those conditions. Damiana also can help control hyperglycemia and is being studied for treatment of diabetes.[42] This herb is useful for any menopause type—especially those types predisposed to high blood sugar and insulin resistance. Take 500 mg, 1 to 3 times a day.

Dong Quai

Dong quai *(Angelica sinensis)* has many functions that make it a valuable herb for women. The Chinese call dong quai the "ginseng for women." It has phytoestrogenic activity and has been used to decrease the symptoms of menopause. Like many phytoestrogens, it has no true estrogen action, so it may be considered safe for women who need to avoid steroid estrogens.[43, 44] It has antioxidant and antitumor activity that also can benefit women needing to avoid steroid estrogens.[45, 46] In addition, dong quai is a hematonic—a blood-building herb used to treat anemia.[47]

Dong quai has mildly sedative, tranquilizing, and analgesic (pain-killing) properties.[48, 49, 50] Its antiinflammatory and antiallergenic actions are very effective. It can be used to decrease sensitivity to dust, animal dander, or pollen and can slow down progression of inflammation and fibrosis in affected lungs.[51, 52, 53] Dong quai also decreases risk for heart disease.[54, 55]

This herb is well known for its ability to moisten the intestines and help move the stool, so some regard it as a mild laxative.[56, 57] It also will increase vaginal lubrication and may increase sexual activity.[58] Dong quai is a good herb for all menopause types that need estrogen. It can be very useful when steroid estrogen replacement must be avoided or is not fully effective. As this herb has sedating and tranquilizing properties, use it cautiously if depression or fatigue is present. In such cases, use an adaptogenic herb concurrently. Sometimes, because of its effect on the intestines, dong quai may increase flatulence. If this happens, take fennel or ginger with the dong quai. Dosages for dong quai are 500 to 750 mg, 1 to 3 times a day.

False Unicorn Root

False unicorn root *(Chamaelirium luteum)* has phytoestrogens that ease the symptoms of decreased estrogen in menopause.[59, 60] It has been used to treat prolapsed uterus and to increase pelvic and vaginal tone.[61, 62] It is a tonic for the uterus and the ovaries.[63–65] It helps with reduced vaginal lubrication and lack of sexual desire.[66] It also has mild diuretic properties, so urine flow may be increased.[67] It can be used for any menopause type that has symptoms of estrogen deficiency. Take 500 mg, 1 to 3 times a day.

Fenugreek

Fenugreek (*Trigonella foenumgraecum*) seed has a significant ability to lower elevated blood sugar levels.[68–70] The seeds also have estrogen-mimetic properties, may increase breast size, and purportedly have aphrodisiac, tonic, and general restorative properties.[71, 72] Fenugreek is mildly adaptogenic and specifically able to help some people adapt to the stress of high altitude and overcome mountain sickness.[73] This herb is useful for all menopause types—especially those types predisposed to high blood sugar and insulin resistance. Take 1 ounce of fenugreek (as a condiment), 1 to 3 times a day.

Ginkgo

Ginkgo (*Ginkgo biloba*) is an herb of great value to the brain. It is most widely known for its ability to decrease memory loss, improve memory, and slow the loss associated with aging, and for the treatment of memory impairment caused by dementia.[74, 75] As well as being able to prevent loss of mental function, it is widely used to enhance learning and improve memorization skills. It is also able to improve mood and can be used in the treatment and prevention of depression.[76-78] Ginkgo increases blood flow to the brain and extremities, making it very useful in the treatment of vascular disorders such as Raynaud's disease and other conditions involving poor blood flow.[79]

Women of all menopause types can use ginkgo, but you should seriously consider it if you have low estrogen or testosterone levels. Take 40 to 80 mg daily. Ginkgo is usually available as a standardized tablet with a specific amount of the active ingredient.

Hops

Hops (*Humulus lupulus*) is best known as a brewing ingredient that gives beer its bitter taste. Some of the compounds that occur naturally in hops have very strong phytoestrogenic activity.[80] Recent research has even suggested that some of the compounds in hops have a preventive effect against breast and ovarian cancer in humans.[81] Hops also has sedative effects and can be used to reduce anxiety and irritability, or to help induce sleep. It is also regarded as a mild antiandrogen, decreasing the effects of testosterone and other androgens.

Due to its potential protective activity against some forms of cancer, hops is a good herb for any menopause type. It is, of course, useful for any type with low estrogens, but is especially helpful in types with excessive androgens. Take 500 to 1,000 mg daily, usually at bedtime to aid in sleep. Divide the daily dose into four doses of 125 to 250 mg each if you want to take it during the day to help relieve stress and anxiety.

Asian Ginseng

Asian ginseng (*Panax ginseng*) is a popular adaptogenic that balances several body functions and helps the body deal with stress.[82] It can be calming to over-stressed women, helping to relieve anxiety, insomnia, and restlessness. At the same time, it can be strengthening to the body, relieving lethargy, fatigue, forgetfulness, abdominal bloating and fullness, uterine prolapse, and muscle weakness.[83] Asian ginseng increases the overall energy and vitality of the body. It is said to have estrogenic activity.[84, 85] *Panax* helps preserve the size and weight of the adrenal glands and increase ACTH secretion by the pituitary gland.[86]

> Asian ginseng is used to enhance heart function, decrease depression, and improve mood, digestion, physical endurance, mental function, and immune function.

This herb can be helpful in enhancing adrenal recruitment. It is also used to enhance heart function, decrease depression, and improve mood, digestion, physical endurance, mental function, and immune function.[87–89] It also can help with glucose metabolism and can decrease mildly elevated blood sugar levels.[90, 91] Thus, this herb can be useful in the management of insulin resistance.

Asian ginseng is appropriate for all menopause types, though it is classically considered to be more estrogenic than Siberian ginseng is. Take 125 to 250 mg in the morning, with a second dose of the same size at noon if needed.

Licorice

Licorice *(Glycyrrhiza glabra)*, an adaptogenic herb that has a major influence on steroid hormone activity, is most well-known for its estrogenlike action. Licorice is believed to alter the metabolism of steroid hormones, especially when used with Asian ginseng.[92] Licorice can produce changes in the steroidogenic pathway. It also exerts some direct, though minimal, action on estrogen and androgen receptors, and has a moderate affinity for cortisol receptors.[93] It contributes to an increase in aldosterone activity. In fact, prolonged use of licorice can cause high blood pressure, sodium retention, and loss of potassium, a sign of increased aldosterone.

Licorice can preserve adrenal function and size of the adrenal gland, and help the body adapt to stress. It also has a beneficial effect on the urinary tract, decreasing bladder infections by increasing local immunity.[94, 95] Licorice also has anti-inflammatory, cancer-preventive, and mild antidepressant properties. This herb is suitable for any menopause type—as long as there is no history or risk of high blood pressure. Take 500 to 1,000 mg in the morning, with a second dose of the same size at noon if needed.

Paeonia

Paeonia *(Paeonia lactiflora)*, also called white peony root *(bai-shao)*, is very helpful in relieving excessive uterine bleeding. It is a traditional Chinese medicine for female disorders, including spontaneous sweating, stomachaches, and headaches as well as abnormal uterine bleeding, dysmenorrhea (menstrual cramps), and leukorrhea (excessive vaginal discharge).[96] It also has muscle-relaxant and antispasmodic actions.[97] Paeonia can be used for any menopause type, especially if you suffer from excessive bleeding. Take 500 mg, 1 to 3 times a day.

Passion Flower

Passion flower *(Passiflora incarnata)* has mild sedative and sleep-inducing properties.[98] It is very helpful for the treatment of irritability, insomnia, muscle tension, and nervous indigestion.[99-102] It has been used to treat cardiac symptoms such as heart palpitations and high blood pressure.[103] Passion flower is a good herb for women, especially women sensitive to medication, because it is effective, yet at the same time, has relatively mild actions and is well tolerated. Passion flower is appropriate for all menopause types, but use it with caution if you suffer from depression. Take 500 to 1,000 mg, 1 to 3 times a day.

Rehmannia

Rehmannia *(Rehmannia glutinosa)* is an herb used for disorders of the kidneys and adrenal glands. It appears to work by preserving adrenal gland function and weight, and helping the body adapt to stress.[104] Rehmannia affects the immune system with antiallergy and antiinflammatory actions, and has been used to treat autoimmune conditions such as rheumatoid arthritis.[105, 106] Rehmannia has the ability to decrease hyperglycemia (elevated blood glucose) and has been used to treat diabetes.[107, 108] It can normalize heart function, lower cholesterol, and increase blood flow to the brain.[109]

Rehmannia is useful in situations where there is debility (weakness) combined with inflammation. It will not increase vitality and energy as robustly as will a ginseng, but it is still considered adaptogenic. It is the herb to try first when inflammation and allergies are present along with fatigue. This herb will not be as stimulating as other adaptogens. Take 1,000 mg in the morning, with a second dose of the same size at noon if needed.

Sage

Sage *(Salvia officinalis)* contains estrogenlike substances that make it useful for women.[110, 111] It has been used to treat a wide range of menopausal symptoms, including hot flashes and mood swings due to hormone changes. It has the ability to decrease perspiration, so it has obvious benefits for its value for relieving hot flashes.[112-114] Sage can be used for any menopause type in doses of 500 mg, 1 to 3 times a day.

St. John's Wort

St. John's wort *(Hypericum perforatum)* is a very popular, widely used nervine with antidepressant actions. It is also helpful in decreasing anxiety, irritability, and nervous fatigue.[115, 116] Its antidepressant action does not take effect for a few weeks to a couple of months after you start using the herb.[117] St. John's wort also can be used to improve digestion due to its bitter qualities. Bitter herbs stimulate the flow of saliva and gastric juices, aiding the digestive process. It can be used for any type of menopause. Take 300 mg of a standardized extract, 1 to 3 times a day.

Sarsaparilla

Sarsaparilla *(Smilax spp.)* was traditionally used to make root beer. Though its reputation as an herb that raises testosterone has not been scientifically proven, it is still widely believed to increase libido. It has a number of steroidlike compounds—many of which may bind to estrogen, progesterone, and testosterone receptors.[118]

Sarsaparilla is an adaptogen, and can help the body adapt to stress.[119] It is also used to balance and regulate hormones.[120] The steroid like compounds in sarsaparilla have anti-inflammatory actions, which are very useful in menopause types with increased inflammation due to a low P:E ratio.[121] Women experiencing any menopause type may take sarsaparilla, but it is best for those women with low or normal testosterone. Since it has adaptogen actions, it is best to take it in the morning, or noon at the latest, so that the 24-hour hormone patterns are preserved. It may be taken as 500 to 1,000 mg, 1 to 2 times daily.

Saw Palmetto

Saw palmetto (*Sabal serrulata*) is mostly popular as anti-androgenic herb that men use to decrease prostate enlargement. It's important to note, however, that the antiandrogen action can also benefit women, and that saw palmetto is currently being used to treat excess androgen conditions in women by a number of physicians. Saw palmetto binds to both androgen receptors as well as estrogen receptors.[122, 123] Saw palmetto is best for any menopause type with high testosterone, and may be taken as 500 to 1,000 mg 1 to 3 times daily.

Schisandra

Schisandra (*Schisandra chinensis*), an adaptogenic herb, has been used to treat insomnia, irritability, and forgetfulness, while at the same time being effective against fatigue and exhaustion.[124] It improves concentration, coordination, vision, hearing, and sense of touch.[125] It is also used to treat spontaneous sweating. Its adaptogenic actions appear to influence the brain the most.

This herb is useful in any menopause type that has decreased nervous system function, especially due to estrogen deficiency. Take 1,000 mg (1 g) in the morning, with a second dose of the same size at noon if needed.

Shepherd's Purse

Shepherd's purse *(Capsella bursa-pastoris)* is best known as a hemostatic herb—an herb that stops bleeding. Though research is not conclusive, this herb is indicated for chronic uterine bleeding.[126, 127] Shepherd's purse also has been used to treat hemorrhoids and chronic diarrhea and has a mild diuretic action.[128, 129] This herb has been quite effective in controlling dysfunctional uterine bleeding in menopausal women, possibly due to its ability to increase uterine tone and cause uterine contraction.[130, 131] It is most effective in menopause types that have dysfunctional uterine bleeding due to progesterone deficiency. Take 500 mg, 1 to 3 times a day.

Siberian Ginseng

Siberian ginseng *(Eleutherococcus senticosus)* is an adaptogen that also enhances the function of the immune system, nervous system, and other systems of the body. It can help maintain adrenal gland size and weight, and as such could help with adrenal recruitment in menopause.[132] Siberian ginseng improves general resistance and enhances the immune system's response to bacterial infections, viral infections, and cancers.[133, 134] Siberian ginseng also increases physical performance and stamina, increases mental awareness and ability to learn, promotes tissue healing, and decreases heart and lung disease.[135, 136]

This herb is appropriate for all menopause types, though it is classically considered to be more androgenic than Asian ginseng is. Some women find Siberian ginseng too stimulating, resulting in anxiety and insomnia. If these effects occur, reduce the dose and/or try Asian ginseng or dong quai instead. Take 500 to 1,000 mg (1 g) in the morning, with a second dose of the same size at noon if needed.

> Siberian ginseng increases physical performance and stamina, increases mental awareness and ability to learn, promotes tissue healing, and decreases heart and lung disease.

Skullcap

Skullcap (*Scutellaria lateriflora*), a calming nervine, is useful in the treatment of nervous tension, stress with exhaustion, muscle spasms, anxiety, insomnia, and heart palpitations.[137–139] It is soothing and restoring to the nervous system.[140] It is useful in menopause types that include irritability, anxiety, and nervous exhaustion. Skull-cap is also mildly diuretic and can help decrease blood pressure.[141] It can have an anti-aphrodisiac effect—lowering the sex drive in some people.[142] Women of all menopause types can use skullcap, but do so with caution if you suffer from depression. Take 500 mg, 1 to 3 times a day.

Valerian and Mexican Valerian

Valerian *(Valeriana officinalis)* and Mexican valerian *(Valeriana mexicana)* are nervines that are safe, gentle, and effective sedatives.[143, 144] Mexican valerian is a bit stronger than *Valeriana officinalis,* but essentially has the same action.[145] Both of these herbs are able to calm and sedate without causing extreme drowsiness and decreased alertness.[146, 147] These herbs can also be used to decrease pain and induce sleep.[148] Valerians are helpful for any condition of excessive nervousness, such as anxiety, nervous muscle tension, nervous headaches, insomnia, nervous upset stomach, and so on.[149–151] These herbs are useful for any menopause type, but you should exercise caution if you suffer from depression. Take 500 mg, 1 to 3 times a day.

Vervain

Vervain *(Verbena officinalis)* is another calming nervine that, like St. John's wort, can be used to improve digestion because of its bitter qualities.[152-154] This herb has a relaxing and toning effect on the nervous system and is useful for the treatment of depression, insomnia, nerve pains, nervous exhaustion, and stress.[155-157] Vervain can have an aphrodisiac effect on some people—increasing their sex drive.[158] It can be used for any menopause type, and is safe and useful in types that involve depression. Take 500 mg, 1 to 3 times a day.

Vitex

Vitex *(Vitex agnus-castus)*—also known as chaste tree, chasteberry, and monk's pepper—was used in the past as an herb to suppress libido in men. Its primary action in women appears to be increasing progesterone levels while lowering estrogen levels, because of its ability to increase luteinizing hormone (LH) while decreasing follicle-stimulating hormone (FSH).[159] This makes it useful as a perimenopausal herb for PMS caused by low levels of progesterone. The effects of vitex on menopausal women have been mixed. Some women appear to benefit, while others have no change, or seem to do worse, with the libido-suppressing action becoming evident to them. This herb is best avoided in menopause types with low or slightly low testosterone, at least until more is learned about this herb. Take 500 to 1,000 mg, 1 to 3 times a day.

Wild Yam

Wild yam *(Dioscorea villosa)* itself does not contain progesterone, nor can the human body make progesterone from wild yam. It takes an elaborate chemical process in a pharmaceutical laboratory to create progesterone from the raw material found in the tuberous root of the wild yam. Other steroid hormones also can be created from the same raw material, but only in a laboratory. You should be aware that "wild yam" creams only contain progesterone if the hormone has been added to the cream. Wild yam, itself, isn't progesterone.

But it has medicinal value as an herb. Wild yam can be used to decrease cramps of the digestive and female reproductive systems.[160–163] I have found it very effective for gallbladder spasms as well. The anti-inflammatory and antispasmodic actions of this herb resemble the similar actions of progesterone. Wild yam has estrogen- and progesterone-mimetic qualities and is of value in all menopause types. Take 500 mg, 1 to 3 times a day.

SUMMARY

As you can see, herbal remedies have a wide range of applications for women of menopausal age. They can be used for the treatment of common menopausal symptoms such as hot flashes and mood swings. Their greatest benefit is their ability to enhance the function of tissues that are fatigued, weakened, or debilitated from the effects of time, stress, and diminished hormone levels. Herbs can be used to revitalize the adrenal glands and ovaries. Additionally, they can be used to enhance the function of the nervous system to relieve stress and preserve or improve memory and learning.

Herbal remedies can be used alone or in combination with other herbs. They also can be used in conjunction with hormone-replacement therapy. As herbs work by restoring normal function, balance, and vitality to tissues, you need to take them for a period of time to allow them to be effective. It's best to take herbs with a specific purpose or goal in mind. Once the goal is obtained, it is often possible to lower the amount of herb and still maintain the benefit.

Here, I have reviewed some of the most popular herbs for woman's health, out of the thousands of herbs used by various cultures throughout the world. As herbal research continues, new herbs and new benefits are sure to be discovered. These healing and nurturing plants are great gifts to all people, and of great benefit to most women.

CHAPTER THIRTEEN

Glandular Extracts and Menopause

Glandular extracts are preparations of specific tissues or glands that are used to restore health and function to the tissue or gland targeted. For example, you can take an adrenal gland from an animal and make an extract from it that can stimulate healing in the adrenal glands of a human.

Glandular extracts are traditionally believed to restore the normal function of and rejuvenate the target tissue. Traditionally, they have been used to strengthen and tonify weak glands and tissues. Glandular extracts are referred to as being trophorestorative—nourishing and restoring to the target tissues.

When the Food and Drug Administration (FDA) was amending its regulations on nutrient-content claims to change the terminology used to describe vitamins, minerals, herbs, and other nutritional substances, it struggled to define what the "other nutritional substances" were. The FDA ruled to categorize glandular extracts as nutritional substances, along with amino acids and nutritional powdered drink mixes.[1]

In 1934, three American researchers who had found that liver extracts were able to cure pernicious anemia, won the Nobel Prize in Medicine. In the acceptance speech, the use of glandular extracts was referred to as organotherapy. Organotherapy was defined as a method of treatment in which a patient who has unsatisfactory function of some organ or tissue is given an extract or portion of that organ or tissue from an outside source.[2] The speaker discussed the use of liver, pancreas, and testes extracts. There is evidence of the practice of organotherapy at an even earlier date—in 1889—and it may go as far back as ancient Egypt.

The use of glandular extracts has grown from the turn of this century to today. In the 1930s and 1940s, articles discussing this form of medicine frequently appeared in medical journals such as the *Lancet*, the *Journal of the American Medical Association*, the *British Medical Journal*, and *Endocrinology*.[3] In fact, glandular therapy has been a major part of conventional endocrinology. Even though thyroid hormone was synthesized in 1927, some clinicians were finding they had better results with dried thyroid gland preparations.[4] Even to this day, many clinicians continue to choose dried gland preparations over synthetic hormones.

DO GLANDULAR EXTRACTS REALLY WORK?

The active constituents of glandular extracts include a variety of enzymes, lipids (fats and oils), and polypeptides (protein fragments). When a person takes an oral glandular extract, the active constituents are absorbed into the bloodstream and may have a definite effect on the tissues of the human body, even though the extracts are derived from animal sources.[5–8]

The ability of intact proteins and large polypeptides to be absorbed into the bloodstream from the human digestive system is debated. Some believed that glandular extracts taken orally were completely broken down into amino acids and fatty acids in the digestive system.

Research supports the view that some small intact proteins do cross the gastrointestinal tract, and this absorption is a physiologically normal process.[9] Both the stomach mucosa (mucous-membrane lining) and the intestinal mucosa are capable of actively transporting intact dietary proteins into the bloodstream.[10] The cells of the mucousal membrane actually engulf large proteins (endocytosis) and transport them from one end of the cell to the next using a microtubular network within the cell.[11, 12] Once these proteins and polypeptides pass through the lining of the small intestine, they enter the systemic circulation and are able to reach other tissues of the body, where they may affect blood pressure, growth factors, hormone secretion, immune function, and nervous system activity.[13, 14]

The body's ability to absorb larger protein molecules and peptides is so important that individuals with diminished absorption of intact protein may be compromised.[15] The requirement for peptides in nutrition is so evident that hospitals routinely use feeding formulas with peptides for critically ill patients.[16, 17] So, there is no doubt that the molecules, enzymes, lipids, and polypeptides within glandular extracts are to some extent absorbed and able to affect hormone, immune, and nerve function.

Health-care practitioners currently interested in the use of glandular extracts include medical doctors, osteopathic physicians, chiropractic physicians, naturopathic physicians, licensed acupuncturists, and nurses, as well as nutritionists and herbalists.

> The molecules, enzymes, lipids, and polypeptides within glandular extracts are to some extent absorbed and able to affect hormone, immune, and nerve function.

Glandular extracts are traditionally used to nourish, strengthen, balance, and restore function to tissues or glands that are in need of this support. They are considered to work best in conjunction with a health program of good nutrition, proper exercise, and adequate rest. Glandular products are currently available as either pure glandular extracts or as part of a mixture that includes other nutrients that work with the extracts. The success of these products is based upon protocols and dosages that have been used for more than 60 years.[18–20]

HOW GLANDULAR EXTRACTS ARE PREPARED

Most glandular products used to enhance and restore gland function are from bovine (cow) sources. The four most popular methods of processing the glandular tissue are freeze-drying, salt precipitation, predigestion, and the azeotrophic method.[21]

Freeze-drying involves quick-freezing the glandular material to −40°F or colder. The material is then subjected to a vacuum, which pulls the water out of it while it is still frozen. Salt precipitation involves blending of glandular material in salt and water and then separating the fat from the mixture, which is dried and powdered. The predigestion method uses enzymes to partially digest the glandular material, which is then freeze-dried and powdered. The azeotrophic method quick-freezes the material, then washes it with a solvent such as ethylene dichloride to remove the fatty tissue. The solvent and water are removed from the material, which is then powdered.

No matter what preparation method is used, it is important that the glandular material comes from livestock free of infection, pesticides, herbicides, antibiotics, and synthetic hormones.

The exact method (or recipe) for preparing glandular extracts is unique to each manufacturer. Many clinicians report success with the use of glandular extracts, independent of manufacturer or preparation method. The relative lack of standardization of processes and extracts, however, makes scientific study of this therapy a challenge.

THE SAFETY OF GLANDULAR EXTRACTS

Any discussion of the use of glandular extracts must be approached with reserve. Due to valid concerns about the spread of slow viral diseases such as bovine spongiform encephalitis (BSE), also known as "mad cow disease," I must caution the reader about the use of raw bovine glandular extracts. BSE is one of many related conditions known as transmissible spongiform encephalopathies (TSEs)—fatal neurological diseases that afflict animals and livestock. As well as BSE, this group of diseases includes chronic wasting disease (CWD) of deer, transmissible mink encephalopathy (TME), and scrapie, which infects sheep. Many believe BSE originated from scrapie. TSEs also have been diagnosed in domestic cats, various wild species of animals, and possibly in ostriches. Similar diseases, such as Creutzfeldt-Jakob disease and kuru, occur in humans.

The discovery in Britain of a new variant of Creutzfeldt-Jakob disease (nvCJD), which causes dementia in humans, was linked to BSE when nvCJD was found to have a similar genetic makeup as BSE. Many believe there is a link between three TSEs: scrapie in sheep, BSE in cattle, and nvCJD in humans. The response by most countries has been to ban the use of ruminant (deer, sheep, cow, etc.) meat by-products (protein concentrates) in feed for sheep and cattle—called a ruminant-to-ruminant feed ban.

Thousands of licensed and skilled clinicians throughout the United States continue to use glandular extracts. Some of the best nutritional supplement companies in the world use adrenal gland and ovarian extracts in their products. Companies that continue to produce and supply glandular extracts receive their material from certified sources, collected from animals free of disease, medication, and additives such as hormone or growth factors commonly used by some livestock companies. The leading producers of glandular supplements have always used material from special herds that were raised with tissue harvesting in mind, so the outbreak of BSE had no impact on them.

One country famous for its disease-free livestock is New Zealand. Though scrapie develops in sheep around the world, a few sheep-producing countries, such as Australia and New Zealand, are free of the disease. New Zealand livestock is also completely free of other TSEs, such as BSE, as well as CWD. These claims are based on long-standing policies designed to prevent the introduction of these diseases, and surveillance programs to detect them. Many regulators, scientists, and academics have explicitly and implicitly confirmed New Zealand's claims of being free from scrapie and BSE.

The United States government responded to the nvCJD in Britain by tightening its already strict import and surveillance policies. On advice of the international BSE Expert Science Panel, the U.S. also imposed a ruminant-to-ruminant feed ban to exclude meat and bone meals containing ruminant protein from feeds given to ruminants. This voluntary feed ban was also enacted as an agreement between the

New Zealand Feed Manufacturers Association and the Ministry of Agriculture. Governmental authority to impose a statutory feed ban (mandatory, no longer voluntary) was enacted as part of the New Zealand Biosecurity Amendment Act in 1997.

> If you choose to use glandular extracts, choose them from a supplier that can certify the product is from a disease-free source.

Thousands of clinicians are confident that they continue to have access to glandular extracts derived from healthy livestock and use them accordingly. Nonetheless, it is important to remember that glandular extracts are basically raw tissue from specific glands in cows. If you choose to use glandular extracts, choose them from a supplier that can certify the product is from a disease-free source. Please make your personal decision on whether to take glandular extracts with this information in mind.

GLANDULAR EXTRACTS FOR LOW HORMONES

Glandular extracts that can be considered for women of menopausal age include, first and foremost, ovarian and adrenal tissue extracts because these are the two endocrine tissues most affected by menopause. With the increased incidence of hypothyroidism in postmenopausal women, it may be appropriate to consider thyroid enhancement as well. Glandular extracts are available for many other glands, including the pituitary, pancreas, and hypothalamus. Numerous non-endocrine tissues, including the heart, brain, lung, and kidney, are also available. As ovarian, adrenal, and thyroid extracts may be most important for women of menopausal age, I limit my discussion here to these three.

Ovarian Extracts

Traditionally, ovarian extracts have been used to raise weak estrogen levels by directly enhancing the function of the ovaries in several female conditions, including PMS, menopause, and infertility. Ovarian extracts can ease menopausal symptoms. Ovarian extracts are not a replacement for hormones because they contain no steroid hormone or, at most, contain only a small trace. They are thought to be beneficial because of their ability to restore balance and to be trophorestorative to the ovary, thereby encouraging the tissue to function normally.

As ovarian extracts can promote increased production of estrogens, women of menopause types that have enough estrogen and not enough progesterone should use ovarian extracts with caution, and should consider progesterone supplementation. Ovarian extracts can increase irritability in some progesterone-deficient women. In addition, since the postmenopausal ovary is still capable of producing testosterone, it follows that ovarian extracts are likely to increase testosterone. Women with high-testosterone menopause types should avoid the use of ovarian extracts, as aggression and agitation have resulted from some of these women taking ovarian extracts.

Ovarian extracts can be taken as a dietary supplement. Start with 1 capsule a day in the morning. After 1 to 2 weeks, increase to 2 capsules a day, if symptoms of low estrogen are not decreasing. After 2 more weeks, increase to 3 capsules a day, if desired. Be cautious with increasing dosages to avoid enhancing ovarian function so much that irritability or agitation result.

Adrenal Extracts

Adrenal gland extracts have been used in cases of low steroid hormones because the adrenal gland is such an important source of the steroid hormones needed during menopause. Recall that production of androstenedione should actually increase in postmenopausal women. This androstenedione is an important precursor for estrogens and for testosterone, which are no longer being made by the ovaries in sufficient quantities.

Adrenal extracts also are used for general adrenal fatigue, which can occur at any age in men or women. The fact that women of menopausal age depend so much upon their adrenal glands makes adrenal fatigue that much more of a problem.

Adrenal fatigue is not to be confused with Addison's disease, a severe disease that ultimately involves loss of adrenal gland function. Adrenal fatigue is best described as a low function or hypofunction. This hypo-adrenal state usually includes symptoms such as weakness, loss of appetite, being easily fatigued, heart palpitations, and low blood pressure, which may show up as slight dizziness on standing. As adrenal fatigue can occur to varying degrees, all of these symptoms may not be present.

Adrenal extracts usually have no steroid hormone in them or, if they do, it is only a small trace. They may be beneficial due to their ability to restore balance and to be trophorestorative to the adrenal gland and restore its normal function.

If you take adrenal extracts, it is important to avoid stimulants such as caffeine. Though not everyone using caffeine and adrenal extracts experiences irritability and nervousness, these side effects occur often enough to advise caution. As caffeine only further stresses an already fatigued adrenal gland, avoiding it is best in all cases of adrenal fatigue anyway.

Although women of any menopause type in which there is a component of fatigue can use adrenal extracts, it is best to exercise caution if you have high testosterone. Adrenal extracts appear to increase testosterone activity in a number of women and have caused agitation in some who already had too much testosterone.

Adrenal glandular extracts can be taken as a dietary supplement. Start with 1 capsule a day in the morning. After 1 to 2 weeks increase to 2 capsules a day, if symptoms persist. After 2 more weeks, increase to 3 capsules a day, if desired. To avoid enhancing adrenal function so much that irritability, agitation, or insomnia results, be cautious when increasing the dosage. Don't increase the dosage in an attempt to get more energy. Though adrenal glandulars can help overcome fatigue, they are not stimulants.

Thyroid Glandular Extracts

True and full-scale hypothyroidism is a serious medical condition that requires medical evaluation and supervision, laboratory work, and conventional thyroid-replacement

✑ USING GLANDULARS

Following is the program I personally use for glandulars:

1. Start with 1 capsule per day in the morning. Remember, you want to preserve the normal 24-hour rhythm of the body.

2. Increase the dosage to 2 capsules each morning if the symptoms persist after 1 to 2 weeks.

3. Increase the dosage to 3 capsules a day if symptoms continue to persist after 2 more weeks. At this point, you can take 2 capsules in the morning and the other capsule no later than noon.

4. Decrease the dosage back to what worked best for you if you feel irritable or agitated or have trouble sleeping.

5. Stay on the dose that works for you for at least 1 month. Some women stay on glandulars for 4 to 6 months, but I encourage weaning after a few months. Glandulars are used to restore function and rejuvenate tissues; therefore, you don't need to take them forever.

6. When you decide to wean yourself from the glandulars, decrease your daily dose by 1 capsule every 2 weeks.

7. Repeat this cycle after a break of at least 1 week, but preferably 1 month. Some women use this program once or twice a year.

therapy. But like the adrenal gland, the thyroid may also have a lesser degree of underfunctioning (hypothyroidism). The thyroid may be working enough that a prescription of thyroid hormone replacement isn't required, but not enough for optimal health and well-being. The existence of a mild form of hypothyroidism has been recognized for more than 50 years.[22] It may present as: dry hair and skin; brittle, thickened, and coarse nails; or premature graying or hair loss. Other symptoms include recurring headaches, fatigue, low energy, dull thinking, dizziness, depression (especially late in the day), constipation, and weight gain. As these are the clinical symptoms of full-blown hypothyroid disease, you should first get an evaluation by your medical doctor.

While the thyroid levels of many people with mild hypothyroidism actually test within the "normal range," they may still feel and look hypothyroid. As with steroid hormone testing, even if laboratory results are in the first quartile, there is no guarantee that it is the best level for the individual. They may do better in a higher quartile. Many physicians are now willing to recognize the validity of the patient's symptoms and treat borderline low thyroid function, even though laboratory results are within "normal" limits.

Women of menopausal age are at increased risk of developing borderline low thyroid function when they take hormone replacement. Recall that estrogen can increase thyroid-binding globulin, which means less thyroid hormone is directly available to the tissues of the body. You may have quite normal thyroid levels, even in the second quartile, and still have a picture of low thyroid function. Usually, the thyroid adjusts to the increased amount of thyroid-binding globulin and raises levels of available thyroid. However, if the thyroid is already "fatigued" or already mildly hypoactive, it may not be able to compensate.

Thyroid tissue extracts are of great value in treating a mild hypothyroid condition. Many of the thyroid glandular extracts have the active thyroid hormones removed—so they are not prescription strength, but still are able to restore balance and be trophorestorative to the thyroid. Women of any menopause type in which there is not anxiety or excessive irritability can use thyroid extracts.

Do not try to use any glandulars as stimulants.

You can take thyroid glandular extracts as a dietary supplement. Start with 1 capsule a day in the morning. After 1 to 2 weeks increase to 2 capsules a day, if symptoms persist. After 2 more weeks, increase to 3 capsules a day if desired. To avoid enhancing thyroid function so much that irritability or insomnia results, be cautious when increasing the dosage. Do not try to use any glandulars as stimulants.

SUMMARY

The most useful glandular extracts for women during menopause are ovarian, adrenal, and thyroid tissue extracts. Proper use of glandulars encourage endocrine tissues to function normally. Ovarian glandulars should not be used in menopause types with adequate estrogen and inadequate progesterone, or in menopause types with excessive testosterone. Glandulars should never be used as stimulants, as they increase irritability and agitation, and they should not be the sole course of action, but work best as part of a program that includes good nutrition, proper exercise, and adequate rest.

CHAPTER FOURTEEN

Hormone-Replacement Therapy

An Overview

One day, my wife was discussing my work with a friend of hers. The friend said, "When I went through menopause, I was started on hormones right away. But it's not as if I had a choice, right?"

In fact, there are many choices available, and it makes sense to look at all of them. It's never a good idea to jump right into hormone-replacement therapy (HRT) without first exploring all the options—and your unique needs. My wife's friend should have received a complete evaluation, including laboratory tests and a careful review of her symptoms, before her doctor gave a prescription for hormones. Only this kind of thorough examination can tell you which hormones you need, if any.

Like my wife's friend, many women get the false impression that hormone therapy is a must for all post-menopausal women. But when you understand the menopause types, you can see why this isn't true. The one-size-fits-all approach won't meet the needs of individual women, nor will the same therapy work for every different menopause type. And many women can restore their bodies' hormonal balance without taking hormones at all. Natural therapies involving herbs, diet, and lifestyle changes can work very effectively to relieve menopausal symptoms and prevent serious health problems. Glandular extracts, as we've seen, are another option, as are precursors.

This is good news for women who can't take supplemental hormones, or would strongly prefer not to. Women who have had breast cancer, or those at higher risk for common complications of hormone therapy as a result of a history of liver or gallbladder disease, may opt not to take hormones. Those with a history of serious medical problems potentially complicated by hormones or their common side effects need to seriously question the use of HRT in any form. And many women simply don't like the idea of taking hormones, either for philosophical reasons or because they're concerned about the possible health risks involved in taking estrogen. For these women, the herbal, nutritional, and lifestyle approaches discussed in other chapters of this book may offer the best therapy.

But hormone therapy has its advantages. Recent advances in medicine are redefining hormone therapy by giving women more options and developing better forms of supplemental hormones. For many women, hormone supplementation may be the best, most effective treatment, especially now that it's no longer a one-size-fits-all formula.

If you're thinking about using some form of HRT, this chapter is for you. I'll tell you about the risks and benefits of taking hormones, the different forms of hormone therapy available to you, and other issues you should be aware of before you make a final decision about hormone therapy.

WHY HORMONE-REPLACEMENT THERAPY?

Hormone-replacement therapy means exactly what it sounds like: giving hormones to replace what the body is no longer able to make. As we've seen, a hormone deficiency can cause extreme discomfort as well as serious long-term health risks. The simplest, and in some ways the most obvious, solution is to correct the deficiency directly by taking a hormone supplement.

We do not hesitate to give insulin to a diabetic child, who would otherwise face disability and premature death. Insulin, as you may know, is a hormone. Of course, menopause is not a disease like diabetes. It's a natural transition and, if it goes smoothly, there won't be any hormone deficiencies. But women who are deficient in one of the three major sex hormones may face serious long-term health problems as a result. Osteoporosis, blood sugar problems, heart disease, some vaginal disorders, certain types of cancer, and prolonged physical discomfort are among the health risks of these hormone deficiencies. Emotional symptoms such as feelings of anxiety and depression can also be severely debilitating. It certainly makes sense to take hormones if it's the best way to bring you back into the balanced state that menopause is naturally meant to be.

For too long, hormone-replacement therapy has focused on estrogen, and little else. Even with all we know about the importance of progesterone and testosterone, it's still common for doctors to focus mainly on estrogen (with synthetic progesterone added to reduce the risk of endometrial cancer). What we really need is a new definition of hormone-replacement therapy. It should be seen as a balancing of all three important hormone levels, with hormone supplements tailored for a woman's individual needs—and suited to her menopause type.

> A hormone deficiency can cause extreme discomfort as well as serious long-term health risks.

The advances in hormone-replacement therapy that are unfolding today may make HRT a valid option for more women than ever. These advances are in the process of totally redefining the therapy.

REDEFINING HORMONE-REPLACEMENT THERAPY

Today, several advances in medicine are changing our definition of hormone-replacement therapy. First, some doctors are becoming acutely aware that women must be properly assessed before making any decisions on HRT. A simple "Do you have hot flashes?" just will not do anymore. The standard of care is coming to be defined as a routine laboratory assessment, pelvic exam, breast exam, and bone evaluation. In writing this book, I hope to help all women and all health-care professionals be even more alert to the importance of identifying the menopause type before deciding on a treatment.

Doctors have known for 20 years that it's important to balance estrogen-replacement therapy with progesterone, to minimize the risk for endometrial cancer. But now, progesterone's true importance in a wide range of menopausal symptoms and health risks is better known, along with the key role played by testosterone.

It's also become clear that women do not need as large a dose of estrogen as the medical profession used to think. By balancing all hormones, it's possible to achieve more with smaller amounts—thus reducing the side effects and risks.

Another advance is the discovery that hormone precursor therapy can be an effective way to raise hormone levels and restore balance. The body can use precursors such as DHEA, androstenedione, and pregnenolone to restore its estrogen, progesterone, and testosterone levels, without the danger of hormonal levels being forced too high as can happen with direct hormone replacement.

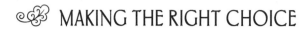 MAKING THE RIGHT CHOICE

Complete and proper assessment focused on your symptoms based on the Menopause Type Questionnaire.

Hormones that are balanced (estrogen, progesterone, and testosterone).

Other hormones or precursors when applicable (DHEA, androstenedione, and pregnenolone).

In-depth evaluation including lab work, pelvic exam, breast evaluation, and bone studies in your evaluation.

Complementary therapies, such as herbs and homeopathy.

Extra vitamins and minerals to optimize the health of all tissues.

Soy and other phytoestrogen-rich foods to decrease symptoms and risks.

A new standard of care for women in menopause is rapidly emerging. Hormone replacement is still an important part of the program, but it's not the be-all and end-all it used to be. If you decide to take hormones, you'll get better results if you think of them as only one part of a complete program that also includes dietary changes if needed, exercise, and stress management.

NEW CHOICES: NATURAL OR SYNTHETIC?

Once you've decided to try hormone-replacement therapy, the next question is whether to choose natural or synthetic hormones. Since the term "natural" can be used in a confusing variety of ways, let me define what I mean by it: A natural hormone is chemically identical to the hormone your body produces. It doesn't matter whether it was made in a laboratory or taken from an animal's body: If a hormone is chemically identical to your body's own hormone, it is usually called "natural."

While "natural" hormones may actually be made in a laboratory, they are exactly like the hormone your body is used to. A "synthetic" hormone is called so not only because it's made in a laboratory, but because it's not identical with your body's own hormone.

Synthetic hormones are a relatively recent phenomenon. Designed in the hope of finding stronger, longer-lasting, more convenient versions of our bodies' own hormones, these synthetic hormones can actually cause more problems than natural ones. Unfortunately, we are now finding that stronger hormones that last longer in the body are not what women need. Think about it: Do you really want a hormonelike chemical that is twice as strong as the one in your body? What about *400 times* as strong?

The researchers who developed many of the synthetic hormones designed them to survive passage through the digestive tract, so they could be taken in a pill form. Natural progesterone, for example, is destroyed during the process of digestion. Until fairly recently, it had to be injected or taken in a skin cream or gel. Scientists developed chemicals called progestins that were similar to progesterone, but could be taken by mouth, in a convenient pill form. Today, progestins are what most doctors prescribe in hormone-replacement therapy. Yet progestins cause more side effects than natural progesterone. They were designed to resist being broken down by the body—but now it's becoming clearer that maybe there are good reasons for letting the body break down hormones in its own way.

Now the industry knows how to make micronized natural hormones. This means that the particles are rendered extremely small, so that they can be absorbed into the bloodstream before they reach the liver, where they would otherwise be broken down. Also, any steroid hormone can be absorbed through the skin, via gels, creams, or patches. These *transdermal* (across/through the skin) methods of treatment also deliver the hormone straight into the bloodstream without it passing through the liver first. Hormones can also be given intravaginally (introduced into the vagina and absorbed through the vaginal walls), sublingually (under the tongue), or transbuccally (held in the side of the mouth and absorbed through the lining of the cheek). Other hormones, such as calcitonin (used in the treatment of osteoporosis), are actually being delivered transnasally (as a nasal spray). Each of these methods is a different kind of what is known as a *drug delivery system*.

It is now possible to take natural hormones in ways that ensure good absorption. These natural hormones are exactly the same as the hormones your body has been making all your life, which means your body is able to react to them in the same way. These hormones have the same strength as the ones your body naturally produces, they bind to receptors the same way, and they can be metabolized the same way.

Please note, however, that each kind of delivery system has its advantages and potential complications. All do not work equally reliably for all individuals or in all circumstances. If you take any form of hormone-replacement therapy, you should do so under the supervision of a qualified health-care provider.

Natural Hormones

The term "natural hormone" deserves a closer look. As I said before, natural hormones are identical to the ones your body makes. A better term might be *bio-identical* rather than "natural." After all, these "natural" hormones are made in a laboratory, often from plants such as soybeans and wild yams.

One of the common types of estrogens used in HRT are conjugated equine estrogens (CEEs). As the name equine (which means horse) implies, CEEs are derived from horses—specifically the urine of pregnant mares. Though this is a "natural" source, there are types of estrogen in CEEs that do not occur naturally in humans.

The word "natural" is overused and frequently misunderstood. It means different things to different people, depending on what is being bought or sold. It is a good idea to ask your doctor or the hormone manufacturer what he or she means by "natural." For the purpose of this book, as I've already explained, my definition of *natural hormone* means a hormone that has the exact same nature, or is bio-identical, to the hormone that occurs naturally in the human body.

Wild Yam: Progesterone and Estradiol

Wild yam is often cited as a source of natural progesterone. This claim is rather misleading. Two points of clarification are needed. First, the wild yam *(Dioscorea villosa)* is actually a cultivated crop, and there is nothing wild about it anymore. Second, the wild yam doesn't contain any progesterone. The root of this plant does contain chemicals that, in a laboratory, can be made into progesterone or any other steroid hormone. But there is simply no way for your body to do these conversions, so you won't get any progesterone by taking plain wild yam.

Almost all wild yam creams contain some added progesterone, which is bio-identical or "natural." If so, the cream may work—but not because it's got the words wild yam extract on the label. Bio-identical progesterone can be made from soybeans, too, but somehow "wild yam cream" sounds more exotic—and more marketable—than "soybean-derived progesterone cream."

There is nothing wrong with this progesterone. In fact, the mass marketing of bio-identical progesterone is probably one of the best things to happen in the history of women's health care. But it is important to recognize that it is not the claims of "wild" or "natural" that make it good, but rather the bio-identical nature of the hormone.

Another bio-identical hormone created from yam and soy is estradiol (17-beta-estradiol). Many of the estradiol products used in hormone-replacement therapy contain this form of estrogen derived from yam or soy which, unlike CEEs, is exactly the same as the estradiol that occurs naturally in a woman's body. Natural wild yam estradiol is available in a micronized form in capsules, as well as in skin patches, creams, and vaginal rings.

❧ "NATURAL" HORMONES: THEN AND NOW

In the early 1930s, progesterone was derived from the gonads and adrenal glands of slaughtered animals. In the 1940s, scientist Russell E. Marker developed a method for converting diosgenin, a substance found in wild yam, into progesterone.[1] Since then, soy and other plants have been used as raw material for the production of other steroid hormones, including estradiol, testosterone, and prednisone.

Synthetic Hormones

Synthetic hormones—hormone supplements that are not bio-identical to the hormones found in the human body—do not act the same way as natural hormones. For example, the synthetic progestogen medroxyprogesterone acetate (Depo-Provera, Provera, Cycrin) has been found to decrease the benefits of estrogen (estradiol) replacement therapy. Estradiol, the strongest naturally-occurring form of estrogen in your body, may play a role in improving blood flow to the heart. Progestogen medroxyprogesterone acetate, taken at a normal dosage, can negate the protective effect of estradiol and possibly leave the coronary arteries more susceptible to disease.[2] Although research suggests that this side effect is likely to occur in a small amount of medroxyprogesterone acetate users, it is still important to understand why it happens.[3]

The potency of ethinyl estradiol, a synthetic estrogen, is about 400 times that of natural estradiol. The synthetic testosterone methyltestosterone is testosterone modified in such a way that it resists being broken down by the liver. This synthetic hormone may increase the risk of liver disease when taken in large doses. It is always wise to follow the example the body has provided when it comes to what type of hormones to take, how much to take, or even when to take them.

Once-a-Day Dosing

When you take hormones—that is, the time of day affects how well the body can use them. There is a well-defined rhythm of hormone production during the day. Steroid hormone levels are naturally highest in the morning to early afternoon, and lowest in the evening to midnight. This 24-hour pattern is called a *circadian rhythm*. Understanding the circadian rhythm of hormones can tell us when to take hormone replacement so that this natural rhythm is preserved.

The ideal way to take estrogen is once a day. The natural daily rhythm of estrogen is such that levels are higher in the day, peaking in the early afternoon, and dropping to the lowest level at midnight.[4, 5] Significantly, in postmenopausal women with low estrogen levels, the 24-hour rhythm is essentially lacking.[6] This lack of circadian rhythm can affect sleep, energy, and mood.

> Steroid hormone levels are naturally highest in the morning to early afternoon, and lowest in the evening to midnight.

When you use estrogen orally in the morning, your levels reach their peak within 4 to 6 hours. That means a morning dose will result in a peak a little earlier than occurs naturally, which is preferable to taking a nighttime dose and having the peak in the middle of the night when levels should be at their lowest.[7, 8] If you take oral estrogen, you may have some fluctuations during the first four weeks as your body adjusts. For this reason, it's best to wait at least a month after starting oral estrogen before you run any hormone tests.

One study using a combination of estrogens found that the blood concentration of estradiol remained within the normal range 24 hours after the last dose.[9] This shows that estrogen levels don't rapidly drop below desired levels between doses, and that once–a-day dosing is enough.

When estradiol is applied topically in a gel, the levels also peak within 4 to 6 hours after application.[10] The peak is not as pronounced as that seen with oral estrogen preparations, most likely because the skin and the layer of fat under the skin act as a reservoir for continuous release of steroid hormones.[11-13] As with oral estrogen, it is advisable to wait at least 4 weeks before testing blood or saliva levels, or making any changes in the dosage when using topical forms of estradiol, because it takes time for a steady state to be reached.

✒ MATCHING YOUR NATURAL PATTERNS

Taking hormones such as estrogen, progesterone, and testosterone every morning allows normal function of hormones that peak at night, such as:

> Melatonin: Required for sleep and many other vital functions (see appendix D).
>
> Growth Hormone: Builds bones, maintains health of skin and other tissues. Commonly called the anti-aging hormone.
>
> Adrenocorticotropic Hormone (ACTH): Keeps adrenal glands functioning on a daily basis. Required for daily production of normal cortisol levels.
>
> Leuteinizing Hormone (LH): Keeps ovaries functioning on a daily basis. Responsible for 24-hour pattern of estradiol.
>
> Thyroid-Stimulating Hormone (TSH): Required for normal, 24-hour pattern of thyroid hormones.

Due to the normally low levels of estrogen during sleep, there is no physiological justification for taking estrogen in the evening, or dividing the dose between morning and evening.

Elevated evening estrogen levels can result in a decreased level of growth hormone when it should be at its highest. Growth hormone levels are usually highest in the evening and during the night, so tissue regeneration and repair can be done while we sleep. This means that evening dosages of estrogen can impair the natural regeneration and repair of the body. For some women, taking estrogen in the evening appears to interfere with melatonin, a hormone your body produces every night to help you sleep, causing disruptions in normal sleep.

Other steroid hormones also have 24-hour rhythms that are best not disturbed when taking hormone replacement. Cortisol has a very pronounced rhythm, with levels highest at about 8:00 A.M. and lowest at about midnight.[14] Progesterone, DHEA, androstenedione, and testosterone also have higher levels in the morning, though their cycles are not as pronounced as cortisol's.[15–17]

ESTROGEN-REPLACEMENT THERAPY

Today, you can choose among several types and forms of estrogen. The most popular types of estrogen used after menopause are: estradiol; two other bio-identical estrogens known as estrone and estriol; conjugated equine estrogens (CEEs), also called PMU estrogens; and ethinyl estradiol.

If you have an intact uterus, whenever you take any type of estrogen you should also take progesterone, or a progestin.[18] (See Risks of Taking Estrogen to follow for more information.) However, it is important to remember that balancing estrogen with progesterone is also required for ideal health of the brain, bones, heart, and other tissues.

Estradiol

Estradiol is the primary estrogen produced by the ovaries before menopause. This is also the type of estrogen used in many estrogen-replacement products. As noted earlier, a bio-identical molecule is produced from wild yam, soybeans, or other plants.

Estradiol is available in many forms, including oral micronized, patches, topical gels or creams, and vaginal rings. Each form appears to have its own advantages and disadvantages. It is important to review the product literature and discuss choices with a health-care professional. The form of estradiol you choose depends largely on personal preference, but your choice may be influenced by other factors such as blood pressure or a desire to relieve vaginal symptoms while keeping hormonal blood levels low.

Oral-Micronized Estradiol

Oral-micronized estradiol is rapidly absorbed, though quite a bit of it is converted to estrone in the gastrointestinal tract and liver.[19–20] Estrone is the main type of estrogen your body naturally produces after menopause (before menopause, estradiol predominates). When you take oral-micronized estradiol, the result tends to be a higher level of estrone than estradiol. However, there is a slower drop in the estradiol level in the blood, believed to be due to the high estrone level acting as a reservoir for estradiol.[21]

So, the result of taking oral estradiol (if your hormone test shows that you need it) is very close to what happens in an ideal menopause, with somewhat higher levels of estrone than estradiol. This is one reason why it may be better to take oral-micronized estradiol—it is bio-identical, and may produce more similar results to those of your own natural hormones.

It's important to realize that, even though CEEs are the leading type of estrogen given to postmenopausal women, there is evidence that oral-micronized estradiol works just as well. Oral-micronized estradiol has been shown to provide many of the benefits attributed to CEE. While it has been less studied than other types of estrogen, research suggests that oral-micronized estradiol is effective in protecting against heart disease and increasing blood flow to the brain.[22, 23]

It is also important to be aware that women do not absorb steroid hormones in an identical way. Some of the factors known to affect absorption include age and body weight.[24]

You need less estrogen as you get older, or as your body weight decreases. Other factors such as gastrointestinal health also may play a role. Individualized and customized estrogen replacement, as is available through compounding pharmacists, may be the best solution to these unique needs. These customized formulas should be based on both symptoms and laboratory test results.

> It is important to be aware that women do not absorb steroid hormones in an identical way.

Also note that oral estrogens can decrease testosterone levels more than topical estrogens, which may show up in both your symptoms and your lab tests.

When starting on oral-micronized estradiol, it is helpful to base the dosage on how strong your menopausal symptoms are. One good method is to correlate your starting dose of micronized estradiol with the number of hot flashes you experience in a day. If you have five or fewer hot flashes per day, start with 1 mg daily. If you're having six or more hot flashes per day, try 2 mg daily. Some women find that they need as much as 3 to 4 mg daily to relieve hot flashes.[25]

Micronized estradiol is considered by many physicians and pharmacists a highly effective and safe form of oral estrogen-replacement therapy, and can be used for any menopausal type involving estrogen deficiency. Oral-micronized estradiol is available as Estrace (0.5 mg, 1 mg, or 2 mg) or as customized capsules from a compounding pharmacist.

Transdermal Estradiol System   A transdermal system is a patch that releases estradiol through a membrane in the patch into the skin at a continuous, controlled rate. You must attach the patch only to intact skin that is free from abrasions or rashes. The estradiol is absorbed easily through the skin into the bloodstream.

Patches are relatively accurate at delivering the prescribed amount of estradiol, and so they are a viable alternative for women who prefer not to take oral estrogen. Research indicates that skin patches are an effective way to take estrogen. One study showed estradiol patch use in postmenopausal women increased the function of heart muscle (cardiac output) while also decreasing blood pressure.[26] Transdermal patches are available as Alora, Climera, Estraderm, Fempatch, and Vivelle. The patches come in two different systems: 0.05 mg/day or 0.1 mg/day.

Transdermal Estradiol and Norethindrone Acetate

This transdermal patch is a combination of estradiol and norethindrone acetate (NETA), a synthetic progesterone. Research indicates that such combination patches are safe and effective, and have the ability to prevent abnormal endometrial growth (endometrial hyperplasia).[27] As with any estrogen and progesterone combined therapy, this combination can decrease symptoms of menopause, including anxiety, depression, sleep disturbances, poor libido, hot flashes, and vaginal atrophy.[28] These patches are available as Estragest™ or Combipatch™ in two different sizes. Each size delivers 0.05 mg/day of estradiol. The 9-square-centimeter (cm²) round patch delivers 0.14 mg/day of norethindrone acetate, while the 16-cm² round patch delivers 0.25/day of norethindrone acetate.

Topical Gel and Cream

You can also get estradiol in the form of a topical gel or cream, available through compounding pharmacists, as customized prescriptions. As noted earlier, topical estradiol does not have as pronounced a peak during absorption. For this reason, women who feel irritable when estradiol peaks occur prefer this form. Topical gels and creams can be used for any estrogen-deficient menopause type. (Gels and creams will *not* tend to reduce your testosterone levels as oral estradiol will. It is also available as Estrogel, a topical estradiol gel.

Estradiol Vaginal Ring   The estradiol vaginal ring was developed to deliver a controlled, very low dose of estradiol to local tissues only, while having very little effect on estrogen levels in the rest of the body.[29, 30] It is effective in easing vaginal dryness and vaginal atrophy and lowering the pH of the vagina to normal.[31, 32] It does not appear to protect against osteoporosis or heart disease, nor help with any mental or emotional symptoms of menopause. Estradiol rings typically deliver a dose of 6.5 to 9.5 mcg (0.065 to 0.095 mg) per 24 hours.[33]

The estradiol vaginal ring offers a good, safe alternative to existing vaginal therapies, with a very low systemic exposure to estradiol.[34-36] Vaginal estradiol rings are available as Estring; one ring lasts about 3 months.

Estrone

Estrone is the estrogen that is naturally dominant in postmenopausal women. Before menopause, your body has significant levels of estrone, but estradiol predominates. When estradiol levels drop during menopause, estrone levels actually increase as some of your estrogen production shifts from the ovaries to the adrenal glands.

Estrone is only half as potent as estradiol, so it may be less stimulating to some cancer cells and to the endometrium. Thus, some doctors consider it safer than estradiol. However, there is evidence that estrone stimulates breast and uterine tissue, and may be linked to cancer.[37] In general, any estrogen supplement carries the same precautions.

Conjugated Equine Estrogens (Premarin)

Conjugated equine estrogens (CEEs) are a mixture of estrogens obtained from pregnant mares' urine (the brand name is Premarin). Sometimes they are referred to simply as "conjugated estrogens."

There is a significant amount of debate concerning the use of CEEs for hormone-replacement therapy. Much of the debate focuses on how ethical it is to continue to use pregnant mares' urine now that we are able to make bio-identical estrogens from yam and soy. And although CEEs do contain estrone that is bio-identical to human estrone, they also contain horse estrogens such as equilenin and equilin. In fact, these horse estrogens can make up between 30% and 45% of the estrogens in the tablet.[38] These horse estrogens do interact with the body, and have potent estrogenic effects, but they're not bio-identical to the human body's own estrogens.[39]

> A 1998 study of 14,601 women showed that when their prescriptions were changed from horse estrogens (Premarin) to plant-based estrogens (Estratab), most women preferred the plant-based estrogen.

A 1998 study of 14,601 women showed that when their prescriptions were changed from horse estrogens (Premarin) to plant-based estrogens (Estratab), most women preferred the plant-based estrogen. After 6 months, 93.5% of the women continued to use the plant-based estrogens. Two-thirds of women who did not go back to CEEs were still using plant-based estrogens 3 years after changing their prescriptions.

In the past, estrogen-replacement therapy involved so many side effects that 50% of women dropped it after a year. Now, the wide range of choices of estrogen types, including bio-identical estrogens, allow HRT with significantly less side effects. Increasing public demand for plant-based bio-identical forms of estrogen may mean the role of horse-urine estrogens is waning. If you do choose to use CEEs, they are available in 0.3-mg, 0.625-mg, 0.9-mg, 1.25-mg, and 2.5-mg strength tablets. CEEs are also available for intravenous or intramuscular injections and as a vaginal cream.

Conjugated Equine Estrogens and Medroxyprogesterone Acetate

Combinations of CEEs and medroxyprogesterone acetate (MPA) are available. These combinations offer the benefits of both estrogens and progesterone in one tablet. However, the estrogens include horse estrogens, and the progesterone is synthetic, which means that they may have more side effects than other, bio-identical choices. This combination is available on either a continuous or a cyclic regimen. The continuous regimen is available in two different strengths as Prempro™. Each contains 0.625 mg of CEEs, mixed with either 2.5 mg or 5 mg of MPA. The cyclic regimen is available as Premphase™. It consists of 0.625 mg of CEEs taken orally for 28 days, with 5 mg of MPA also taken on days 15 through 28.

Esterified Estrogens

Esterified estrogens are plant-based estrogens synthesized from soy and wild yam plant sources. Esterified estrogens deliver primarily estrone. One study showed that a 0.3-mg daily dose was sufficient to result in positive bone and lipid changes, without causing abnormal growth of the endometrium.[40] This study is encouraging but, at present, most evidence indicates the need to treat all forms of estrone with the same caution as any other type of estrogen. In general, the same health risks apply. Women with an intact uterus shouldn't take estrone without a progestogen (any natural or synthetic substance that produces some or all of the effects of progesterone). I also strongly recommend a qualified health-care provider's supervision, with yearly evaluation.

Esterified estrogen is available in 0.3-mg, 0.625-mg, 1.25-mg, and 2.5-mg tablets as Estratab or Menest.

Esterified Estrogens and Methyltestosterone

This combination of esterified estrogens and methyltestosterone offers the benefits of both estrogen and testosterone in one tablet. (Keep in mind that women with an intact uterus should always take a progestogen along with any type of estrogen. This combination doesn't provide any synthetic or natural progesterone.)

The combination is available as Estratest tablets (1.25 mg of esterified estrogens and 2.5 mg of methyl-

testosterone) and Estratest H.S. tablets (0.625 mg of esterified estrogens and 1.25 mg of methyltestosterone).

Estropipate Tablets

Estropipate tablets were formerly known as piperazine
estrone sulfate. For this preparation, estrone is synthesized from soybeans or wild yams and is bio-identical to
human estrone. The purified estrone is then made more
soluble as a sulfate and stabilized with a molecule called
piperazine. Estropipate tablets are available as Ogen or
Ortho-Est in 0.75-mg, 1.5-mg, or 3 mg-tablets. These
tablets come in dosages of 0.625 mg, 1.25 mg, or 2.5 mg.

Estriol

Estriol has gained popularity as a "new estrogen" in recent years. Actually, its use is not new—it has been used
in Europe for years. It is most popular and most effective
in the treatment of thinning vaginal tissue (vaginal atrophy) and urinary symptoms. Estriol is actually a metabolite (a breakdown product of estradiol and estrone that is
excreted from the body) and is not produced by the
ovaries and adrenal glands. It is one of about 40 metabolites of estradiol and estrone; and the one that is receiving
a lot of attention as a useful treatment for menopause.

The estrogenic action of estriol is much weaker than
that of estradiol and estrone. (Estriol is about one-tenth
as potent as estradiol.)[41] This means it may have less of a

stimulating effect on cancers. As estriol has such a weak estrogenic influence, oral doses of estriol are effective for the treatment of vaginal atrophy and urinary symptoms at a dose small enough to avoid abnormal changes in the uterine lining.[42]

While some authors say estriol is safer, let's not go overboard. It does have an estrogenic effect, so proper dosing is still important. Overall, estriol carries the same precautions and risk profile as any other hormone-replacement therapy. Perhaps in time, estriol will scientifically be proven safer. Such evidence does not currently exist, however. As always, if you have an intact uterus, you should take a progestogen with any type of estrogen—even estriol.

For some women, estriol is also able to improve symptoms of hot flashes and sweating.[43] However, most women need some estradiol added to their estriol to get this benefit.

Oral-Micronized Estriol   Oral estriol decreases vaginal dryness and has a noticeably beneficial effect on the vaginal lining.[44] Preliminary laboratory research demonstrated that estriol had an antioxidant effect on LDL ("bad") cholesterol, but its effect was less potent than that of estradiol.[45] So, estriol could possibly decrease the risk of heart disease in postmenopausal women, though more research is needed.

The ability of estriol to prevent osteoporosis is still open to debate. One study found that about half of post-menopausal women treated with calcium and estriol had significant improvement in bone density.[46] But it might have been the calcium and not the estriol that caused the improvements. A more recent study found that estriol was unable to maintain bone mass or prevent osteoporosis.[47]

Oral-micronized estriol is available through a compounding pharmacist. Estriol capsules are dispensed in doses ranging from 2 to 5 mg, or occasionally higher. Doses above 5 mg may cause nausea in some women. If 2 to 5 mg of estriol is not effective, consider adding a little estradiol, or using estrogen-mimetic herbs, phytoestrogens, or homeopathic treatments.

Estriol Vaginal Cream

As mentioned above, estriol is most popular for its ability to treat vaginal dryness and thinning, and urinary symptoms such as incontinence and urinary tract infections. Estriol vaginal cream is one of the best treatments for these conditions.[48–53] It may also be helpful to restore the vagina's normal pH, and thus help prevent vaginal infections.[54, 55]

> Estriol is most popular for its ability to treat vaginal dryness and thinning, and urinary symptoms such as incontinence and urinary tract infections.

The typical dose is an initial 3.5 mg of estriol cream daily for a week or two. Then, after the symptoms are somewhat relieved, you can switch to a much lower dosage of 0.03 to 0.05 mg used 1 to 7 days per week, as needed. Estriol vaginal creams are available through compounding pharmacists.

Tri-Estrogen and Bi-Estrogen Compounds

Estriol is increasingly being used as part of a triple estrogen, or tri-estrogen, compound. Licensed physicians prescribe tri-estrogens and bi-estrogens, which are dispensed by compounding pharmacists. The three estrogens are formulated in various ways. A common formula has 80% estriol, 10% estrone, and 10% estradiol. The advantage is that these formulas allow a woman to use a much lower dosage of estradiol, the most powerful type of estrogen, while still getting enough of the weaker estrogens to relieve vaginal dryness and other symptoms. Tri-estrogen compounds also seem to be effective against hot flashes and heart disease.[56-59] The usual dose is 2.5 mg of tri-estrogen a day, but can range from 1.25 to 5.0 mg a day.

As oral estradiol is converted to estrone in the digestive system, some compounds contain no estrone. These bi-estrogen compounds are 80 to 90% estriol and 10 to 20% estradiol. Estrone levels are already higher than estradiol levels in most postmenopausal women, so a bi-estrogen compound may be more beneficial in maintaining estradiol levels, while keeping estrone levels from climbing higher. A bi-estrogen dose ranges from 1.25 to 5.0 mg per day.

Risks of Taking Estrogen

The most well known risk associated with estrogen replacement is that, if taken alone, it greatly increases the risk for uterine cancer. Before menopause, estrogen and progesterone work together to orchestrate the menstrual cycle. Without enough progesterone, the uterine lining expands but doesn't shed in a monthly period. Taking estrogen alone can lead to a dangerous buildup of tissue in the uterine lining.

For this reason, whenever estrogen is prescribed for a postmenopausal woman with an intact uterus, progesterone or a synthetic equivalent should also be prescribed. Adding progesterone to estrogen therapy virtually eliminates any added risk for uterine cancer.

Taking estrogen also seems to increase the risk for at least certain types of breast cancer, but the evidence isn't as clear as with the endometrial cancer risk. A major women's health study recently found evidence that taking estrogen increased the risk for only certain types of breast cancer. At present, women who have ever had breast cancer are advised by most physicians not to take estrogen.

About 10% of women who take supplemental estrogen experience side effects. The most frequent are bloating (fluid retention), nausea, breast tenderness, migraines, and headaches.[60] The stronger synthetic estrogens cause more side effects than bio-identical estrogens.

Estrogen-replacement therapy also increases the risk for gallbladder disease.[61, 62] Even though higher dosages of estrogen (as in birth control pills) can cause the formation of dangerous blood clots in the blood vessels, the lower dosages used for postmenopausal women don't seem to do this.[63, 64] But women taking estrogen-replacement therapy should probably still be careful about taking any other medication or nutritional supplement that could promote blood clotting. For example, taking calcium without adequate magnesium may do this, so some clinicians believe it is best to take one part magnesium for every two parts calcium while on estrogen replacement.[65]

Other possible side effects and risks include fluid retention with weight gain, abnormal uterine bleeding, increased vaginal secretions, and breast tenderness and swelling. There can also be a drop in testosterone, resulting in decreased libido, depression, and other symptoms of low testosterone. Though any type of estrogen in too high a dose can cause these side effects, women are reporting fewer symptoms on the lower doses of bio-identical estrogens. This is especially true when these natural estrogens are balanced with progesterone and testosterone.

A patient recently said to me, "Oh yeah, I know all the risks, but with my family history for osteoporosis, it's better I take the estrogen." Taking estrogen is indeed a valid choice, but "knowing the risks" is not enough. And remember, progesterone and testosterone also help prevent osteoporosis. Any woman taking any form of estrogen should be closely monitored by her health-care professional. Any case of persistent or recurring vaginal bleeding must be investigated, with diagnostic testing to make sure there is no risk of cancer. All forms of estrogen carry increased risk of endometrial cancer. The risk may be lower with some forms of estrogen, but there is still a risk. Routine monitoring should also include breast evaluation.

PROGESTERONE-REPLACEMENT THERAPY

Progesterone was added to estrogen-replacement therapy when it became clear that, taken alone, estrogen could cause endometrial cancer. As mentioned earlier, at first, the only way to take progesterone was in either a skin cream or an injection, because it would be destroyed in the digestive tract if taken orally. But then scientists developed the progestins, chemicals similar to your body's natural progesterone—but not quite identical to it. Perhaps because they're slightly different from your body's own progesterone, progestins cause uncomfortable side effects in many women. But the convenience of taking them in a pill made them very popular in spite of their side effects.

Today, several different types of progesterone and progestin are used to relieve menopausal imbalances. Bio-identical progesterone is available in skin creams, gels, and pills. Synthetic forms of progesterone fall into two classes: some are derived from progesterone, while others are made from testosterone. It's important to know which kind you're taking, since the testosterone-derived progestins may also tend to raise your levels of testosterone.

Medroxyprogesterone acetate (Depo-Provera Provera, Cycrin), megestrol acetate (Megace), cyproterone acetate, and various forms of 17-hydroxyprogesterone are all derived from progesterone.[66-69] Testosterone-derived progestins include norethisterone acetate, norethindrone (Micronor, Norlutin, Nor-QD), norethynodrel, norgestrel (Ovrette), norgestinate ethynodiol diacetate, levonorgestrel, desogestrel, and gestodene (compounded

under various trade names).[70–73] Of these, medroxyprogesterone acetate (Depo-Provera, Provera, Cycrin) and
norethindrone acetate (Aygestin, Norlutate) are the most
common prescriptions for postmenopausal women. These
will be discussed below.

There are several factors to consider before starting
on any progesterone therapy. The dosage should be
based on reviewing your medical and family history, taking into account your present
health and weight. Women
with diabetes and/or those
who are overweight and at
high risk for diabetes should
use any form of progesterone
cautiously, including natural
progesterone. Since stress can
deplete progesterone, women
who are basically healthy, but
under a lot of stress, may
need more natural proges-
terone. Your dosage should be based on your laboratory
test results, your symptoms, and your doctor's recommendation. You can evaluate your symptoms with the
Menopause Types Questionnaire (see chapter 3).

Women with diabetes and/or those who are over-weight and at high risk for diabetes should use any form of pro-gesterone cautiously, in-cluding natural progesterone.

Natural Progesterone

The adrenal glands and the ovaries naturally produce
progesterone. As discussed earlier, the bio-identical
progesterone used in many hormone-replacement prod-

ucts is produced from wild yam, soybeans, or other plants. This progesterone is commonly referred to as natural progesterone. Even though it is synthesized from plant sources, it is chemically identical to your body's own progesterone. Natural progesterone will produce fewer side effects than synthetic progestogens.

Various forms of natural (bio-identical) progesterone are available, including oral micronized, topical creams, vaginal gels, and progesterone-releasing intrauterine devises.

Oral-Micronized Progesterone

Only about 10% of oral-micronized progesterone is absorbed into the bloodstream.[74] Oral doses usually need to be much higher than the doses used in skin creams. The absorption rate improves as you grow older, which is one reason that older women need lower dosages.[75] (Other reasons are that older women have decreased rates of metabolism and digestive function.)

Within 2 to 6 hours after taking micronized progesterone by mouth, you'll have higher levels of progesterone and its metabolites throughout your body.[76, 77] There is tremendous variability in the amount of progesterone absorbed after taking oral-micronized progesterone. This variability appears to be as much as 40 times different from woman to woman.[78, 79] Some women do very well on 25 mg of micronized progesterone, while others need much higher doses to absorb a similar amount.

Since there is no way to know in advance how well you'll absorb progesterone, you should always check your progesterone level every six months when taking oral-micronized progesterone. Likewise, given the highly variable rate of absorption and thereby highly variable effects, you should only use this therapy under the supervision of a physician.

Overall, oral progesterone is safe. To date, no significant detrimental changes in hormones or other laboratory tests have been proven.[80] No side effects concerning blood clotting or blood pressure have been reported, as they have been with synthetic progestogens.[81]

But taking too much progesterone isn't good for you. As with any hormone, levels above the normal range are dangerous. High progesterone levels can affect blood sugar, while the metabolites of even normal dosages can make you feel depressed. (See Risks of Taking Progesterone or Progestins to follow.)

Oral-micronized progesterone is suitable for hormonal-replacement therapy in any menopause type that involves a progesterone deficiency. Taking oral-micronized progesterone with food helps the body to absorb it, making it about twice as effective than if you take it on its own.[82] Oral-micronized progesterone is available as Prometrium (100-mg capsules) or in customized dosages from a compounding pharmacist. Doses range from 25 to 400 mg/day, though the required dose may be higher for some women.

Topical Progesterone Cream   In the 1970s, progesterone creams were recommended by physicians for the treatment of thinning of the tissues of the vulva, and for excessive itching.[83, 84] Researchers noticed that women using progesterone creams developed higher blood levels of progesterone, but the effect of progesterone therapy on the whole body wasn't widely recognized until the 1980s.[85, 86]

Physicians, pharmacists, and researchers now recognize that transdermal creams and gels are effective ways to raise your body's levels of progesterone.[87]

Topical progesterone creams are absorbed more effectively than oral progesterone is, so it's sometimes better to use progesterone in a skin cream or gel than in a pill. You need only 10% of the oral dose to get the same effect. Instead of taking 100 to 400 mg per day in a pill, the progesterone creams require only 10 to 40 mg per day.

Early research reported that progesterone is much more readily absorbed when applied on the breast than when applied on other tissues.[88] However, I have noted a number of cases in which breast pain and engorgement result from applying progesterone on the breast. A number of pharmacists and physicians have reported similar findings, even when the progesterone is applied on the arms. The current recommendation is to apply progesterone cream on the abdomen.

Many forms of progesterone creams are available. Unfortunately, many of them are marketed as "wild yam creams"—as if to imply that they are wild yam extracts. As noted previously, the body cannot turn the chemicals in wild yam into progesterone. Only a laboratory can make progesterone out of wild yam (or soybeans, for that matter). For any progesterone cream to be effective, it must have pharmacy-grade progesterone in the cream, and not just an extract of wild yam. Many "wild yam" creams do actually contain progesterone; if they do, the amount should be listed on the label. You need to know exactly how much to use, so choose a product that gives clear information about the amount of progesterone it contains. Compounding pharmacists are an excellent source for progesterone creams that supply a specific and consistent amount of progesterone per dose. A dose of 10 to 40 mg of cream should be taken in the morning, as discussed in the section Once-a-Day Dosing earlier in this chapter.

Vaginal Progesterone Gel   A vaginal gel is another effective method of administering natural progesterone. There are several advantages to using a gel. It is very well absorbed by the body, and you don't need to take very much to have a significantly good effect. As with oral and topical methods of treatment, micronized progesterone delivered via the vagina protects against endometrial cancer.[89] A study showed that a vaginal dose of 90 mg of progesterone per day was as effective as 300 mg per day of micronized progesterone taken orally.[90, 91] Dosages as low as 45 mg every other day seem to be effective enough to protect against endometrial cancer.[92]

This reflects another advantage of the vaginal gel: like skin creams or patches, it delivers the progesterone into the blood without going through the liver. Even doses as low as 45 mg of progesterone administered vaginally every other day can eliminate the proliferative effects of estrogen treatment in postmenopausal women. The benefit of vaginal progesterone gel is that it can provide protection to the endometrium without causing such a pronounced systemic effect.[93] Vaginal progesterone gel is available as Crinonein, an 8% gel containing 90 mg of micronized progesterone per application, or a 4% gel containing 45 mg of micronized progesterone per application.

Progesterone-Releasing Intrauterine Device   You may think of intrauterine devices (IUDs) as a form of birth control, but they can also be used to deliver natural progesterone to postmenopausal women. The use of IUDs decreased dramatically in the 1970s after the Dalkin shield IUD was found to increase the risk for pelvic inflammatory disease (PID) and other serious problems.[94] Since then, safer IUDs have been developed and introduced on the market. Progestasert is one of the two progesterone-releasing IUDs currently approved for use in the United States, the other being Paragard, a copper "T" IUD.[95, 96]

> You may think of intrauterine devices (IUDs) as a form of birth control, but they can also be used to deliver natural progesterone to postmenopausal women.

Women using progesterone-releasing IUDs may have a lower risk of developing PID than do users of other kinds of IUDs.[97] The progesterone released from the IUD acts locally on the endometrium to uniformly suppress endometrial proliferation while barely penetrating to the deeper portions of the endometrium.[98–100] This localized effect of progesterone can decrease the risk of uterine cancer.

Research found that the use of the progesterone-releasing IUD resulted in significant relief of menorrhagia (excessive uterine bleeding), and could be a valuable treatment for this condition.[101] Both the amount and duration of menstrual blood loss is decreased, making the device a valid option for women who must avoid systemic progesterone, but have menorrhagia and risk of anemia.[102, 103]

Synthetic Progesterone

As noted, a synthetic progesterone may be synthesized from progesterone or from testosterone. Of the many synthetic progestogens available, norethindrone acetate and medroxyprogesterone acetate are two examples of hormones commonly used in menopause. With the advances made in our understanding of natural progesterone over the last few decades, an increasing number of women are choosing natural progesterone over synthetic progestogens. However, these hormones are still widely used by some physicians.

Norethindrone Acetate (Aygestin, Micronor)   Norethindrone acetate (NETA) is a synthetic form of progesterone that is synthesized from testosterone. Like other progestins, NETA has been shown to be effective in preventing endometrial cancer in women taking estrogen-replacement therapy.[104] The minimum effective dosage of norethindrone acetate given cyclically appears to be 2.5 mg, or 1 mg per day in continuous NETA therapy.[105–108]

NETA also has been shown to be beneficial to bone and heart health. The addition of NETA to estrogen treatment produces a significant increase in bone mineral density, resulting in a decreased incidence of osteoporosis.[109] Though NETA diminishes some of estrogen's helpful effects on blood lipids, it appears to improve others.[110]

Norethindrone acetate is available as Aygestin and Micronor. The cyclical dose is about 2.5 mg/day for days 16 through 25. The continuous dose is 1 mg/day. It is also available in transdermal patches in combination with estradiol, as noted earlier.

Medroxyprogesterone Acetate (Depo-Provera, Provera, Cycrin)   Medroxyprogesterone acetate (MPA) is a synthetic derived from progesterone. As with other progestins, MPA has been shown to be effective at reducing the risk of endometrial cancer.[111, 112] MPA will reduce hot flashes in up to 90% of women and can be used as an alternative to estrogen therapy in menopausal women when estrogen use is undesirable.[113–116] MPA also can decrease the rate of bone loss, and may be an appropriate therapy for the prevention and treatment of osteoporosis.[117, 118]

High doses of MPA have been used in the treatment of some forms of breast cancer.[119–121] When given with estrogen, MPA is less likely to cause a drop in HDL ("good") cholesterol than norethindrone acetate or levonorgestrel are.[122, 123] This is because nonandrogenic progestogens like MPA do not negate the beneficial effects of long-term estrogen therapy on the blood lipids of postmenopausal women.[124]

Research has observed these same effects—endometrial protection, reduction of hot flashes, osteoporosis protection, and breast cancer treatment—with oral-micronized progesterone and with other 17-hydroxyprogesterone-derived progestogens. These effects are most likely due to the basic activity of progesterone, which is still present in its synthetic forms. However, you may recall from chapter 10 that MPA has antiestrogenic, antiandrogenic, and antiprogestogenic properties. Natural progesterones might be a much better choice.

MPA is available as Provera and Cycrin in 2.5-mg, 5-mg, or 10-mg tablets. It is also available in various injections such as Depo-Provera, or in transdermal patches in combination with estradiol, as noted earlier.

Risks of Taking Progesterone or Progestins

The greatest risk involved in taking progesterone, or any progestogen, is that you'll develop an imbalance in your progesterone-to-estrogen ratio. (See chapter 5 for a discussion of the P:E ratio, and its importance.) Insulin resistance is one of the chief concerns. Too much progesterone can also decrease the muscle tone of the urinary system, and result in urinary stress incontinence.[125]

TESTOSTERONE-REPLACEMENT THERAPY

Though the use of testosterone in women of menopausal age was overlooked for many years, testosterone is now considered an important hormone for menopausal women.[126-130] In low-testosterone menopause types, the use of testosterone can restore sex drive (libido) and other signs of healthy sexuality such as sexual desire, fantasies, satisfaction, and ability to achieve orgasm.[131-136] Testosterone-replacement therapy appears to be especially beneficial to women who have had a hysterectomy, either with or without removal of the ovaries.

✍ WATCHING YOUR P:E RATIO

If you take supplemental estrogen or progesterone, you need to make sure that your progesterone-to-estrogen (P:E) ratio remains in balance. As we saw in chapter 5, a high P:E ratio can increase your risk for insulin resistance, and all of its accompanying health risks.

Feelings of depression, brought on by low testosterone, can be relieved with proper testosterone-replacement therapy. The effect is not the same as with antidepressant medications. There is less of the "high" or euphoria that gives a false sense of "everything is going to be all right," that is sometimes associated with antidepressant medications. Instead, women report increased confidence and diminished insecurity when a testosterone deficiency is corrected.

It is worth noting that you should receive prompt medical evaluation to exclude any treatable medical cause if you are suffering from a severe mood disorder. Although feelings of depression or despair can be related to menopause, it is important to be sure that there is not a more specific mood disorder at play.

If your testosterone level gets too high, you may have a permanent increase in facial and body hair that persists even after your testosterone level returns to normal. If you take testosterone, be very careful not to take too much. Check your testosterone level every six months until it stabilizes, then follow up with yearly tests. Another reason to monitor your testosterone level and make sure it doesn't get too high is to protect against insulin resistance.

> In low-testosterone menopause types, the use of testosterone can restore sex drive (libido) and other signs of healthy sexuality.

The effect of testosterone therapy on cardiovascular health is mixed. Though androgens such as testosterone lower total cholesterol and LDL ("bad") cholesterol levels, they also lower the HDL ("good") cholesterol level, and can actually promote atherosclerosis (thickening and hardening of the arteries).[137, 138] When testosterone is given with estrogen, however, the opposite effect is created and atherosclerosis decreases.[139, 140] Testosterone therapy also can increase bone density, thus decreasing the risk of osteoporosis.[141, 142]

When testosterone is taken orally, the liver rapidly breaks it down. Topical testosterone bypasses the liver, and has been effective for a number of women. Modifying the testosterone into methyltestosterone, a synthetic hormone, protects it against rapid breakdown by the liver, as noted earlier. However, methyltestosterone has been linked to increased incidence of liver cancer when taken in large doses; therefore, avoid large doses if you choose methyltestosterone.

As with all forms of hormone-replacement therapy, testosterone replacement should be based on a review of your medical and family history, consideration of your present health and weight, and an examination of both your laboratory test results and your symptoms. The most common forms of testosterone used by women of menopausal age are natural testosterone (usually administered topically) and methyltestosterone (used topically or orally).

Natural Testosterone

Natural (bio-identical) testosterone is least effective when taken orally. It is commonly used in the form of a topical gel or cream. A typical dose is 2.5 to 5 mg/day. Caution: In some women, topical testosterone can increase hair growth on the site where it is applied. If you use topical testosterone, follow the directions on the packet as to where to apply it.

Methyltestosterone

Methyltestosterone can be taken orally or topically, and is one of the most commonly used forms of testosterone for postmenopausal women. As I explained above, methyltestosterone can be taken orally because the liver does not break it down as readily as natural testosterone. However, it has been linked to increased incidence of liver cancer when taken in large doses. I have not seen liver problems linked to the usual dose taken by women. The typical dose ranges from 1.25 to 5 mg/day.

HORMONAL PRECURSORS

Before coming to a final decision on the use of hormones to manage your menopause, it is a good idea to first take a look at hormonal precursors.

⚜ HOW SAFE IS METHYLTESTOSTERONE?[143–146]

A typical dose of methyltestosterone for women is 1.25 to 5 mg a day, but keep in mind that any hormone in excess is dangerous.

In the late 1970s, medical journals reported an increased incidence of liver disease and liver cancer in transsexual females taking 150 mg of methyltestosterone a day (30 to 120 times the typical dose).

Recently, a medical journal reported that a study of 641 menopausal women taking 1.25 to 2.5 mg of methyltestosterone a day showed no liver disease or liver cancer. They concluded that therapy which included methyltestosterone was found to be safe in regard to liver health.

DHEA is a precursor of both estrogen and testosterone, so it is no surprise that some of the reported benefits of taking DHEA sound like the effects of taking estrogen and testosterone. These benefits include an increased libido, decreased vaginal dryness, decreased shrinking of breasts, improved memory, increased energy, reduced body fat, and improved skin tone. If these benefits match those of taking testosterone and estrogen, it is because in some women estrogen and testosterone levels increase after taking DHEA supplements. However, this effect does not take place in all women.

There is no guarantee that taking DHEA will result in increased testosterone or estrogen. Yes, it does work for some women. And I do encourage the use of DHEA as a precursor if your saliva hormone test reveals that your DHEA level is low. But if your DHEA level is already adequate, or if trying DHEA does not cause an increase in estrogen and testosterone, then I discourage the use of DHEA as a precursor of these hormones. If you take DHEA, it is always a good idea to monitor your estrogen and testosterone levels.

Androstenedione is also a precursor of testosterone and estrogens. Androstenedione appears to be more readily converted into estrogens and testosterone than DHEA does, so we will probably see more attention given to this precursor. However, the same truth applies to androstenedione and DHEA: There is no guarantee that the body will make estrogen and testosterone out of them. As with DHEA, it is wise to monitor estrogen and testosterone levels when taking androstenedione.

Though we talk about progesterone as a hormone in its own right, it is a hormone that also acts as a precursor for estrogen and testosterone—which is why we sometimes hear exaggerated claims about what progesterone can do. In some women, progesterone is converted into testosterone and estrogen, so the effects can extend beyond those normally seen with progesterone replacement. But again, it does not always work this way. Many women taking progesterone experience no improvement, or even a worsening, of their symptoms. When taking progesterone, in any form, monitor your estrogen, testosterone, and progesterone levels. The same holds true for supplementation with pregnenolone, which is a precursor to progesterone.

Your personal hormone replacement should always be based upon both your lab results and your symptoms, which are evaluated with the Menopause Type Questionnaire.

Each of these precursors has effects of its own, even if they are not converted to estrogen, testosterone, or progesterone. They are involved in maintaining a healthy immune system, building bones, helping the body to manage stress, and preserving function of the brain and nerves. Therefore, checking their levels periodically and keeping them within normal range is a healthy practice.

IS HORMONE-REPLACEMENT THERAPY RIGHT FOR YOU?

Hormone-replacement therapy involves supplementing estrogen, progesterone, and testosterone with the goal of restoring normal function and balance. Though some women will not require hormone replacement because they are able to maintain proper levels of these hormones, for other women, hormone-replacement therapy is a valid option. Your personal hormone replacement should always be based upon both your lab results and your symptoms, which are evaluated with the Menopause

Type Questionnaire in chapter 3. Determine the potential for increased risks and side effects by also taking into account your personal medical history and the medical history of your mother and blood relatives.

Remember that, if chosen, hormone-replacement therapy will always be part of your complete health program. Adequate rest and exercise, a healthful diet with good supplements, herbs, glandulars, and homeopathy are all important components in the restoration and maintenance of your optimal health based on your menopause type.

Conclusion

The Future of Menopause: How to Prepare

In an ideal menopause, the adrenal glands are able to take over some of the hormone-producing function of the ovaries, so that estrogen, progesterone, and testosterone remain at healthy levels, even after you have stopped menstruating. With a healthy menopause, you go through a phase of adjustment during which you may have a few symptoms, if any, but they do not cause debilitating discomfort, and you do not develop any long-term health problems.

How can you prepare ahead of time, so that you are more likely to have an ideal menopause? There are several lifestyle choices that make having a healthy menopause much more probable. You can optimize your health by eating well, exercising, and reducing your stress level.

If you have premenstrual syndrome (PMS), you should use diet, herbs, and other remedies (such as acupuncture and homeopathy) to balance your hormones before you go into menopause. Women with a history of PMS tend to have a more difficult menopause. One study found that women who suffered from PMS had more psychological and physical symptoms during perimenopause.[1] PMS can be caused by many factors, including hormonal imbalances and the need for specific fatty acids, vitamins, or minerals.

While balancing your hormones so that you no longer have PMS, you can begin to take care of your adrenal glands. An ideal menopause can occur when the adrenal glands are able to increase production of androstenedione (the precursor to estrogen and testosterone) and maintain adequate production of progesterone.

One of the main ways you can support your adrenal glands is by making sure your diet is fully meeting your body's needs for nutrition. Every vitamin and mineral is required at some point in the production of steroid hormones and, therefore, in the maintenance of adrenal gland health. Vitamin C, pantothenic acid (B_5), and zinc are called "the adrenal gland vitamins," but, in fact, you need the whole range of vitamins and minerals in order for your adrenal glands to function optimally. Enzymes in the glands use these nutrients to produce the various hormones.

Women who frequently go on weight-loss diets are particularly at risk for adrenal insufficiency due to inadequate nutrition. The same goes for women who eat a lot of junk food and tend to snack rather than eat healthy, balanced meals. The simplest course of action is taking a multivitamin every day, but for overall health, eating a highly nutritious diet is crucial. Vitamin pills alone won't be able to compensate for the damage caused by eating junk food and drinking sodas all day. And no pill can give you the psychological satisfaction of eating healthful food.

The enzymes within the adrenal glands and ovaries that make the various hormones are very sensitive to drugs and toxins. Alcohol and tobacco can significantly decrease your body's ability to make certain hormones. People who have had toxic exposures and are chemically sensitive often develop severely decreased adrenal function. There are numerous cases in which women have gone into premature and overnight menopause after exposure to a toxin such as solvent or paint fumes. So, to have a healthy and timely menopause, avoid exposure to toxic solvents and chemicals by choosing less toxic cleaning agents and wearing protective gloves if you must use such a cleaning agent. Take every measure to prevent inhalation of solvents, as in paint fumes. Use very good ventilation. If you can smell it, you can inhale it—right into your body.

> Take every measure to prevent inhalation of solvents, as in paint fumes. Use very good ventilation. If you can smell it, you can inhale it—right into your body.

Sleep is also very important. The proper function of the adrenal glands and ovaries depends on the release of hormones that occurs while you sleep. Chronically depriving yourself of sleep will result in decreased production of adrenal and ovarian hormones. If there is so much to do that you are sacrificing sleep, then you need to make some lifestyle changes. If you have difficulty sleeping, seek natural help to regulate your sleep pattern; a natural solution may be as simple as using herbs to relax you before bedtime.

Other measures that increase overall health—a diet rich in whole foods, avoiding processed foods and additives, a moderate exercise program, relaxation techniques, and stress management—help your adrenal glands function well. The various herbs and glandular extracts listed in this book may be used as adrenal tonics as needed or as part of an adrenal gland enhancing program.

The adrenal glands are designed to respond to intermittent stress. But these days, many women are dealing with the double stress of raising a family and working full time, within the context of a rapidly changing world. This may be amplifying the "normal" level of stress to the point where chronic burnout sets in.

Women who have had severe crises or trauma are particularly at risk for adrenal fatigue. If you are going through a stressful time, it is doubly important to eat properly, take vitamins, and get enough sleep and relaxation. Exercise can be very useful for discharging tension, and relaxation techniques such as yoga, prayer, and meditation can deeply relax the body and mind.

By taking good care of yourself before menopause, you maximize your chances of having a healthy transition.

CHAPTER FIFTEEN

THE NEED FOR A STANDARD
OF PRACTICE

There is not yet a standard of practice for doctors to measure hormone levels before giving women hormones for
menopausal symptoms. The phrase "standard of practice"
is actually a medical/legal term that means that certain
tests or therapies are considered standard in the practice of
medicine. If those standards are not followed, it may be
considered substandard medicine. For instance, it is a standard of practice to routinely test thyroid function before
any patient is placed on thyroid medication, and to routinely test for thyroid function thereafter, especially when
the patient is hospitalized or has significant medical problems. No patient on thyroid medication would be denied
routine monitoring—the risks are too great. Likewise, no
man over forty with complaints suggesting prostate problems would be denied a prostate test (PSA)—again, because the risks are too great. But menopausal women are
regularly given hormones without prior hormone testing.

Standard of practice also means that medical services are made available and covered by routine medical
insurance. I was appalled recently when an insurance
company explicitly stated they would pay for any medication "except progesterone." No doubt they were reacting
to the overzealous use of progesterone, but requiring the
doctor to test the woman before ordering is a more hu-
mane solution than a blanket policy that denies coverage
of this hormone to all women.

The standard of care for women should include routine assessment of hormones as needed and insurance

coverage for hormones if they are necessary. Anything less is unacceptable.

THE FUTURE OF MENOPAUSE TREATMENT

From where we stand now, we can look at the way menopause was treated 20, 10, or even 5 years ago and wonder why it took so long to realize that progesterone and testosterone are also very important hormones for women. When I look at today's medical research—which is finally recognizing women's need for testosterone—I can't help but wonder why they didn't figure this out decades ago, especially because physiology books have always said the ovaries make testosterone. Likewise, it is unbelievable that decades have gone by with progesterone being for the most part ignored, even though we have known for years that it was more than a hormone to support pregnancy. But that's how medicine was practiced. The wheels of progress turned slowly and medical advances took place far from the public eye.

Today, the practice of medicine is no longer immune from public evaluation and scrutiny. Health-care consumers are no longer passive patients. The public is reading books and newsletters containing medical information and research analysis that, until recently, were only available to physicians. The delivery of health care can be, and has been, affected by public requests and demands for services. The strongest proof of this is the continued growth of complementary and alternative medicine.

In a recent survey, it was found that 62% of those surveyed had used alternative medicine.[2] Another survey found that two-thirds to three-fourths of physicians surveyed were at least moderately interested in using alternative therapies with their patients.[3] A survey of 60 nurses who work with cancer patients found that 63% believed alternative medicine could be useful in the treatment of cancer patients, and 32% would sometimes suggest alternative medicine to the patients.[4]

A recent issue of a pharmacist journal reported that pharmacists should initiate discussion with women of all ages to help prevent, recognize, and treat osteoporosis. It advised pharmacists to take a more active role in assessing calcium, vitamin D, caffeine, alcohol, and phosphate intakes, along with exercise, and presenting the risks and benefits of hormone-replacement therapy to women.[5]

The traditional model of practicing medicine and health care by the "medical school textbooks" is rapidly eroding. Doctors, nurses, pharmacists, and other health-care practitioners are more willing to embrace new ways of diagnosing and treating health conditions—including menopause. The oversights and mistakes that have taken place in recent years should serve to remind us to stay on guard for extreme and unbalanced approaches to working with menopause.

So what is the future of menopause treatment? The future is ripe with change. Previous works by other authors have opened our eyes to the importance of progesterone and testosterone. This book, and no doubt others, will guide us to restoring hormonal balance and harmony. But what follows after we come to center?

After reviewing ongoing research and analyzing the trends in hormone assessment, I can say with full confidence that we will be hearing a lot more about food and herbs for the treatment of menopause as ongoing research comes to completion. Conventional medicine will embrace these nonmedical choices. The many other adrenal hormones affected by menopause, such as androstenedione (which has been discussed in this book), will also receive increased attention, as will growth hormone and other pituitary hormones. Routine testing of hormones will become more readily available as technology advances. Normal hormonal patterns, particularly the circadian (24-hour) rhythm of hormones, will also be a focus of study. These circadian rhythms tell us so much more than mere hormone levels do; they reveal the proper function of the adrenal glands and ovaries at a precise and subtle level.

> As ongoing research comes to light, there will be a shorter time between discovery and allowing women to benefit from that discovery.

As ongoing research comes to light, there will be a shorter time between discovery and allowing women to benefit from that discovery. The public is becoming so interested in medical findings that many news shows and mainstream publications routinely include a section on health. As encouraging as this is, it is important to look at the big picture. The body is too complex to be "fixed" or "cured" by a single pill or a single hormone. As we are all unique individuals, there will be some remedies that work for some people, but not for others. We need to remember that there are many types of menopause and that the future of menopause must involve new ways of helping you, the woman of menopause age, to understand and manage your unique menopause type.

Estrogen

Natural Estrogens and Estrogen Metabolites

Two estrogens are naturally created in the steroidogenic pathway of the body, estradiol and estrone. These two estrogens are further changed (metabolized) by the liver and other tissues of the body into about 40 metabolic products called metabolites.[1] These metabolites include estriol and epiestriols. Though estriol is actually a by-product of metabolism, it has been used as part of estrogen-replacement therapy because it is much weaker than estradiol and estrone, yet has enough of an estrogenic effect to give some relief to women with symptoms of low estrogen.

Another group of estrogen metabolites is the catechol estrogens. The catechol estrogens are formed from estradiol and estrone and have a chemical structure that is part estrogen and part *catecholamine*.[2] Catecholamines are molecules that appear to influence the release of hormones from the pituitary gland and hypothalamus.[3] Research has associated the catechol estrogen 4-hydroxyestradiol with increased uterine and breast cancer, and the catechol 2-hydroxyestradiol with anticancer properties, a decreased risk of heart disease, decreased inflammation, and other beneficial actions discussed below.[4, 5] In fact, 2-hydroxyestradiol has even been called the "good" estrogen.[6]

When thinking about estrogens, it is important to remember that even though there are only two estrogens produced by the ovaries and adrenal glands, some metabolites are just as important—if not more so. After reviewing estradiol and estrone, I will discuss estriol and 2-hydroxyestradiol in more detail.

ESTRADIOL

Estradiol is the most potent of the estrogens that occur naturally in a woman's body. During the reproductive years, it is the principal estrogen produced by the ovaries. Estradiol is the specific estrogen responsible for the normal monthly cycle. This hormone also affects bone, blood vessel, heart, brain, and skin health and function, as well as many other tissues and organs. When acting upon the tissues, organs, and bones of your body, estradiol is 12 times stronger than estrone and 80 times stronger than estriol.[7] Estradiol is the estrogen to which all other estrogen activity is compared.

Estradiol is responsible for your growth and development as a woman. It develops the structure of your reproductive organs and maintains their function. It increases the amount of fat in subcutaneous tissues, particularly breasts, buttocks, and thighs, and increases hipbone formation resulting in the characteristic female skeletal development.

By the time you reach menopausal age, estradiol has been occurring naturally in your body for decades. As noted earlier, estradiol is produced in the steroidogenic pathway from either testosterone or estrone. Normal blood levels before menopause are from 40 to 350 pg (picograms)/ml, but drop to about 13 pg/ml in menopause.[8] Before menopause, the predominant producer of estradiol is the ovaries, but the adrenal glands—and during pregnancy, the placenta—also manufacture it. Since the adrenal glands only contribute to about 4% of estradiol production before menopause, it is evident that the adrenal glands are not a significant source of primary estradiol production after menopause. The major source of estradiol in postmenopausal women is from the conversion of estrone to estradiol by an enzyme called aromatase, present in adipose (fat) cells throughout the body.

The Use of Oral Estradiol

The use of oral-micronized estradiol in estrogen-replacement therapy is increasing, though other forms of estrogen are still widely used. Oral estradiol (even micronized) will result in higher estrone levels than estradiol levels due to the metabolic conversion of estradiol by the intestinal mucosa and the liver.[9, 10] Due to its increased interaction with the liver, oral estradiol also reduces LDL ("bad") cholesterol concentrations and increases the HDL ("good") cholesterol.[11]

However, oral estrogens can cause increased production of sex-hormone-binding globulin, corticosteroid-binding globulin, and thyroxin-binding globulin.[12] High levels of these globulins can make it more difficult for the cells of the body to gain access to estrogens and testosterone, cortisol and progesterone, or thyroid hormones, respectively. The greatest concern is when there are borderline low levels of these hormones and they get "caught up" in the globulins so that less of the hormone is available to the cells of the body. As a salivary hormone test reveals how much of the hormone is bio-available, it is one of the best ways to assess hormone levels when you are taking estrogen supplements (see chapter 4). This test makes it possible to take advantage of oral estradiol's ability to improve the HDL/LDL ratio of cholesterol and at the same time manage its effect on binding globulins by monitoring hormonal levels.

The use of transdermal (across/through the skin) estradiol does not produce such a rise in the estrone level as its oral counterpart does, but it also does not demonstrate the same beneficial effect on HDL/LDL cholesterol.[13, 14] Transdermal estradiol applied daily reaches its peak within 4 to 6 hours after application, and reaches a steady state after 3 to 5 days of use.[15]

One of the concerns about oral estradiol replacement is that it may increase blood pressure because of its effect on the renin-angiotensin system, which controls blood pressure.[16, 17] But some data suggest natural estrogens have less of an effect on the renin-angiotensin system than do conjugated and synthetic estrogens.[18] Additionally, transdermal gels or patches do not affect the renin-angiotensin system.[19] Of course, you should monitor your blood pressure, but you need not avoid estrogen-replacement therapy now that transdermal and natural micronized estradiol preparations are available.

ESTRONE

Before menopause, estradiol levels are higher than estrone levels. In the postmenopausal woman, the reverse is true—estrone levels are higher than estradiol levels. The primary cause is decreased estradiol production by the ovaries, but other factors are involved, as well. With adrenal recruitment, there is increased production of the androgen androstenedione by the adrenal glands. This androstenedione is converted to estrone by an aromatase enzyme in fat cells of the body. In postmenopausal women, 95% of androstenedione is produced by the adrenal glands, while the ovaries produce only 5%.[20] It should be evident now that healthy adrenal glands are crucial during menopause.

Recall that in the steroidogenic pathway (see Appendix E), the arrows between estradiol and estrone go both ways, signifying that estrone can be converted to estradiol and estradiol converted to estrone. This conversion leans more heavily toward estrone, with 15% of estradiol being converted to estrone but only 5% of estrone being converted to estradiol.[21] The conversion of estradiol to estrone takes place in the liver and other tissues. Some of the estrone is converted back to estradiol by the aromatase enzymes in fat tissue, but with less estradiol being made by the ovaries, estrone levels still dominate in the menopausal woman. Since the aromatase enzyme is present in fat tissue, there is increased conversion of androstenedione to estrone with increased body fat. This resulting increase in estrogen levels gives the benefits that come with adequate estrogen levels during menopause. A higher risk of certain cancers also accompanies these increased estrogen levels, however. I discuss a way to decrease these risks in the section on how to increase the good estrogen metabolites later in this appendix.

Although estrone is only about 8% as strong as estradiol, for many women it has enough estrogenic activity to actually prevent the occurrence of menopausal symptoms. When the body is functioning as it was designed to, menopause marks a transition from estradiol as the dominant estrogen to estrone as dominant. Estrone is not capable of maintaining fertility, however. Once the body switches from estradiol to estrone, the ability to carry a child has ended.

ESTRIOL

Estriol is one of the principal metabolites of estradiol and estrone, and is formed primarily in the liver. The liver is responsible for metabolizing and detoxifying many compounds in the body. By converting estradiol and estrone to estriol, the liver makes these molecules less active, which is important because too much estradiol and estrone can be toxic to the body. Since estriol is only 8% as potent as estradiol and only 14% as potent as estrone, it has a very weak effect on the tissues of the body. By binding to the estrogen receptors on cells throughout the body, it does not allow the stronger estradiol or estrone to bind. Since its effect on the cells is so weak and it blocks stronger estrogens from the cells, it can actually be considered to have both estrogenic and antiestrogenic properties. The estrogenic properties are estriol's natural effect, weak as it is, which decreases some of the symptoms of low estrogen. However, estriol is so weak compared to the stronger estrogens that it diminishes the estrogen response, resulting in a relatively antiestrogenic effect.[22]

The metabolic conversion of estradiol and estrone to estriol is accomplished through a process called hydroxylation, in which hydrogen and oxygen molecules create a new molecule with different properties. Epiestriols are isomers of estriol, which have the same composition but a slightly different arrangement of the atoms. The presence of estriol and epiestriols indicates the liver has the ability to properly metabolize and detoxify. Like most metabolites, estriol is excreted through the urine as well as through the bile. Decreased urinary excretion of estriol relative to estrone and estradiol excretion has been associated with increased risk of breast cancer.[23] In contrast to estradiol and estrone, which are considered to have cancer-promoting properties, estriol is not considered cancer causing. It may, in fact, have anticancer properties, likely due to its ability to bind to estrogen receptors and therefore prevent the more cancer-promoting estrogens from binding.[24, 25] In a study of postmenopausal women with endometrial cancer, their estradiol levels were higher while their estriol levels were lower as compared to women without endometrial cancer, suggesting that low estriol levels play a role in endometrial cancer.[26]

Estriol has become increasingly popular as a component in estrogen-replacement therapy because some research has associated low estriol levels with increased risk of breast and uterine cancer.[27–29] As noted, the current theory is that estriol decreases estradiol and estrone activity by competing with them for estrogen receptor sites, in effect, preventing estradiol and estrone from stimulating these sites.[30] This idea was first presented because, in some experiments on uterine growth, estriol was only weakly active, and partially inhibited the effects of estradiol.

Research has shown that estriol behaved as an estrogen with low potency not because of a failure to stimulate tissues as much as estradiol does, but because it failed to sustain the growth of cancer cells.[31] However, continuously high estriol levels are as active as estradiol and are less likely to have any significant protective action. This suggests that the protective function of estriol is seen only when estriol is in the normal range and that excessive estriol levels should be avoided.

Human studies indicate an excellent tolerance of oral estriol doses ranging from 10 to 200 micrograms per kilogram of body weight per day, which is the dosage used to correct the subnormal estriol levels that some authors have associated with elevated risk of breast cancer.[32] However, tissue of women receiving oral estriol has up to 90 times as much of a metabolite called 16-hydroxyestrone.[33] 16-hydroxyestrone is a metabolite of estriol, as well as other estrogens, and is associated with increased risk of breast and cervical cancers.[34–36] Fortunately, 16-hydroxyestrone production can be decreased by dietary changes and supplements, which are discussed at the end of this appendix.[37]

2-HYDROXYESTRADIOL AND 2-HYDROXYESTRONE

Another group of metabolites formed from estradiol and estrone are the catechol estrogens. Like estriol, these molecules are formed by hydroxylation, in which hydrogen and oxygen molecules create a new molecule with different properties. In fact, some of the many actions of estradiol may not be caused by estradiol itself, but may result from the action of estrogen metabolites including catechol estrogens.[38]

There are four catechol estrogens of concern: 2-hydroxyestradiol, 4-hydroxyestradiol, 2-hydroxyestrone, and 4-hydroxyestrone. Research suggests that the protective action of estrogens against atherosclerosis and osteoporosis may be due to the ability of catechol estrogens to inhibit inflammatory molecules called leukotrienes.[39]

Of the four catechol estrogens, the two metabolites 2-hydroxyestradiol and 2-hydroxyestrone have the most beneficial properties. These two catechols are created in the body by a process called 2-hydroxylation. One researcher reports that for every experiment in which 2-hydroxylation was increased, protection against cancer was achieved, and even decreased the growth of some existing cancers.[40]

Compared to estradiol, 2-hydroxyestradiol and 2-methoxyestradiol (which is made from 2-hydroxyestradiol) are much more potent in inhibiting abnormal growth of cardiac fibroblasts (CFs). These CFs are increased in postmenopausal women and are associated with the greater risk of hypertension and myocardial infarction that we see in women of this age group.[41] The ability of these metabolites to decrease the risk of high blood pressure and heart disease is enhanced by the concurrent use of progesterone, which is a perfect illustration of why a proper balance of hormones is crucial. It is important to note that estrone and estriol do not decrease abnormal growth of CFs and may be less effective in protecting postmenopausal women against cardiovascular disease.[42]

Another feature of 2-hydroxyestradiol and 2-hydroxyestrone is their antioxidant activity, which is actually better than vitamin E.[43] Their antioxidant activity decreases the free-radical damage (oxidation) to lipids in the blood such as LDL, as well as lipids on cell membranes.[44, 45] When lipids are oxidized, they become lipid peroxides. Because one of the mechanisms of coronary atherosclerosis and increased risk of heart disease is increased lipid peroxides, 2-hydroxyestrone and 2-hydroxyestrone decrease risk of heart disease.[46, 47] By decreasing lipid peroxides on cell membranes, they may play a role in decreasing cell degeneration and inflammation.

The estradiol metabolite 4-hydroxyestradiol does not have the beneficial properties of the other catechol estrogens, and is actually considered to play a role in the development of uterine and breast cancers.[48–50] Fortunately, since it is the elevated ratio of 4-hydroxyestradiol to 2-hydroxyestradiol that is implicated in the development of these cancers, increasing 2-hydroxyestradiol can decrease these risks. Increased 2-hydroxyestradiol and 2-hydroxyestrone also decreases the activity of 16-hydroxyestrone, thereby decreasing cancer risks.[51] So, the goal is to increase 2-hydroxyestradiol and 2-hydroxyestrone without increasing 4-hydroxyestradiol or 16-hydroxyestrone.

ESTROGENS AND XENOESTROGENS

The word "estrogen" is actually a generic term for any substance, whether it is natural or synthetic, that has a similar biological and physiological effect to the hormone estradiol. The word "estrogenic" is often used to describe the actions of a substance as being "estrogenlike." For example, some plastics and pesticides have estrogenic properties that interfere with normal estrogen function in the body. These estrogenlike plastics, pesticides, and similar chemicals are sometimes referred to as "xenoestrogens." The root word *xeno* means "different," which is a good description because these chemicals are so different from anything that occurs in nature that the body has a very difficult time breaking them down.

Xenoestrogens are just some of the many toxins that we are exposed to from our food and the environment. The general term used to describe these toxins is "xenobiotics" (meaning, different [for our] living organisms). So the proper approach to xenoestrogens is to recognize them more as toxins than as estrogens and assist the body in breaking down and eliminating these toxins—that is, doing whatever can be done to promote detoxification in the body.

Detoxification can be supported by lifestyle changes, such as decreasing alcohol intake, avoiding tobacco, eating a healthful diet, and maintaining proper bowel function.[52] Other measures such as herbs, enzymes, antioxidants and other nutrients, special fasts, and even saunas can be employed to promote detoxification. The book *Total Wellness*, by Dr. Joseph Pizzorno, is a very comprehensive resource for information on detoxification.

HOW ESTROGENS WORK

Estrogens work by crossing the cell membrane into the cell and attaching to estrogen receptors on the nucleus of the cell. Each type of estrogen has a different ability to attach itself (receptor affinity) and to stay attached to the receptor on the nucleus (nuclear retention). The stronger the receptor affinity and longer the nuclear retention time, the more potent the physiological action of the estrogen. Estradiol not only has a strong receptor affinity, but also increases the affinity of the receptor for estradiol.[53] In contrast, estrone and estriol may decrease estradiol binding by lowering the cell's affinity for estradiol. Estrone and estriol have only slightly lower receptor affinity than estradiol.

Estradiol varies significantly in its nuclear retention time. While estradiol has a nuclear retention time of 6 to 24 hours, estriol's is only 1 to 4 hours, with estrone higher than estriol, but still lower than estradiol.[54] This means that once estradiol attaches itself to a cell, it sticks to it longer and has a stronger influence than estriol does.

TABLE 5

Potency of Various Estrogen Preparations Relative to Estradiol

Estrogen Preparation and Relative Potency	
Estradiol	1.0
Estrone	0.083
Estriol	0.0125
Conjugated Estrogens	2.17
Ethinyl Estradiol	419.00
Piperazine Estrone Sulfate	0.8

The longer an estrogen occupies a receptor, the stronger its influence will be. Thus, the estrogenic potency of a substance is determined by the duration of its occupation of receptors.[55] Levels of a specific estrogen also can affect the duration of its influence on a cell. In fact, if estriol levels are in excess of normal nonpregnant levels for long periods of time, they can have the same effect on cells as estradiol does. Research has demonstrated that continuously high estriol is as active as estradiol and less likely to exert any significant protective action.[56] At normal physiological dosages, estradiol remains the most potent of the naturally occurring estrogens in the human body. However, conjugated estrogens (such as Premarin) and synthetic estrogens are more potent than estradiol. Table 5 lists substances commonly used in estrogen replacement, and their estrogenic potency relative to estradiol.[57, 58]

INCREASING THE GOOD ESTROGEN METABOLITES

It should be clear now that the many benefits of estrogen replacement come from proper metabolism of the estrogens, while the problems associated with estrogen replacement, such as increased cancer risk, are associated with improper metabolism of estrogens. The objective then is to direct the metabolism of estrogens so that there are increased amounts of the good estrogen metabolites.

The two estrogen metabolites 2-hydroxyestradiol and 2-hydroxyestrone have the most beneficial properties. These two catechols are created in the body by a process called 2-hydroxylation. This process can be enhanced by dietary intake of broccoli and other members of the cruciferous family, which contain a substance called indole-3-carbinol (I3C).[59, 60] When the process of 2-hydroxylation is increased by intake of I3C, both 2-hydroxyestradiol and 2-hydroxyestrone levels increase. This results in decreased cancer risk and can even decrease the growth rate of some existing cancers.[61]

As there is a limit to the amount of estrogen that can be in the body at any given time, when estrogens are encouraged to be metabolized into 2-hydroxyestradiol and 2-hydroxyestrone, there will be a decrease in other metabolites.[62] The ability of I3C to increase the process of 2-hydroxylation is so specific that it does not increase 16-hydroxyestrone.[63] In fact, in one study, after intake of about 3 mg of I3C for each pound of body weight, the levels of nearly all other estrogen metabolites were lower, including levels of estradiol, estrone, estriol, and 16-hydroxyestrone.[64]

Since estrogen levels are higher in obese women, there are concerns of increased risk for cancers. The benefits of I3C for obese women are similar to those for non-obese women. A study in which women took 400 mg of purified I3C for 2 months, found that I3C increased the process of 2-hydroxylation in obese women.[65] This response indicates reduced estrogen-dependent cancer risk.

The amounts of purified I3C used in various studies have ranged from 400 mg/day to about 3 mg per pound of body weight each day. When whole vegetables were used, the dose was 500 grams a day of broccoli—a pretty hefty dose of about a pound a day![66]

Another way to get the benefits of I3C is to use diindolylmethane (DIM). DIM is a metabolite of I3C and also has the ability to increase good estrogen metabolites by stimulating 2-hydroxylation. I3C and DIM are indicated for all menopause types.

Progesterone

Progestogen (or progestin) is the name for the group of substances that have actions similar to the progesterone that naturally occurs in the body. In addition to progesterone, the other naturally occurring progestogen is 17-hydroxyprogesterone, which is explained in chapter 5. The 17-hydroxyprogesterone molecule is considered to have no progesteronelike activity. However, it can be synthetically modified and made into various progestogens which do have progesteronelike activity.[1] The most popular progestogen in this group is medroxyprogesterone acetate.

This group of progestogens is mostly used in women using estrogen replacement to prevent the development of endometrial cancer. Other synthetic progesterones, such as norethinodrone, are made by altering the testosterone molecule, and are used in birth control pills as well as during menopause.[2] More information on commonly used progestogens can be found in chapter 14, which discusses progesterone in detail.

Throughout the book, the word progesterone is used to describe the naturally occurring molecule. When medroxyprogesterone or another progestogen is being discussed, it is mentioned by name.

HOW PROGESTOGENS WORK

Progestogens enter the cell the same way that estrogens do. They cross the cell membrane into the cell and attach themselves to progesterone receptors on the nucleus of the cell. Just as each type of estrogen has a different ability to attach itself (receptor affinity), progestogens have different affinities for progesterone receptors. Some of the synthetic progesterones have a stronger affinity for progesterone receptors than does naturally occurring progesterone.[3] The synthetic progesterones derived from testosterone (and used in birth control) appear to have a greater affinity than natural progesterone, while progesterone has a greater affinity than medroxyprogesterone acetate, which is commonly administered to women in menopause.[4]

In many ways, the effects of synthetic progestogens mimic the effects of natural progesterone. There are some indications that natural micronized progesterone is more beneficial than synthetic progestogens. Research is showing that natural progesterone may possess better cardiac-protection properties.[5, 6] Some of the effects of progesterone on the nervous system are due to metabolites of natural progesterone. When we realize that the body has been using natural progesterone since before it was born, it is not difficult to understand that when menopause occurs the body may need supplementation with natural progesterone.

Testosterone
and the Androgens

The word "androgen" is used to describe the group of steroid hormones that are similar to testosterone. In women, the ovaries and the adrenal glands create these androgens. Additionally, there are various metabolites of androgens, just as there are with estrogens and progestogens. The hormones that are produced in the ovaries and adrenal glands include testosterone, androstenedione, androstenediol, dehydroepiandrosterone (DHEA), and dehydroepiandrosterone-sulfate (DHEA-S). There are many metabolites of these androgens, but the most important one (to our current knowledge) is dihydrotestosterone (DHT), a more potent form of testosterone.

The term androgen also is applied to any substance, whether natural or synthetic, that has similar biological and physiological effects as testosterone. In this book, the word "androgenic" is used to describe the actions of a substance as being "androgenlike." The group of progestogens synthesized from testosterone still has some androgenic activity. Numerous synthetic drugs also have androgenic activity. The root word for androgen means "male forming" or "male-like," so these are hormones with "male-like" activity.

Anabolic is another word commonly used to describe the actions of testosterone and similar substances. Anabolic refers to tissue-building activity, not necessarily male-like activity. Recall that estrogen has anabolic activity as well. As most male hormones are anabolic as well as androgenic, it is appropriate to use the word anabolic to describe them, but it is an incomplete description.

HOW TESTOSTERONE WORKS

In the same fashion as estrogens and progesterone, testosterone works by crossing the cell membrane into the cell and attaching itself to androgen receptors on the nucleus of the cell. Androgen receptors have been found in every tissue where estrogen and progesterone receptors have been noted. The presence of these receptors in some tissues is a recent discovery, particularly their presence in women. Based on clinical findings of testosterone deficiency and the resulting improvements when testosterone is replaced, it is fair to say that testosterone affects virtually every tissue in the female body.

All the naturally occurring androgens—testosterone, androstenedione, androstenediol, and DHEA, as well as dihydrotestosterone—bind to androgen receptors. Research indicates that different androgens have different effects on the receptors, in the same way that different types of estrogen have different effects on estrogen receptors. However, in some tissues, the effects of testosterone and dihydrotestosterone appear to be the same.[1] And, as estradiol causes an increase in the number of progesterone receptors, dihydrotestosterone is able to increase the number of androgen receptors on its own.[2]

Although much more research is needed to determine the role of androgen receptors in women, we know enough now to say that the functions of testosterone and other androgens in the female body require a more in-depth look into their actions.

See Appendix D, which further discusses the androgens DHEA and androstenidione.

Other Important Hormones

Though estrogen, progesterone, and testosterone are, without question, the major players in hormone balancing during menopause, there are many other hormones that also can be affected in postmenopausal women. Some of these hormones, such as DHEA and cortisol, share the same steroidogenic pathway as estrogen, progesterone, and testosterone. The changes seen in DHEA and cortisol are partly due to the changes taking place in the adrenal glands during menopause. Other hormones—such as melatonin, insulin, thyroid, and growth hormone—are produced in different tissues but are still affected by changes that the whole body is experiencing.

An overview of the changes taking place in other hormones will give additional insights into why some types of menopause bring about such different symptoms and such different risks for disease than other menopause types. So even though the changes that occur in these following hormones do not happen to all women in menopause, they can happen more often in certain menopause types. Knowing your type will help you decide if you need to monitor these hormones as well as estrogen, progesterone, and testosterone.

DHEA

Dehydroepiandrosterone (DHEA) is one of the androgens produced in the adrenal glands. Levels are higher in the morning and lower in the evening. As mentioned earlier, it is a precursor to other androgens such as testosterone, as well as to estrogens. DHEA affects metabolism of fats, carbohydrates, and proteins in the body.[1] The actual DHEA hormone itself only lasts about 30 minutes in the body, because most of it is converted to the more stable form dehydroepiandrosterone-sulfate (DHEA-S).[2,3] DHEA-S is the source of DHEA that is converted to androgens and estrogens.[4,5]

Like cortisol, DHEA can help the body handle stress when it is balanced with cortisol.[6, 7] DHEA also contributes to normal REM (rapid eye movement) sleep, and may help with memory and learning, possibly decreasing symptoms of dementia in Alzheimer's patients.[8, 9] Proper levels of DHEA may enhance immune function and decrease the incidence and severity of autoimmune diseases such as systemic lupus erythematosus.[10–13] Research has noted low DHEA levels in individuals with other autoimmune diseases, such as rheumatoid arthritis.[14–16]

DHEA may be helpful in decreasing obesity, though there is considerable debate on its effectiveness.[17–19] Although low DHEA has been noted in some people with hypertension, this is thought to be because the steroid pathway is making more aldosterone instead of DHEA, and it is the high aldosterone causing the problem.[20] However, there is clear evidence of increased risk of coronary atherosclerosis and heart disease with low DHEA-S levels.[21] This may be in part to the ability of DHEA to lower LDL ("bad") cholesterol levels.[22] Another reason may be because DHEA prevents and reduces insulin resistance, and helps stabilize blood sugar.[23–30]

However, excess DHEA in women is a form of androgen excess, which could actually increase the risk of insulin resistance.[31, 32] So it is best that women do not take too much DHEA, but rather aim for normal levels, and closely monitor themselves for signs of excess DHEA or other androgens, such as acne, oily skin, or facial hair.

Research has also noted low DHEA levels in individuals with hypothyroidism.[33] Though the low DHEA may be due to the low thyroid function, some researchers view DHEA as able to enhance thyroid function.[34] As hypothyroidism has serious effects on the body, it is best to consult your doctor for monitoring and treatment of your thyroid condition, and avoid trying to change thyroid function with DHEA.

Numerous studies also report low DHEA levels in individuals with Alzheimer's disease, bladder cancer, stomach cancer, prostate cancer, and lung cancer.[35–39] Higher levels of DHEA have been noted in postmenopausal women with some forms of breast cancer.[40] This may be due more to hyperinsulinemia or abnormal estrogen metabolism than to a direct effect of DHEA. See chapter 5 for more on androgens and breast cancer.

DHEA levels decline gradually with age. By the time a person is in his or her seventies, DHEA levels are much lower than they were at 25 or 30 years old.[41–43] This may be a sign of progressive weakening of the adrenal glands, an important consideration for postmenopausal women who depend on these glands to make up for decreased ovary function. As one of the most important hormones produced by the adrenal glands, you should have your DHEA (along with cortisol) levels evaluated if adrenal fatigue is suspected. Your DHEA level should also be evaluated whenever estradiol or testosterone levels are low, because it is a precursor of these hormones.

CORTISOL

Cortisol is an important hormone secreted by the adrenal glands. Since cortisol can affect how the body uses glucose, protein, and fats, it influences the normal function of virtually every tissue in the body. Cortisol levels are highest in the early morning and lowest at night. When cortisol levels are lowest at night, REM sleep takes place. Rising cortisol levels in the morning decrease REM sleep and bring on wakefulness.[44, 45] Proper cortisol rhythm allows rejuvenating sleep, mental health, and proper patterns in the levels of other hormones such as melatonin. Research has noted abnormal cortisol rhythms in people with depression and other mood disorders.[46–50]

Cortisol levels can increase significantly any time of the day if the body is under stress. These elevated levels can continue as long as the stress continues.[51, 52] The ability of the body to increase cortisol levels as needed is important because the elevated levels help the body adapt to the stress. However, chronic stress can result in loss of the normal daily rhythm, and eventual fatigue of the adrenal glands. This is thought to be due to continual oversecretion of cortisol, which wears the body down over time and results in symptoms of exhaustion. Some forms of chronic fatigue, with low blood pressure, dizziness, and increased aches and pain, occur when cortisol levels finally drop. Raising this cortisol back to normal increases energy and vigor.[53–55]

Chronic excessive cortisol levels can result in suppression of the immune system, high blood pressure, and increased risk of heart disease.[56–61] Research also reports increased occurrence of obesity with high cortisol levels.[62–64] This may be due, in part, to the adverse effect high cortisol has on normal insulin activity.[65, 66] Higher cortisol levels also can suppress thyroid function, leading to hypothyroidism, and cause or worsen osteoporosis.[67–70]

When the body increases cortisol levels as a response to stress, it does so at the expense of progesterone, estradiol, and testosterone. As the steroidogenic pathway reveals (see Appendix E), cortisol shares a common pathway with these other hormones. Since the need of the body to tolerate stress is so important, steroidogenesis will shift hormone production toward more cortisol, resulting in less progesterone, testosterone, and estradiol. For the postmenopausal woman, proper nutrition and support of the adrenal glands is especially important, because levels of progesterone, testosterone, and estradiol are probably already lower due to menopause.

Cortisol is a major steroid produced by the adrenal glands that is of major importance to the body. Low cortisol, high cortisol, or abnormal cortisol rhythms can lead to numerous adverse health conditions, including depression, insomnia, heart disease, stress, obesity, and chronic fatigue. Shifts in cortisol production also can affect progesterone, testosterone, and estradiol levels. For this reason, you should check your cortisol levels when there is a significant drop in other steroid hormones.

PREGNENOLONE

The most significant thing to say about pregnenolone is that it is the precursor to every other steroid hormone, including estrogens, androgens, and progesterone, as well as cortisol and aldosterone. Due to its recognized role as a precursor, interest in using pregnenolone as a precursor for the other hormones is increasing. This may be an appropriate option, but there is no guarantee that any precursor will become any specific hormone. Even if pregnenolone does not work as a precursor, however, it has its own beneficial effects on the body.

Pregnenolone is best described as a "neurosteroid"—a steroid hormone that affects the nervous system. Research reports low pregnenolone levels in individuals suffering from depression, and a decrease in symptoms of depression when levels are restored.[71, 72] This beneficial effect may be due to the ability of pregnenolone to act as a neurotransmitter and affect the function of other neurotransmitters.[73]

The greatest effect of pregnenolone on the brain may be increased memory. Pregnenolone has demonstrated an ability to maintain memory in a number of studies.[74-76] As pregnenolone levels appear to decrease with age, the link between poor memory and aging may be due in part to pregnenolone. Increasing the pregnenolone levels in animals has been shown to decrease age-related loss of memory.[77] The ability of pregnenolone to enhance memory in older humans looks promising, especially if it is used as part of a comprehensive program designed to help preserve memory.[78, 79]

Research also discovered significantly lower levels of pregnenolone, as well as DHEA and testosterone, in the blood and the fluid around joints (synovial fluid) of individuals with a wide range of inflammatory joint diseases. These conditions included rheumatoid arthritis, psoriatic arthritis, ankylosing spondylitis, reactive arthritis, post-traumatic arthritis, and arthritis due to regional enteritis, which is a chronic bowel disease.[80] Research as long ago as the late 1940s and early 1950s first suggested pregnenolone in the treatment of arthritis and other autoimmune conditions.[81]

As promising as pregnenolone appears to be, especially for memory enhancement and preservation, further research would be greatly welcomed. If you take this supplement, caution is advised because abnormal increases of other hormones could cause considerable problems.

ANDROSTENEDIONE

For postmenopausal women, androstenedione may be the most important androgen secreted by the adrenal glands. As discussed in chapter 5, androstenedione production increases considerably during postmenopause. The amount of androstenedione produced by healthy postmenopausal adrenal glands is over five times the amount produced before menopause. This increase is an important part of adrenal recruitment, and is how the body compensates for the ovaries' decreased estradiol production.

Though the primary role of androstenedione is as a precursor for other hormones, it does have its own effect on the body. Androstenedione can directly attach to androgen receptors and may help promote proper function of certain tissues, such as bone. Though this hormone is increasingly popular, there is much we still need to learn about its direct effect on numerous tissues in the body.

We do know that, in women, excessive androstenedione can cause insulin resistance, which is typical of any androgen excess. It is now also clear that androstenedione levels are vital for proper health in postmenopausal women. As crucial as this hormone is for the continued production of estrogen, however, you must closely monitor supplementation in order to prevent insulin resistance and the increased risk of heart disease that accompanies that condition. Monitor estrogen and testosterone levels to ensure that you are getting the desired effect of supplementation. Ideally, you should check your androstenedione level before you start taking the supplement.

MELATONIN

Melatonin is the hormone that promotes proper sleep. It is important for falling asleep and for staying asleep during the night.[82] The body's temperature decreases at night when melatonin levels rise, which may help the body sleep.[83, 84] The pineal gland, a small endocrine gland located inside the skull, produces melatonin. Melatonin is not a steroid hormone—the pineal gland synthesizes it from the amino acid tryptophan after exposure to darkness.[85] Though the retina of the eye and the lining of the digestive system may also make small amounts of melatonin, their contribution to total melatonin levels is minor.[86]

The light and dark cycle of the day affects the 24-hour rhythm of melatonin, with levels at their lowest during the day and highest at about 2:00 or 3:00 in the morning.[87, 88] Nighttime exposure to light can rapidly decrease melatonin levels.[89] Natural exposure to morning light is required to lower daytime melatonin levels.

Melatonin is so sensitive to light that a great way to treat insomnia is to take 1 to 5 mg of melatonin at bedtime and then expose yourself to bright light in the morning. This combination effectively treats difficulty in both falling asleep and staying asleep.[90] Melatonin also can be used in this way to adjust to new time zones after air travel and reduce the symptoms of jet lag.[91]

Exposure to electromagnetic fields such as television and computer screens also can decrease melatonin levels.[92–95] Some people seem to be more sensitive than others and wind up with sleeping problems. If you cannot avoid exposure to electromagnetic fields, you might want to consider melatonin supplementation.

In addition to helping with sleep, melatonin can decrease the risk of cardiovascular disease by curtailing atherosclerosis, promoting healthy cholesterol levels, and decreasing platelet clumping.[96–98] Melatonin also appears to strengthen the immune system.[99–101] It acts as a potent antioxidant, helping the body scavenge free radicals and protecting cells and tissues throughout the body, including the brain.[102–107]

Perhaps of greatest interest to women is the relationship melatonin has with estrogen. Melatonin can make breast cancer cells resistant to the cancer-causing effects of estrogen by decreasing growth stimulatory factors and making cancer less invasive.[108–110] Thus, melatonin can have a protective effect on women taking estrogens by making cells less likely to become stimulated into becoming cancerous.

Just as melatonin decreases the effect of estrogen on cells, estrogen can affect melatonin. Estrogen can cause a significant decrease in the secretion of melatonin by the pineal gland.[111, 112] So, it is best to take estrogen supplements in the morning. This way, melatonin levels will not drop in the middle of the night while the estrogen is being absorbed.

Many drugs, foods, and herbs can affect melatonin levels. Substances that increase melatonin levels include, of course, melatonin, and also its precursor, tryptophan or 5-hydroxy-tryptophan. Drugs that can stimulate melatonin production include Thorazine, fluvoxamine, desipramine, clorgyline, or tranylcypromine.[113–118] One herb that is believed to raise melatonin levels is St. John's wort (*Hypericum perforatum*). Foods that are high in melatonin or melatonin precursors, such as oats, sweet corn, rice, ginger, tomatoes, bananas, and barley, can also raise melatonin levels.

Substances that decrease melatonin levels come from a wide variety of drug classes including NSAIDs (nonsteroidal anti-inflammatory drugs), beta-blockers, calcium–channel blockers, antihypertensives, antianxiety drugs, antidepressants, and steroids, as well as commonly utilized substances such as caffeine, tobacco, and alcohol. The current list of melatonin-decreasing substances includes:[119–127]

Acetaminophen
Alcohol
Alprazolam
Aspirin
Atenolol
Benzerazide
Bepridil
Caffeine
Clonidine
Dexamethasone
Diazepam
Diltiazem
Filodipine
Flunitrazepam
Fluoxetine
Ibuprofen
Indomethacin
Interleukin-2

Isradapine
Luzindole
Methylcobal
   amine
Metoprolol
Nicotine
Nicardipine
Nifedipine
Nimodipine
Nisoldipine
Nitrendipine
Prazosin
Propanolol
Reserpine
Ridazolol
Tobacco
Vitamin B$_{12}$

Exercise during the evening also can decrease melatonin levels. Conversely, daytime exercise can increase melatonin levels at night.[128–132] Though melatonin can offer many benefits to the postmenopausal woman, side effects—such as nightmares, hypotension, sleep disorders, and abdominal pain—are possible.[133] There is also some concern that melatonin may affect steroid hormone function.[134] I have seen a few cases in which women taking high doses of melatonin showed signs of decreased adrenal and ovarian function but, to date, no research studies clearly support this finding. As with all hormones, moderation and proper monitoring are in order when using melatonin supplements.

THYROID HORMONES

The thyroid secretes a number of different hormones. Of these, T3 is the most active, with T4 being a larger, but less-active hormone. Blood tests for these hormone levels involve looking at the entire amount of T3 or T4, but there is also a small amount of each hormone that is more available to the cells. This is called the "free" part of the hormone and is the most active form of each hormone. The free form provides valuable information about how much of the hormone can reach the body's cells. Many times the free amount of T4 will be measured in what is called a "free T4" test or fT4 for short.

Another important test is the thyroid-stimulating-hormone test. The thyroid-stimulating hormone, or TSH, is secreted by the pituitary gland to stimulate thyroid activity; the level of TSH shows how thyroid hormones are being balanced or regulated by the body. A high TSH means the body is not satisfied with the amount of thyroid hormone available to the tissues, so the pituitary is trying to stimulate more hormone production. A low TSH means the body is getting too much thyroid hormone and the last thing it wants is more, so the pituitary gland decreases TSH as much as possible to decrease more hormone production.

In the past, it was thought that thyroid hormone-replacement therapy caused increased risk of osteoporosis. This was because women taking thyroid hormones showed increased bone loss. It is now well established that the increased osteoporosis was due to excessive thyroid hormone replacement.

When thyroid-replacement therapy is so high that it suppresses TSH, it means there is too much thyroid. This excessive thyroid can result in increased postmenopausal bone loss.[135-136] The increased loss of bone can be avoided if thyroid hormone levels are not so high that they decrease TSH.[137] TSH is a hormone secreted by the pituitary gland to stimulate thyroid gland activity in the normal, healthy thyroid; therefore, there should always be some TSH in the blood. When thyroid hormone replacement is at too high a level and TSH is suppressed below normal levels, a mild form of hyperthyroidism has been created.[138] This mild hyperthyroidism with suppressed TSH is what causes the increased bone loss, and also can affect the heart in some people.[139] Excessive thyroid hormone can cause bone loss in *pre*menopausal women, as well.[140]

Oral estrogen-replacement therapy can negate the bone-dissolving effect of thyroid hormones if estrogen levels are low.[141, 142] However, estrogens can cause a moderate increase in blood levels of T4 and thyroid-binding globulin, the protein that carries the thyroid hormone through the blood.[143] Unfortunately, some physicians have interpreted this as a result of too much thyroid supplementation. Estrogens cause no significant change in levels of TSH, fT4, or T3.[144] Women on oral estrogen-replacement therapy should use fT4 and TSH to monitor thyroid levels. The T4 levels are falsely elevated and should not be measured in these women. Thyroid levels should never be increased to the point that they suppress TSH.

GROWTH HORMONE AND IGF-1

The pituitary gland secretes growth hormone, which then acts upon the liver, creating insulinlike growth factor-1 (IGF-1) and other growth agents. IGF-1 then acts on various tissues of the body to increase growth. The greatest concern for the postmenopausal women regarding growth hormone and IGF-1 is the effect that too much of these hormones have on the body. Though there is a current movement to use growth hormone and IGF-1 as supplements, the promoters of the movement fail to give sufficient warning regarding the fact that high levels can induce insulin resistance and increase the risk of developing certain cancers. However, in 1998, the American Association of Clinical Endocrinologists, the group of physicians who specialize in the endocrine system, issued a health alert calling for "responsible use" of human growth hormone. They pointed out that the proper way to test for growth hormone deficiency is not a single blood test, but a test to evaluate whether the pituitary gland can release growth hormone when stimulated.[145] They also pointed out, as have others, that much more research is needed on this hormone, and caution is advised in its use.

Considering that growth hormone and IGF-1 production is increased by testosterone and progesterone, and controlled by estradiol, it might be wiser to balance the three major hormones first, and let the body control the levels of growth hormone and IGF-1.

INSULIN

As discussed in previous chapters, the greatest risk for postmenopausal women concerning insulin is the development of insulin resistance due to an imbalance of estrogens, progesterone, and androgens, especially testosterone. It is a relative lack of estradiol, and/or a relative excess of progesterone or testosterone, that will bring on insulin resistance and hyperinsulinemia.

The conditions and health risks that develop due to hyperinsulinemia include increased risk of heart disease, increased risk of breast cancer, increased occurrence of non-insulin–dependent diabetes, and high blood pressure.

Since proper management of estrogen, testosterone, and progesterone levels are one way to prevent and control hyperinsulinemia, you should get an assessment of these hormones by a skilled clinician if hyperinsulinemia is a possibility.

The Steroidogenic Pathway

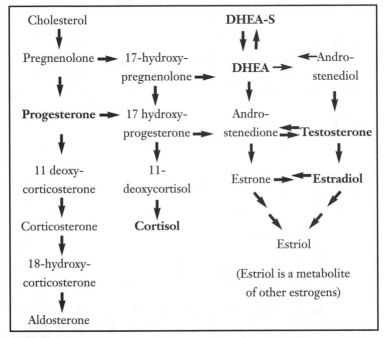

The Steroidogenic Pathway—Also showing estriol, which is a metabolite of other estrogens.

As discussed extensively in chapter 5, the steroidogenic pathway illustrates how cholesterol is converted to pregnenolone, progesterone, DHEA, testosterone, and estrogens. Looking at the steroidogenic pathway can help you appreciate the complex relationships between hormones. Scientific and educational websites that discuss the steroidogenic pathway in great detail include:

> www.icgeb.trieste.it/p450/steroid_list.html
> www.genome.ad.jp/dbget-bin/show_pathway?MAP00140
> www.yourmenopausetype.com

Notes

Chapter 1

Wilson RA. *Feminine Forever.* New York, NY: M. Evans & Co., 1966.

Chapter 2

No notes.

Chapter 3

No notes.

Chapter 4

1. Bhagavan NV. *Medical Biochemistry.* Boston: Jones and Bartlett Publishers, 1992: 737–738.
2. Hofman LA. Steroid hormones in saliva. *Diagnostic Endocrinol Metab* 16(9): 265–273, 1998.
3. Worthman CM, et al. Sensitive salivary estradiol essay for monitoring ovarian function. *Clin Chem* 36: 1769–1773, 1990.
4. Mandel ID. The diagnostic uses of saliva. *J Oral Pathol Med* 19: 119–125, 1990.
5. Choe JK, et al., Progesterone and estradiol in the saliva and plasma during the menstrual cycle. *Am J. Obstet. Gynecol.* 147: 557, 1983.
6. Hofman LA. Steroid hormones in saliva. *Diagnostic Endocrinol Metab* 16(9): 265–273, 1998.
7. Same as 5.
8. Adekunle AO, et al., Progesterone in saliva as an index of ovarian function. *Int. J. Gynecol. Obstet* 28: 45–51, 1989.
9. Walker RF, et al., Radioimmunoassay or progesterone in saliva: application to the assessment of ovarian function. *Clin Chem* 25/12: 2030–2033, 1979.
10. Walker S, et al., The role of salivary progesterone in studies of infertile women. *Br Obstet. Gynecol* 88: 1009–1015, 10/1981.
11. Riad-Fahmy D, et al., Steroids in saliva for assessing endocrine function. *Endocr Rev* 3(4): 367-95, 1982.
12. Berthonneau J, et al., Salivary oestradiol in spontaneous and stimulated menstrual cycles. *Hum Reprod* 4(6): 625–628, 1989.
13. Osredkar J, et al., Salivary free testosterone in hirsutism. *Ann Clin Biochem* 26(6): 522–526, 1989.

14. Campbell BC, Ellison PT. Menstrual variation in salivary testosterone among regularly cycling women. *Horm Res* 37(4–5): 132–136, 1992.
15. Navarro MA, et al., Salivary testosterone in postmenopausal women with rheumatoid arthritis. *J Rheumatol* 25(6): 1059–1062, 1998.
16. Bojali II. Sero-salivary progesterone correlation. *Int J Gynaecol Obstet* 45(2): 125–131, 1994.
17. Bolaji II, et al., Assessment of bioavailability of oral micronized progesterone using a salivary progesterone enzymeimmunoassay. *Gynecol Endocrinol* 7(2): 101–110, 1993.

Chapter 5

1. Schiff I, Walsh B. Menopause. IN: Becker KL, eds. *Principles and Practice of Endocrinology and Metabolism*. Philadelphia: JB Lippincott, 1995: 920.
2. Phillips JI, Davies I. A comparative morphometric analysis of the component tissues of the urethra in young and old female C57BL/ICRFAt mice. *Invest Urol* 18(8): 422–425, 1981.
3. Brincat M, et al., Long-term effects of the menopause and sex hormones on skin thickness. *Br J Obstet Gynaecol* 92(3): 256–259, 1985.
4. Grosman N, et al., The effect of oestrogenic treatment on the acid mucopolysaccharide pattern in skin of mice. *Acta Pharmacol Toxicol* 30(5): 458–464, 1971.
5. Grosman N. Study on the hyaluronic acid–protein complex, the molecular size of hyaluronic acid and the exchangeability of chloride in skin of mice before and after oestrogen treatment. *Acta Pharmacol Toxicol* 33(3): 201–208, 1973.
6. Guyton AC. *Textbook of Medical Physiology*. Philadelphia: WB Saunders, 1986: 975–976.
7. Smith RNJ, Studd JWW. Estrogens and depression in women. IN: Lobo RA, ed. *Treatment of the Postmenopausal Woman, Basic and Clinical Aspects*. Philadelphia: Lippincott-Raven Publishers, 1996.
8. Jacobs DM, et al., Cognitive function in nondemented older women who took estrogen after menopause. *Neurology* 50(2): 368–373, 1998.
9. Sherwin BB. Estrogen effects on cognition in menopausal women. *Neurology* 48(5 suppl 7): S21–S26, 1997.
10. Kampen DL, Sherwin BB. Estrogen use and verbal memory in healthy postmenopausal women. Department of Psychology, McGill University, Montreal, Quebec, Canada. *Obstet Gynecol* 83(6): 979–983, 1994.
11. Rice MM, et al., Estrogen replacement therapy and cognitive function in postmenopausal women without dementia. *Am J Med* 103(3A): 26S–35S, 1997.
12. Sherwin BB. Estrogenic effects on memory in women. *Ann N Y Acad Sci* 743: 213–230; discussion 230–231, 1994.
13. Altieri M, Bogousslavsky J. [Brain dysfunction in climacteric and prevention]. [Article in German] *Schweiz Rundsch Med Prax* 86(36): 1378–1382, 1997.
14. Henderson VW. Estrogen, cognition, and a woman's risk of Alzheimer's disease. *Am J Med* 103(3A): 11S–18S, 1997.
15. Sherwin BB. Estrogen effects on cognition in menopausal women. *Neurology* 48(5 suppl 7): S21–S26, 1997.
16. Jacobs DM, et al., Cognitive function in nondemented older women who took estrogen after menopause. *Neurology* 50(2): 368–373, 1998.
17. Christiansen C. Treatment of Osteoporosis. IN: Lobo RA, ed. *Treatment of the Postmenopausal Woman, Basic and Clinical Aspects*. Philadelphia: Lippincott-Raven Publishers, 1996: 96.

18. Tohme JF, et al., Osteoporosis. IN: Becker, KL, ed. *Principles and Practice of Endocrinology and Metabolism*. Philadelphia: JB Lippincott, 1995: 567–585.
19. Gaby AR. *Preventing and Reversing Osteoporosis*. Rocklin, CA: Prima Publishing, 1994.
20. Mano H, et al., Mammalian mature osteoclasts as estrogen target cells. *Biochem Biophys Res Commun* 223(3): 637–642, 1996.
21. Hughes DE, et al., Estrogen promotes apoptosis of murine osteoclasts mediated by TGF-beta. *Nat Med* 2(10): 1132–1136, 1996.
22. Tremollieres F, et al., [Postmenopausal bone loss. Role of estrogens]. [Article in French] *Presse Med* 21(19): 903–906, 1992.
23. Yamaguchi M, Matsui T. Zinc enhancement of 17-beta-estradiol's anabolic effect in osteoblastic MC3T3-E1 cells. *Calcif Tissue Int* 60(6): 527–532, 1997.
24. Slootweg MC, et al., Estrogen enhances growth hormone receptor expression and growth hormone action in rat osteosarcoma cells and human osteoblast-like cells. *J Endocrinol* 155(1): 159–164, 1997.
25. Stepan J, et al., [Comparison of the effectiveness of 17-beta-estradiol and calcitonin in women with postmenopausal bone loss]. [Article in Czech] *Cas Lek Cesk* 136(8): 242–248, 1997.
26. Koka S, et al. Estrogen inhibits interleukin-1 beta-induced interleukin-6 production by human osteoblast-like cells. *J Interferon Cytokine Res* 18(7): 479–483, 1998.
27. Heikkinen AM, et al. Postmenopausal hormone replacement therapy and autoantibodies against oxidized LDL. *Maturitas* 29(2): 155–161, 1998.
28. Haines CJ, et al. An examination of the effect of combined cyclical hormone replacement therapy on lipoprotein(a) and other lipoproteins. *Atherosclerosis* 119(2): 215–222, 1996.
29. Espeland MA, et al. Effect of postmenopausal hormone therapy on lipoprotein(a) concentration. PEPI Investigators. Postmenopausal Estrogen/Progestin Interventions. *Circulation* 97(10): 979–986, 1998.
30. Wouters MG, et al. Plasma homocysteine and menopausal status. *Eur J Clin Invest* 25(11): 801–805, 1995.
31. Nasr A, Breckwoldt M. Estrogen replacement therapy and cardiovascular protection: lipid mechanisms are the tip of an iceberg. *Gynecol Endocrinol* 12(1): 43–59, 1998.
32. Sudhir K, et al. Estrogen supplementation decreases norepinephrine-induced vasoconstriction and total body norepinephrine spillover in perimenopausal women. *Hypertension* 30(6): 1538–1543, 1997.
33. Sacks FM, et al. Sex hormones, lipoproteins, and vascular reactivity. *Curr Opin Lipidol* 6(3): 161–166, 1995.
34. Mauvais-Jarvis P, Kuttenn F. [Is progesterone insufficiency carcinogenic?] [Article in French] *Nouv Presse Med* 4(5): 323–326, 1975.
35. Gorodeski IG, et al. Decreased Ratio of Total Progesterone to Total Estradiol Receptor Levels in Endometria of Women with Adult Dysfunctional Uterine Bleeding. *Gynecol. Obstet. Invest.* 22: 22–28, 1986.
36. Mauvais-Jarvis P, et al. [Progesterone administered by percutaneous route: an antiandrogen locally useful]. [Article in French] *Ann Endocrinol* 36(2): 55–62, 1975.
37. Amadeo M. Antiandrogen treatment of aggressivity in men suffering from dementia. *J Geriatr Psychiatry Neurol* 9(3): 142–145, 1996.
38. Cooper AJ, et al. A double-blind placebo controlled trial of medroxyprogesterone acetate and cyproterone acetate with seven pedophiles. *Can J Psychiatry* 37(10): 687–693, 1992.

39. Tsang DC. Policing "perversions": Depo-Provera and John Money's new sexual order. University of California, Irvine 92713, USA. *J Homosex* 28(3–4): 397–426, 1995.

40. Cooper AJ. Progestogens in the treatment of male sex offenders: a review. *Can J Psychiatry* 31(1): 73–79, 1986.

41. Cordoba OA, Chapel JL. Medroxyprogesterone acetate antiandrogen treatment of hypersexuality in a pedophiliac sex offender. *Am J Psychiatry* 140(8): 1036–1039, 1983.

42. Glick ID, Bennett SE. Psychiatric complications of progesterone and oral contraceptives. *J Clin Psychopharmacol* 1(6): 350–367, 1981.

43. Hessemer V, Bruck K. Influence of menstrual cycle on shivering, skin blood flow, and sweating responses measured at night. *J Appl Physiol* 59(6): 1902–1910, 1985.

44. Harvell J, et al. Changes in transepidermal water loss and cutaneous blood flow during the menstrual cycle. *Contact Dermatitis* 27(5): 294–301, 1992.

45. Same as 43.

46. Same as 34.

47. Rapkin AJ, et al. Progesterone metabolite allopregnanolone in women with premenstrual syndrome. *Obstet Gynecol* 90(5): 709–714, 1997.

48. Backstrom T. Symptoms related to the menopause and sex steroid treatments. *Ciba Found Symp* 191: 171–180, 1995.

49. Lancel M, et al. Progesterone induces changes in sleep comparable to those of agonistic GABAA receptor modulators. *Am J Physiol* 271(4 Pt 1): E763–E772, 1996.

50. Putnam CD, et al. Inhibition of uterine contractility by progesterone and progesterone metabolites: mediation by progesterone and gamma amino butyric acid A receptor systems. *Biol Reprod* 45(2): 266–272, 1991.

51. Bitran D, et al. Anxiolytic effect of progesterone is associated with increases in cortical allopregnanolone and GABAA receptor function. *Pharmacol Biochem Behav* 45(2): 423–428, 1993.

52. Gron G, et al. Assessment of cognitive performance after progesterone administration in healthy male volunteers. *Neuropsychobiology* 35(3): 147–151, 1997.

53. Herzog AG. Reproductive endocrine considerations and hormonal therapy for women with epilepsy. *Epilepsia* 32(suppl 6): S27–S33, 1991.

54. Galli R, et al. Circulating levels of anticonvulsant metabolites of progesterone in women with partial epilepsy in the intercritical phase. *Ital J Neurol Sci* 17(4): 277–281, 1996.

55. de Wit H, Rukstalis M. Acute effects of triazolam in women: relationships with progesterone, estradiol and allopregnanolone. *Psychopharmacology* 130(1): 69–78, 1997.

56. Smith SS, et al. Withdrawal from 3alpha-OH-5 alpha-pregnan-20-one using a pseudopregnancy model alters the kinetics of hippocampal GABAA-gated current and increases the GABAA receptor alpha4 subunit in association with increased anxiety. *J Neurosci* 18(14): 5275–5284, 1998.

57. Block AJ, et al. Sleep-disordered breathing and nocturnal oxygen desaturation in postmenopausal women. *Am J Med* 69(1): 75–79, 1980.

58. Bayliss DA, et al. Progesterone stimulates respiration through a central nervous system steroid receptor-mediated mechanism in cat. *Proc Natl Acad Sci U S A* 84(21): 7788–7792, 1987.

59. Pickett CK, et al. Progestin and estrogen reduce sleep-disordered breathing in postmenopausal women. *J Appl Physiol* 66(4): 1656–1661, 1989.
60. Bayliss DA, Millhorn DE. Central neural mechanisms of progesterone action: application to the respiratory system. *J Appl Physiol* 73(2): 393–404, 1992.
61. Same as 59.
62. Bayliss DA, et al. The stimulation of respiration by progesterone in ovariectomized cat is mediated by an estrogen-dependent hypothalamic mechanism requiring gene expression. *Endocrinology* 126(1): 519–527, 1990.
63. Chen SW, et al. The hyperphagic effect of 3 alpha-hydroxylated pregnane steroids in male rats. *Pharmacol Biochem Behav* 53(4): 777–782, 1996.
64. Lett BT, et al. Chlordiazepoxide counteracts activity-induced suppression of eating in rats. *Exp Clin Psychopharmacol* 5(1): 24–27, 1997.
65. Verhaar HJ, et al. A comparison of the action of progestins and estrogen on the growth and differentiation of normal adult human osteoblast-like cells in vitro. *Bone* 15(3): 307–311, 1994.
66. Chen L. Induction of osteocalcin gene expression in vitro by progesterone. *J Tongji Med Univ* 17(2): 72–74, 1997.
67. MacNamara P, Loughrey HC. Progesterone receptor A and B isoform expression in human osteoblasts. *Calcif Tissue Int* 63(1): 39–46, 1998.
68. Chen L, Foged NT. Differentiation of osteoblast in vitro is regulated by progesterone. *J Tongji Med Univ* 16(2): 83–86, 1996.
69. MacNamara P, et al. Progesterone receptors are expressed in human osteoblast-like cell lines and in primary human osteoblast cultures. *Calcif Tissue Int* 57(6): 436–441, 1995.
70. Heersche JN, et al. The decrease in bone mass associated with aging and menopause. *J Prosthet Dent* 79(1): 14–16, 1998.
71. Wei LL, et al. Evidence for progesterone receptors in human osteoblast-like cells. *Biochem Biophys Res Commun* 195(2): 525–532, 1993.
72. Pensler JM, et al. Sex steroid hormone receptors in normal and dysplastic bone disorders in children. *J Bone Miner Res* 5(5): 493–498, 1990.
73. Tremollieres FA, et al. Progesterone and promegestone stimulate human bone cell proliferation and insulin-like growth factor-2 production. *Acta Endocrinol* 126(4): 329–337, 1992.
74. Ribot C, Tremollieres F. [Sex steroids and bone tissue]. [Article in French] *Ann Endocrinol* 56(1): 49–55, 1995.
75. Barengolts EI, et al. Effects of progesterone on serum levels of IGF-1 and on femur IGF-1 mRNA in ovariectomized rats. *J Bone Miner Res* 11(10): 1406–1412, 1996.
76. Same as 65.
77. Tremollieres F, et al. [Postmenopausal bone loss. Role of progesterone and androgens]. [Article in French] *Nouv Presse Med* 21(21): 989–993, 1992.
78. Bowman BM, Miller SC. Elevated progesterone during pseudopregnancy may prevent bone loss associated with low estrogen. *J Bone Miner Res* 11(1): 15–21, 1996.
79. Barengolts EI, et al. Effects of progesterone on postovariectomy bone loss in aged rats. *J Bone Miner Res* 5(11): 1143–1147, 1990.
80. Fujimaki T, et al. Effects of progesterone on the metabolism of cancellous bone in young oophorectomized rats. *J Obstet Gynaecol* 21(1): 31–36, 1995.
81. Slootweg MC, et al. Oestrogen and progestogen synergistically stimulate human and rat osteoblast proliferation. *J Endocrinol* 133(2): R5–R8, 1992.
82. Prior JC. Progesterone as a bone-trophic hormone. *Endocr Rev* 11(2): 386–398, 1990.
83. Sherwin BB. Sex hormones and psychological functioning in postmenopausal women. *Exp Gerontol* 29(3–4): 423–430, 1994.

Notes 349

84. Leiblum S, et al. Vaginal atrophy in the postmenopausal woman. The importance of sexual activity and hormones. *JAMA* 249(16): 2195–2198, 1983.
85. Hodgins MB, et al. An immunohistochemical study of androgen, oestrogen and progesterone receptors in the vulva and vagina. *Br J Obstet Gynaecol* 105(2): 216–222, 1998.
86. Hall D. Lichen sclerosus: early diagnosis is the key to treatment. *Nurse Pract* 21(12 Pt 1): 57–8, 61–62, 1996.
87. Khastgir G, Studd J. Hysterectomy, ovarian failure, and depression. *Menopause* 5(2): 113–122, 1998.
88. Sands R, Studd J. Exogenous androgens in postmenopausal women. *Am J Med* 98(1A): 76S–79S, 1995.
89. Persky H, et al. Plasma testosterone level and sexual behavior of couples. *Arch Sex Behav* 7(3): 157–173, 1978.
90. Brincat M, et al. Sex hormones and skin collagen content in postmenopausal women. *Br Med J (Clin Res Ed)* 287(6402): 1337–1338, 1983.
91. Brincat M, et al. Decline in skin collagen content and metacarpal index after the menopause and its prevention with sex hormone replacement. *Br J Obstet Gynaecol* 94(2): 126–129, 1987.
92. Pochi PE, et al. Age-related changes in sebaceous gland activity. *J Invest Dermatol* 73(1): 108–111, 1979.
93. Slayden SM. Risks of menopausal androgen supplementation. *Semin Reprod Endocrinol* 16(2): 145–152, 1998.
94. Kaaks R. Nutrition, hormones, and breast cancer: is insulin the missing link? *Cancer Causes Control* 7(6): 605–625, 1996.
95. Berrino F, et al. Serum sex hormone levels after menopause and subsequent breast cancer. *J Natl Cancer Inst* 88(5): 291–296, 1996.
96. Juricskay S, et al. Urinary steroids at time of surgery in postmenopausal women with breast cancer. *Breast Cancer Res Treat* 44(1): 83–89, 1997.
97. Lipworth L, et al. Serum steroid hormone levels, sex hormone-binding globulin, and body mass index in the etiology of postmenopausal breast cancer. *Epidemiology* 7(1): 96–100, 1996.
98. Same as 97.
99. Same as 95.
100. Zeleniuch-Jacquotte A, et al. Relation of serum levels of testosterone and dehydroepiandrosterone sulfate to risk of breast cancer in postmenopausal women. *Am J Epidemiol* 145(11): 1030–1038, 1997.
101. Wakley GK, et al. Androgen treatment prevents loss of cancellous bone in the orchidectomized rat. *J Bone Miner Res* 6(4): 325–330, 1991.
102. Saito H, Yanaihara T. Steroid formation in osteoblast-like cells. *J Int Med Res* 26(1): 1–12, 1998.
103. Kasperk CH, et al. Androgens directly stimulate proliferation of bone cells in vitro. *Endocrinology* 124(3): 1576–1578, 1989.
104. Gasperino J. Androgenic regulation of bone mass in women. A review. *Clin Orthop* 311: 278–286, 1995.
105. Nakano Y, et al. The receptor, metabolism and effects of androgen in osteoblastic MC3T3-E1 cells. *Bone Miner* 26(3): 245–259, 1994.
106. Takeuchi K, Guggino SE. 24R,25-(OH)2 vitamin D_3 inhibits 1alpha,25-(OH)2 vitamin D_3 and testosterone potentiation of calcium channels in osteosarcoma cells. *J Biol Chem* 271(52): 33335–33343, 1996.
107. Bruch HR, et al. Androstenedione metabolism in cultured human osteoblast-like cells. *J Clin Endocrinol Metab* 75(1): 101–105, 1992.
108. Takeuchi M, et al. Androgens directly stimulate mineralization and increase androgen receptors in human osteoblast-like osteosarcoma cells. *Biochem Biophys Res Commun* 204(2): 905–911, 1994.

109. Lea CK, et al. Androstenedione treatment reduces loss of cancellous bone volume in ovariectomised rats in a dose-responsive manner and the effect is not mediated by oestrogen. *J Endocrinol* 156(2): 331–339, 1998.
110. Nishimura S. [Role of testosterone propionate and insulin in the regeneration and growth of bone]. [Article in Japanese] *Meikai Daigaku Shigaku Zasshi* 19(3): 291–309, 1990.
111. Somjen D, et al. Regulation of proliferation of rat cartilage and bone by sex steroid hormones. *J Steroid Biochem Mol Biol* 40(4–6): 717–723, 1991.
112. Brincat M, et al. Sex hormones and skin collagen content in postmenopausal women. *Br Med J (Clin Res Ed)* 287(6402): 1337–1338, 1983.
113. Davis SR, Burger HG. Use of androgens in postmenopausal women. *Curr Opin Obstet Gynecol* 9(3): 177–180, 1997.
114. Tremollieres F, et al. [Postmenopausal bone loss. Role of progesterone and androgens]. [Article in French] *Presse Med* 21(21): 989–993, 1992.
115. Adami S, et al. Effect of hyperandrogenism and menstrual cycle abnormalities on bone mass and bone turnover in young women. *Clin Endocrinol* 48(2): 169–173, 1998.
116. Crook D, Seed M. Endocrine control of plasma lipoprotein metabolism: effects of gonadal steroids. *Baillieres Clin Endocrinol Metab* 4(4):851–875, 1990.
117. Sarrel PM. Cardiovascular aspects of androgens in women. *Semin Reprod Endocrinol* 16(2): 121–128, 1998.
118. Same as 117.
119. Yue P, et al. Testosterone relaxes rabbit coronary arteries and aorta. *Circulation* 91(4): 1154–1160, 1995.
120. White CM, et al. The pharmacokinetics of intravenous testosterone in elderly men with coronary artery disease. *J Clin Pharmacol* 38(9): 792–797, 1998.
121. Rako S. Testosterone deficiency: a key factor in the increased cardiovascular risk to women following hysterectomy or with natural aging? *J Womens Health* 7(7): 825–859, 1998.
122. Proudler AJ, et al. Aging and the response of plasma insulin, glucose and C-peptide concentrations to intravenous glucose in postmenopausal women. *Clin Sci* 83(4): 489–494, 1992.
123. Spencer CP, et al. Is there a menopausal metabolic syndrome? *Gynecol Endocrinol* 11(5): 341–355, 1997.
124. Bruning PF, et al. Insulin resistance and breast-cancer risk. *Int J Cancer* 52(4): 511–516, 1992.
125. Same as 94.
126. Stoll BA. Diet and exercise regimens to improve breast carcinoma prognosis. *Cancer* 78(12): 2465–2470, 1996.
127. Stoll BA. Essential fatty acids, insulin resistance, and breast cancer risk. *Nutr Cancer* 31(1):72–77, 1998.
128. Ciampelli M, Lanzone A. Insulin and polycystic ovary syndrome: a new look at an old subject. *Gynecol Endocrinol* 12(4): 277–292, 1998.
129. Gamayunova VB, et al. Comparative study of blood insulin levels in breast and endometrial cancer patients. *Neoplasma* 44(2): 123–126, 1997.
130. Lindheim SR, et al. A possible bimodal effect of estrogen on insulin sensitivity in postmenopausal women and the attenuating effect of added progestin. *Fertil Steril* 60(4): 664–667, 1993.
131. Same as 122.
132. Colacurci N, et al. Effects of hormone replacement therapy on glucose metabolism. *Panminerva Med* 40(1): 18–21, 1998.
133. Wu J, et al. [The effects of ethinyl estradiol on glucose metabolism in postmenopausal women]. [Article in Chinese] *Chung Hua Fu Chan Ko Tsa Chih* 32(9): 528–531, 1997.
134. Same as 130.

135. Kumagai S, et al. The effects of oestrogen and progesterone on insulin sensitivity in female rats. *Acta Physiol Scand* 149(1):91–97,1993.

136. Puah JA, Bailey CJ. Effect of ovarian hormones on glucose metabolism in mouse soleus muscle. *Endocrinology* 117(4): 1336–1340, 1985.

137. Andersson B, et al. Estrogen replacement therapy decreases hyperandrogenicity and improves glucose homeostasis and plasma lipids in postmenopausal women with non-insulin–dependent diabetes mellitus. *J Clin Endocrinol Metab* 82(2): 638–643, 1997.

138. Cagnacci A, et al. Effects of low doses of transdermal 17 beta-estradiol on carbohydrate metabolism in postmenopausal women. *J Clin Endocrinol Metab* 74(6): 1396–1400, 1992.

139. Same as 122.

140. Sutter-Dub MT, Dazey B. [Role of progesterone in the insulin-resistance during pregnancy in the rat]. [Article in French] *Ann Endocrinol* 1979 Jan–Feb; 40(1): 37–38.

141. Sutter-Dub MT. Effects of pregnancy and progesterone and/or oestradiol on the insulin secretion and pancreatic insulin content in the perfused rat pancreas. *Diabete Metab* 5(1): 47–56, 1979.

142. Leturque A, et al. [Insulin resistance during pregnancy]. [Article in French] *Ann Endocrinol* 41(6): 573–578, 1980.

143. Ri K. [Study on insulin resistance in rats treated with estrogen and progesterone—assessment with the euglycemic glucose clamp technic]. [Article in Japanese] *Nippon Naibunpi Gakkai Zasshi* 63(6): 798–808, 1987.

144. Sutter-Dub MT, et al. Progesterone and insulinresistance in the pregnant rat. I. In vivo and in vitro studies. *Diabete Metab* 7(2): 97–104, 1981.

145. Sutter-Dub MT, Vergnaud MT. Progesterone and insulin resistance. III. Time-course study of progesterone action on differentially labelled 14C-glucose utilization by adipose tissue and isolated adipocytes of the female rat. *J Physiol (Paris)* 77(6–7): 797–802, 1981.

146. Same as 136.

147. Elkind-Hirsch KE, et al. Hormone replacement therapy alters insulin sensitivity in young women with premature ovarian failure. *J Clin Endocrinol Metab* 76(2): 472–425, 1993.

148. Colacurci N, et al. Effects of hormone replacement therapy on glucose metabolism. *Panminerva Med* 40(1): 18–21, 1998.

149. Same as 130.

150. Kalkhoff RK. Metabolic effects of progesterone. *Am J Obstet Gynecol* 142(6 Pt 2): 735–738, 1982.

151. Same as 136.

152. Falkner B, et al. Gender differences in insulin-stimulated glucose utilization among African-Americans. *Am J Hypertens* 7(11): 948–952, 1994.

153. Khaw KT, Barrett-Connor E. Fasting plasma glucose levels and endogenous androgens in non-diabetic postmenopausal women. *Clin Sci* 80(3): 199–203, 1991.

154. Same as 125.

155. De Pergola G, et al. The free testosterone to dehydroepiandrosterone sulphate molar ratio as a marker of visceral fat accumulation in premenopausal obese women. *Int J Obes Relat Metab Disord* 18(10): 659–664, 1994.

156. Same as 137.

157. Same as 124.

158. Haffner SM, Valdez RA. Endogenous sex hormones: impact on lipids, lipoproteins, and insulin. *Am J Med*; 98(1A): 40S–47S, 1995.

159. Givens JR, et al. Adrenal function in hirsutism I. Diurnal change and response of plasma androstenedione, testosterone, 17-hydroxyprogesterone, cortisol, LH and FSH to dexamethasone and ½ unit of ACTH. *J Clin Endocrinol Metab* 40(6): 988–1000, 1975.
160. McKenna TJ, et al. Variable clinical and hormonal manifestations of hyperandrogenemia. *Metabolism* 33(8): 714–717, 1984.
161. Satta MA, et al. An unusual hormone pattern in a virilized woman affected by Sertoli-Leydig cell tumor. Report of a case. *Acta Pathol Jpn* 39(11): 755–758, 1989.
162. Prelevic GM, et al. Effects of a low-dose estrogen-antiandrogen combination (Diane-35) on clinical signs of androgenization, hormone profile and ovarian size in patients with polycystic ovary syndrome. *Gynecol Endocrinol* 3(4): 269–280, 1989.
163. Cedeno J, et al. Effect of ketoconazole on plasma sex hormones, lipids, lipoproteins, and apolipoproteins in hyperandrogenic women. *Metabolism* 39(5): 511–517, 1990.
164. Same as 152.
165. Same as 163.
166. Tajima C, et al. Midluteal progesterone/estradiol ratio as an indicator of pregnancy potential. *Folia Endocrinol.* 65: 1278–1285, 1989.
167. Kamada S, et al. Influence of progesterone/estradiol ratio on luteal function for achieving pregnancy in gonadotropin therapy. *Horm Res* 37(suppl 1): 59–63, 1992.
168. Same as 167.
169. Same as 167.
170. Gorodeski I, et al. Decreased ratio of total progesterone to estradiol receptor levels in endometria of women with adult dysfunctional uterine bleeding. *Gynecol. Obstet. Invest.* 22: 22–28, 1986.
171. London RS, et al. Endocrine parameters and alpha-tocopherol therapy of patients with mammary dysplasia. *Cancer Res* 41(9 Pt 2): 3811–3813, 1981.
172. Seeman MV. Psychopathology in women and men: focus on female hormones. *Am J Psychiatry* 154(12): 1641–1647, 1997.
173. Senior J, Whalley ET. Variation in the estrogen–progesterone ratio and its effects on plasma kininogen levels in the rat. *J. Reprod. Fert.* 41, 425–433, 1974.
174. Domenico CR. The Kallikrein-Kinin system. IN: Becker KL, ed. *Principles and Practice of Endocrinology and Metabolism.* Philadelphia: JB Lippincott, 1421–1424, 1995.

Chapter 6

1. Ciampelli M, Lanzone A. Insulin and polycystic ovary syndrome: a new look at an old subject. *Gynecol Endocrinol* 12(4): 277–292, 1998.
2. Gamayunova VB, et al. Comparative study of blood insulin levels in breast and endometrial cancer patients. *Neoplasma* 44(2): 123–126, 1997.

Chapter 7

1. Adami S, et al. Effect of hyperandrogenism and menstrual cycle abnormalities on bone mass and bone turnover in young women. *Clin Endocrinol* 48(2): 169–173, 1998.
2. Andersson B, et al. Estrogen replacement therapy decreases hyperandrogenicity and improves glucose homeostasis and plasma lipids in postmenopausal women with non-insulin–dependent diabetes mellitus. *J Clin Endocrinol Metab* 82(2): 638–643, 1997.

Chapter 8
No notes.

Chapter 9
No notes.

Chapter 10

1. Schmidt JB. Other antiandrogens. *Dermatology* 196(1): 153–157, 1998.
2. Sandow N. Rxlist—The Internet Drug Index. Hyperlink: "http://www.rxlist.com", 1995.
3. Veldhuis JD, Dufau ML. Steroidal regulation of biologically active luteinizing hormone secretion in men and women. *Hum Reprod* 8(suppl 2): 84–96, 1993.
4. Di Silverio F, et al. Effects of long-term treatment with *Serenoa repens* (Permixon) on the concentrations and regional distribution of androgens and epidermal growth factor in benign prostatic hyperplasia. *Prostate* 37(2): 77–83, 1998.
5. Ducrey B, et al. Inhibition of 5 alpha-reductase and aromatase by the ellagitannins oenothein A and oenothein B from Epilobium species. *Planta Med* 63(2): 111–114, 1997.
6. Borvendeg J, et al. Antiestrogens, antiandrogens. *Acta Physiol Hung* 84(4): 405–406, 1996.
7. Miossec P, et al. [Inhibition of steroidogenesis by ketoconazole. Therapeutic uses]. [Article in French] *Ann Endocrinol* 58(6): 494–502, 1997.
8. Tsafriri A, et al. Effects of ketoconazole on ovulatory changes in the rat: implications on the role of a meiosis-activating sterol. *Mol Hum Reprod* 4(5): 483–489, 1998.
9. Duke, JA. *Handbook of Phytochemical Constituents of GRAS Herbs and Other Economic Plants*. Boca Raton, FL: CRC Press, 1992.
10. Same as 6.
11. Same as 7.
12. Same as 8.
13. Latrille F, et al. A comparative study of the effects of ketoconazole and fluconazole on 17-beta estradiol production by rat ovaries in vitro. *Res Commun Chem Pathol Pharmacol* 64(1): 173–176, 1989.
14. Same as 2.
15. Barbieri RL, et al. Nicotine, cotinine, and anabasine inhibit aromatase in human trophoblast in vitro. *J Clin Invest* 77(6): 1727–1733, 1986.
16. Kadohama N, et al. Tobacco alkaloid derivatives as inhibitors of breast cancer aromatase. *Cancer Lett* 75(3): 175–182, 1993.
17. Di Silverio F, et al. Evidence that *Serenoa repens* extract displays an antiestrogenic activity in prostatic tissue of benign prostatic hypertrophy patients. *Eur Urol* 21(4): 309–314, 1992.
18. Same as 5.
19. Same as 14.
20. Erickson GF, et al. Morphology and physiology of the ovary. IN: Becker KL, ed. *Principles and Practice of Endocrinology and Metabolism*. Philadelphia: JB Lippincott, 1995: 1873.
21. Gu Y, et al. Inhibitory effect of gossypol on steroidogenic pathways in cultured bovine luteal cells. *Biochem Biophys Res Commun* 169(2): 455–461, 1990.

22. Kono H, et al. Effects of progesterone and gossypol on monoamine oxidase activity in human term placental explant. *Tohoku J Exp Med* 163(1): 39–45, 1991.
23. Huang HF, Wang M. [Effects of gossypol acetate, danazol, progesterone and GnRH-A on estrogen and progesterone receptors of human endometrial cells]. [Article in Chinese] *Chung Kuo Chung Hsi I Chieh Ho Tsa Chih* 14(6): 325, 352–353, 1994.
24. Yang YQ, Wu XY. Antifertility mechanisms of gossypol acetic acid in female rats. *J Reprod Fertil* 80(2): 425–429, 1987.
25. Duke, JA. *Handbook of Phytochemical Constituents of GRAS Herbs and Other Economic Plants.* Boca Raton, FL: CRC Press, 1992.

Chapter 11

1. Neve J. Clinical implications of trace elements in endocrinology. *Biol Trace Elem Res* 32: 173–185, 1992.
2. Nielsen FH. Biochemical and physiologic consequences of boron deprivation in humans. *Environ Health Perspect* 102(suppl 7): 59–63, 1994.
3. Naghii MR, Samman S. The role of boron in nutrition and metabolism. *Prog Food Nutr Sci* 17(4): 331–349, 1993.
4. Beattie JH, Peace HS. The influence of a low-boron diet and boron supplementation on bone, major mineral and sex steroid metabolism in postmenopausal women. *Br J Nutr* 1993 May; 69(3): 871–884, 1993.
5. Same as 3.
6. Hunt CD, et al. Dietary boron modifies the effects of vitamin D_3 nutrition on indices of energy substrate utilization and mineral metabolism in the chick. *J Bone Miner Res* 9(2): 171–182, 1994.
7. Same as 3.
8. Baeksgaard L, et al. Calcium and vitamin D supplementation increases spinal BMD in healthy, postmenopausal women. *Osteoporos Int* 8(3): 255–260, 1998.
9. Rossier MF, et al. Sources and sites of action of calcium in the regulation of aldosterone biosynthesis. *Endocr Res* 22(4): 579–588, 1996.
10. Hori H, et al. Effects of GnRH on protein kinase C activity, Ca2+ mobilization and steroidogenesis of human granulosa cells. *Endocr J* 45(2): 175–182, 1998.
11. Mathias SA, et al. Modulation of adrenal cell functions by cadmium salts. 4. Ca(2+)-dependent sites affected by CdCl2 during basal and ACTH-stimulated steroid synthesis. *Cell Biol Toxicol* 14(3): 225–236, 1998.
12. Matsuki M, et al. Effects of calcium channel blockers on steroidogenesis stimulated by ACTH and CAMP in isolated rat adrenal cells. *Horm Metab Res* 28(8): 374–376, 1996.
13. Carr BR, et al. The role of calcium in steroidogenesis in fetal zone cells of the human fetal adrenal gland. *J Clin Endocrinol Metab* 63(4): 913–917, 1986.
14. Same as 13.
15. Tsang BK, Carnegie JA. Calcium-dependent regulation of progesterone production by isolated rat granulosa cells: effects of the calcium ionophore A23187, prostaglandin E2, dl-isoproterenol and cholera toxin. *Biol Reprod* 30(4): 787–794, 1984.
16. Seelig MS. Increased need for magnesium with the use of combined oestrogen and calcium for osteoporosis treatment. *Magnes Res* 3(3): 197–215, 1990.
17. McCarty MF. Anabolic effects of insulin on bone suggest a role for chromium picolinate in preservation of bone density. *Med Hypotheses* 45(3): 241–246, 1995.
18. Sugino N, et al. Hormonal regulation of copper-zinc superoxide dismutase and manganese superoxide dismutase messenger ribonucleic acid in the rat

corpus luteum: induction by prolactin and placental lactogens. *Biol Reprod* 59(3): 599–605, 1998.

19. Sugino N, et al. Differential regulation of copper-zinc superoxide dismutase and manganese superoxide dismutase in the rat corpus luteum: induction of manganese superoxide dismutase messenger ribonucleic acid by inflammatory cytokines. *Biol Reprod* 59(1): 208–215, 1998.

20. Tamate K, et al. The role of superoxide dismutase in the human ovary and fallopian tube. *J Obstet Gynaecol* 21(4): 401–409, 1995.

21. Ishikawa M. [Oxygen radicals-superoxide dismutase system and reproduction medicine]. [Article in Japanese] *Nippon Sanka Fujinka Gakkai Zasshi* 45(8): 842–848, 1993.

22. Mason KE. A conspectus of research on copper metabolism and requirements of man. *J Nutr* 109(11): 1979–2066, 1979.

23. Lindeman RD. Trace minerals: hormonal and metabolic interrelationships. IN: Becker KL, ed. *Principles and Practice of Endocrinology and Metabolism.* Philadelphia: JB Lippincott, 1995.

24. Same as 18.

25. Same as 19.

26. Same as 20.

27. Same as 21.

28. Same as 22.

29. Hollowell JG et al. Iodine nutrition in the United States. Trends and public health implications: iodine excretion data from National Health and Nutrition Examination Surveys I and III (1971–1974 and 1988–1994). *J. Clin Endocrinol Metab* 83 (10): 3401–3408, 1998.

30. Smyth PP, et al. A direct relationship between thyroid enlargement and breast cancer. *J Clin Endocrinol Metab* 81(3): 937–941, 1996.

31. Smyth PP. Thyroid disease and breast cancer. *J Endocrinol Invest* 16(5): 396–401, 1993.

32. Kondo K, et al. Effects of maternal iodine deficiency and thyroidectomy on basal neuroendocrine function in rat pups. *J Endocrinol* 152(3): 423–430, 1997.

33. Black SM, et al. Regulation of proteins in the cholesterol side chain cleavage system in JEG-3 and Y-1 cells. *Endocrinology* 132(2): 539–545, 1993.

34. Boyd GS, et al. Cholesterol metabolism in the adrenal cortex. *J Steroid Biochem* 19(1C): 1017–1027, 1983.

35. Barbieri RL, et al. Cotinine and nicotine inhibit human fetal adrenal 11 beta-hydroxylase. *J Clin Endocrinol Metab* 69(6): 1221–1224, 1989.

36. Snyder GD, et al. Nitric oxide inhibits aromatase activity: mechanisms of action. *J Steroid Biochem Mol Biol* 58(1): 63–69, 1996.

37. Suckling KE, et al. In vitro regulation of bovine adrenal cortical acyl-CoA: cholesterol acyltransferase and comparison with the rat liver enzyme. *Biochim Biophys Acta* 753(3): 422–429, 1983.

38. Mikosha AS, et al. [Properties of adrenocortical isocitrate dehydrogenase]. [Article in Russian] *Vopr Med Khim* 27(6): 736–739, 1981.

39. Scheen AJ. Perspective in the treatment of insulin resistance. *Hum Reprod* 12 (suppl 1): 63–71, 1997.

40. Seelig MS. Increased need for magnesium with the use of combined oestrogen and calcium for osteoporosis treatment. *Magnes Res* 3(3): 197–215, 1990.

41. Gaby, AR. *Preventing and Reversing Osteoporosis.* Rocklin CA: Prima Publishing, 1994.

42. Sasaki J, et al. Detection of manganese superoxide dismutase mRNA in the theca interna cells of rat ovary during the ovulatory process by in situ hybridization. *Histochemistry* 102(3): 173–176, 1994.

43. Same as 38.
44. Same as 38.
45. Nomura T, et al. Expression of manganese superoxide dismutase mRNA in reproductive organs during the ovulatory process and the estrous cycle of the rat. *Histochem Cell Biol* 105(1): 1–6, 1996.
46. Begin-Heick N, Deeks JR. Hypercorticism and manganese metabolism in brown adipose tissue of the obese mouse. *J Nutr* 117(10): 1708–1714, 1987.
47. Weiss SL, Sunde RA. Selenium regulation of classical glutathione peroxidase expression requires the 3' untranslated region in Chinese hamster ovary cells. *J Nutr* 127(7):1304–1310, 1997.
48. Paszkowski T, et al. Selenium dependent glutathione peroxidase activity in human follicular fluid. *Clin Chim Acta* 236(2): 173–180, 1995.
49. Kamada H, Ikumo H. Effect of selenium on cultured bovine luteal cells. *Anim Reprod Sci* 46(3–4): 203–211, 1997.
50. Brichard SM, et al. Long term improvement of glucose homeostasis by vanadate treatment in diabetic rats. *Endocrinology* 123(4): 2048–2053, 1988.
51. Poucheret P, et al. Vanadium and diabetes. *Mol Cell Biochem* 88(1–2): 73–80, 1998.
52. Reddy RL, et al. Effects of vanadyl sulphate on ornithine decarboxylase and progesterone levels in the ovary of rat. *Biochem Int* 18(2): 467–474, 1989.
53. Hayashi Y, Kimura T. Vanadium inhibits ACTH-mediated but not cyclic AMP-dependent adrenal steroidogenesis. Mol Cell *Endocrinol* 44(1): 17–24, 1986.
54. Hayashi Y, Kimura T. Inhibition by vanadyl of adenylate cyclase activation reactions in rat adrenal membranes. *Biochem Biophys Res Commun* 130(3): 945–951, 1985.
55. Same as 54.
56. Sandhoff TW, et al. Transcriptional regulation of the rat steroidogenic acute regulatory protein gene by steroidogenic factor 1. *Endocrinology* 139(12): 4820–4831, 1998.
57. Lindeman RD. Trace minerals: hormonal and metabolic interrelationships. IN: Becker KL, ed. *Principles and Practice of Endocrinology and Metabolism.* Philadelphia: JB Lippincott, 1995.
58. Uria JA, Werb Z. Matrix metalloproteinases and their expression in mammary gland. *Cell Res* 8(3): 187–194, 1998.
59. Slootweg MC, et al. Estrogen enhances growth hormone receptor expression and growth hormone action in rat osteosarcoma cells and human osteoblast-like cells. *J Endocrinol* 155(1): 159–164, 1997.
60. Omura T, Morohashi K. Gene regulation of steroidogenesis. *J Steroid Biochem Mol Biol* 53(1–6): 19–25, 1995.
61. Taneja SK, Kaur R. Pathology of ovary, uterus, vagina and gonadotrophs of female mice fed on Zn-deficient diet. *Indian J Exp Biol* 28(11): 1058–1065, 1990.
62. Lipman TO, Vitamins: hormonal and metabolic interrelationships. IN: Becker Kl, ed. *Principles and Practice of Endocrinology and Metabolism.* Philadelphia: JB Lippincott, 1995.
63. Strumilo SA, et al. Effect of oxythiamine on adrenal thiamine pyrophosphate-dependent enzyme activities. *Biomed Biochim Acta* 43(2):159–163, 1984.
64. Strumilo SA, et al. [Enzyme activity of thiamine pyrophosphate in the rat after oxythiamine administration]. [Article in Russian] *Biull Eksp Biol Med* 96(11): 42–44, 1983.
65. Neher R, Milani A. Pyruvate and thiamine pyrophosphate potentiate cyclic nucleotide-induced steroidogenesis in isolated rat adrenocortical cells. *J Steroid Biochem* 18(1): 1–6, 1983.
66. Vinogradov VV, et al. [Thiamine prevention of the corticosteroid reaction afer surgery]. [Article in Russian] *Probl Endokrinol* 27(3): 11–16, 1981.

67. Shelygina NM, et al. [Influence of vitamins C, B₁, and B₆ on the diurnal periodicity of the glucocorticoid function of the adrenal cortex in patients with atherosclerotic cardiosclerosis]. [Article in Russian] *Vopr Pitan* 2: 25–29, 1975.

68. Hastings MM, Van JL. Sodium deprivation during thiamin deficiency in rats: hormonal, histological, and behavioral responses. *J Nutr* 111(11): 1955–1963, 1981.

69. Same as 62.

70. Pinto JT, et al. Adriamycin-induced increase in serum aldosterone levels: effects in riboflavin-sufficient and riboflavin-deficient rats. *Endocrinology* 127(3): 1495–1501, 1990.

71. Hanukoglu I, Rapoport R. Routes and regulation of NADPH production in steroidogenic mitochondria. *Endocr Res* 21(1–2): 231–241, 1995.

72. Same as 33.

73. Benelli C, et al. Effect of thyroidectomy on pregnenolone and progesterone biosynthesis in rat adrenal cortex. *J Steroid Biochem* 16(6):749–754, 1982.

74. Lipman TO. Vitamins: hormonal and metabolic interrelationships. IN: Becker KL, ed. *Principles and Practice of Endocrinology and Metabolism.* Philadelphia: JB Lippincott, 1995.

75. Vinogradov VV, et al. [Mechanisms of the antilipemic action of niacin]. [Article in Russian] *Vopr Pitan* 1: 36–40, 1978.

76. Vinogradov VV, et al. [Further comment on the lipotropic action of niacin]. [Article in Russian] *Vopr Pitan* 2: 34–40, 1979.

77. Pietrzik K, et al. [Influencing of acetylation and corticosterone biosynthesis through long-term pantothenic acid deficiency in rats]. [Article in German] *Int J Vitam Nutr Res* 45(3): 251–261, 1975.

78. Tarasov IUA, et al. [Adrenal cortex functional activity in pantothenate deficiency and the administration of the vitamin or its derivatives]. [Article in Russian] *Vopr Pitan* 4: 51–54, 1985.

79. Schwabedal PE, et al. Pantothenic acid deficiency as a factor contributing to the development of hypertension. *Cardiology* 72(suppl 1): 187–189, 1985.

80. Same as 78.

81. Bermond P. Therapy of side effects of oral contraceptive agents with vitamin B₆. *Acta Vitaminol Enzymol* 4(1–2): 45–54, 1982.

82. el-Zoghby SM, et al. Functional capacity of the tryptophan-niacin pathway in the premenarchial phase and in the menopausal age. *Am J Clin Nutr* 28(1): 4–9, 1975.

83. Haspels AA, et al. Disturbance of tryptophan metabolism and its correction during oestrogen treatment in postmenopausal women. *Maturitas* 1(1): 15–20, 1978.

84. Wolf H, et al. Effect of natural oestrogens on tryptophan metabolism: evidence for interference of oestrogens with kynureninase. *Scand J Clin Lab Invest* 40(1): 15–22, 1980.

85. Jovanovic-Peterson L, Peterson CM. Vitamin and mineral deficiencies which may predispose to glucose intolerance of pregnancy. *J Am Coll Nutr* 15(1): 14–20, 1996.

86. Chan MM, Kare MR. Effect of vitamin B₆ deficiency on preference for several taste solutions in the rat. *J Nutr* 109(2): 339–344, 1979.

87. Same as 67.

88. Steegers-Theunissen RP, et al. Study on the presence of homocysteine in ovarian follicular fluid. *Fertil Steril* 60(6): 1006–1010, 1993.

89. Same as 81.

90. Same as 82.

91. Mgongo FO, et al. The influence of cobalt/vitamin B₁₂ deficiency as a "stressor" affecting adrenal cortex and ovarian activities in goats. *Reprod Nutr Dev* 24(6): 845–854, 1984.

92. Mgongo FO, et al. Effects of cobalt deficiency on the ovarian function in the East African short-horned goat. *Beitr Trop Landwirtsch Veterinarmed* 23(2): 207–216, 1985.

93. Ross R. Factors influencing atherogenesis. In: Hurst JW, Schlant RC, Rackley CE, Sonnenblick EH, Wenger NK, eds. *The Heart, Arteries and Veins.* New York: McGraw-Hill, 1990: 877–923.

94. Stampfer MJ, et al. A prospective study of plasma homocysteine and risk of myocardial infarction in US physicians. *JAMA* 268(7): 877–881, 1992.

95. Miller AL, Kelly GS. Homocysteine metabolism: nutritional modulation and impact on health and disease. *Alt Med Rev* 2(4): 234–254, 1997.

96. Same as 88.

97. Illnerova H: Entrainment of mammalian circadian rhythms in melatonin production by light. *Pineal Res Rev* 6: 173–217, 1988.

98. Reiter RJ: Action spectra, dose response relationships and temporal aspects of light's effects on the pineal gland; The medical and biological effects of light. *Ann NY Acad Sci* 453: 215–230, 1985.

99. Nakamura T, et al. Transient fluctuation of serum melatonin rhythm is suppressed centrally by vitamin B_{12}. *Chronobiol Int* 14(6): 549–560, 1997.

100. Okawa M, et al. Vitamin B_{12} treatment for sleep-wake rhythm disorders. *Sleep* 13: 1–23, 1990.

101. Mayer G, et al. Effects of vitamin B_{12} on performance and circadian rhythm in normal subjects. *Neuropsychopharmacology* 15: 456–464, 1996.

102. Kohsaka M. [Non-24-hour sleep-wake syndrome]. [Article in Japanese] *Nippon Rinsho* 56(2): 410–415, 1998.

103. Same as 18.

104. Same as 19.

105. Kwaśniewska A, et al. Folate deficiency and cervical intraepithelial neoplasia. *Eur J Gynaecol Oncol* 18(6): 526–530, 1997.

106. Same as 96.

107. Mohanty D, Das KC. Effect of folate deficiency on the reproductive organs of female rhesus monkeys: a cytomorphological and cytokinetic study. *J Nutr* 112(8): 1565–1576, 1982.

108. Azhar S, et al. Alteration of the adrenal antioxidant defense system during aging in rats. *J Clin Invest* 96(3): 1414–1424, 1995.

109. Same as 108.

110. Laney PH, et al. Plasma cortisol and adrenal ascorbic acid levels after ACTH treatment with a high intake of ascorbic acid in the guinea pig. *Ann Nutr Metab* 34(2):85–92, 1990.

111. Doulas NL, et al. Effect of ascorbic acid on guinea pig adrenal adenylate cyclase activity and plasma cortisol. *J Nutr* 117(6):1108–1114, 1987.

112. Musicki B, et al. Endocrine regulation of ascorbic acid transport and secretion in luteal cells. *Biol Reprod* 54(2):399–406, 1996.

113. Byrd JA, et al. Effect of ascorbate on luteinizing hormone stimulated progesterone biosynthesis in chicken granulosa cells in vitro. *Comp Biochem Physiol Comp Physiol* 104(2): 279–281, 1993.

114. Gruber KA, et al. Vitamin A: not required for adrenal steroidogenesis in rats. *Science* 191(4226): 472–475, 1976.

115. Rapoport R, et al. Antioxidant capacity is correlated with steroidogenic status of the corpus luteum during the bovine estrous cycle. *Biochim Biophys Acta* 1380(1): 133–140, 1998.

116. Same as 115.

117. Schweigert FJ, Zucker H. Concentrations of vitamin A, beta-carotene and vitamin E in individual bovine follicles of different quality. *J Reprod Fertil* 82(2): 575–579, 1988.

118. Rodgers RJ, et al. The physiology of the ovary: maturation of ovarian granu-losa cells and a novel role for antioxidants in the corpus luteum. *J Steroid Biochem Mol Biol* 53(1–6): 241–246, 1995.

119. Young FM, et al. The antioxidant beta-carotene prevents covalent cross-linking between cholesterol side chain cleavage cytochrome P450 and its electron donor, adrenodoxin, in bovine luteal cells. *Mol Cell Endocrinol* 109(1): 113–118, 1995.

120. Jackson PS, et al. Endocrine and ovarian changes in dairy cattle fed a low beta-carotene diet during an oestrus synchronisation regime. *Res Vet Sci* 1(3): 377–383, 1981.

121. Talavera F, Chew BP. Comparative role of retinol, retinoic acid and beta-carotene on progesterone secretion by pig corpus luteum in vitro. *J Reprod Fertil* 82(2): 611–615, 1988.

122. Graves-Hoagland RL, et al. Relationship of plasma beta-carotene and vita-min A to luteal function in postpartum cattle. *J Dairy Sci* 72(7): 1854–1858, 1989.

123. Same as 122.

124. Bindas EM, et al. Reproductive and metabolic characteristics of dairy cattle supplemented with beta-carotene. *J Dairy Sci* 67(6): 1249–1255, 1984.

125. Folman Y, et al. Fertility of dairy heifers given a commercial diet free of beta-carotene. *Br J Nutr* 41(2): 353–359, 1979.

126. Wang JY, et al. Effect of beta-carotene supplementation on reproductive performance of lactating Holstein cows. *J Dairy Sci* 71(1): 181–186, 1988.

127. Wang JY, et al. Effect of supplemental beta-carotene on luteinizing hor-mone released in response to gonadotropin-releasing hormone challenge in ovariectomized Holstein cows. *J Dairy Sci* 71(2): 498–504, 1988.

128. Folman Y, et al. The effect of dietary and climatic factors on fertility, and on plasma progesterone and oestradiol-17 beta levels in dairy cows. *J Steroid Biochem* 19(1C): 863–868, 1983.

129. Szulc P, et al. Serum undercarboxylated osteocalcin is a marker of the risk of hip fracture in elderly women. *J Clin Invest* 91(4):1769–1774, 1993.

130. Tuppurainen MT, et al. Does vitamin D strengthen the increase in femoral neck BMD in osteoporotic women treated with estrogen? *Osteoporos Int* 8(1): 32–38, 1998.

131. Somjen D, et al. Pretreatment with 1,25(OH)2 vitamin D or 24,25(OH)2 vi-tamin D increases synergistically responsiveness to sex steroids in skeletal-derived cells. *J Steroid Biochem Mol Biol* 55(2): 211–217, 1995.

132. Graafmans WC, et al. The effect of vitamin D supplementation on the bone mineral density of the femoral neck is associated with vitamin D receptor genotype. *J Bone Miner Res* 12(8): 1241–1245, 1997.

133. Baeksgaard L, et al. Calcium and vitamin D supplementation increases spinal BMD in healthy, postmenopausal women. *Osteoporos Int* 8(3): 255–260, 1998.

134. Hallworth RB. Prevention and treatment of postmenopausal osteoporosis. *Pharm World Sci* 20(5): 198–205, 1998.

135. Willhite L. Osteoporosis in women: prevention and treatment. *J Am Pharm Assoc* 38(5): 614–623; discussion 623–4, 1998.

136. Trang HM, et al. Evidence that vitamin D_3 increases serum 25-hydroxyvita-min D more efficiently than does vitamin D_2. *Am J Clin Nutr* 68(4): 854–858, 1998.

137. Kadowaki S, Norman AW. Time course study of insulin secretion after 1,25-dihydroxyvitamin D_3 administration. *Endocrinology* 117(5): 1765–1771, 1985.

138. Billaudel BJ, et al. Effect of 1,25 dihydroxyvitamin D_3 on isolated islets from vitamin D_3-deprived rats. *Am J Physiol* 258(4 Pt 1): E643–E648, 1990.

139. Bourlon PM, et al. Influence of vitamin D_3 deficiency and 1,25 dihydroxyvitamin D3 on de novo insulin biosynthesis in the islets of the rat endocrine pancreas. *J Endocrinol* 160(1): 87–95, 1999.
140. Same as 139.
141. Allegra V, et al. Glucose-induced insulin secretion in uremia: role of 1 alpha,25(HO) 2vitamin D_3. *Nephron* 68(1): 41–47, 1994.
142. Zofkova I, Stolba P. Effect of calcitriol and trifluoperazine on glucose stimulated B cell function in healthy humans. *Exp Clin Endocrinol* 96(2):185–191, 1990.
143. Nyomba BL, et al. Pancreatic secretion in man with subclinical vitamin D deficiency. *Diabetologia* 29(1): 34–38, 1986.
144. Stumpf WE. Vitamin D—soltriol the heliogenic steroid hormone: somatotrophic activator and modulator. Discoveries from histochemical studies lead to new concepts. *Histochemistry* 89(3): 209–219, 1988.
145. Barnes MM, Smith AJ. The effects of vitamin E deficiency on some enzymes of steroid hormone biosynthesis. *Int J Vitam Nutr Res* 45(4): 396–403, 1975.
146. Aten RF, et al. Ovarian vitamin E accumulation: evidence for a role of lipoproteins. *Endocrinology* 135(2): 533–539, 1994.
147. Rapoport R, et al. Antioxidant capacity is correlated with steroidogenic status of the corpus luteum during the bovine estrous cycle. *Biochim Biophys Acta* 1380(1): 133–140, 1998.
148. London RS, et al. The effect of alpha-tocopherol on premenstrual symptomatology: a double-blind study. II. Endocrine correlates. *J Am Coll Nutr* 3(4): 351–356, 1984.
149. London RS, et al. Endocrine parameters and alpha-tocopherol therapy of patients with mammary dysplasia. *Cancer Res* 41(9 Pt 2): 3811–3813, 1981.
150. Guthrie N, et al. Inhibition of proliferation of estrogen receptor-negative MDA-MB-435 and -positive MCF-7 human breast cancer cells by palm oil tocotrienols and tamoxifen, alone and in combination. *J Nutr* 127(3): 544S–548S, 1997.
151. Nesaretnam K, et al. Tocotrienols inhibit the growth of human breast cancer cells irrespective of estrogen receptor status. *Lipids* 33(5): 461–469, 1998.
152. Wener KM, et al. The effect of estradiol-induced hypothalamic pathology on sulfated glycoprotein-2 (clusterin) expression in the hypothalamus. *Brain Res* 745(1–2): 37–45, 1997.
153. Desjardins GC, et al. Vitamin E protects hypothalamic beta-endorphin neurons from estradiol neurotoxicity. *Endocrinology* 131(5): 2482–2484, 1992.
154. Desjardins GC, et al. Estradiol is selectively neurotoxic to hypothalamic beta-endorphin neurons. *Endocrinology* 132(1): 86–93, 1993.
155. Brawer JR, et al. Pathologic effect of estradiol on the hypothalamus. *Biol Reprod* 49(4): 647–652, 1993.
156. Same as 148.
157. Same as 150.
158. Yang SL, et al. Effects of long-term estradiol exposure on the hypothalamic neuron number. *Acta Endocrinol* 29(6): 543–547, 1993.
159. Brawer JR, et al. Ovary-dependent degeneration in the hypothalamic arcuate nucleus. *Endocrinology* 107(1): 274–279, 1980.
160. Chan AC. Vitamin E and atherosclerosis. *J Nutr* 128(10): 1593–1596, 1998.
161. Williams JC, et al. Dietary vitamin E supplementation inhibits thrombin-induced platelet aggregation, but not monocyte adhesiveness, in patients with hypercholesterolaemia. *Int J Exp Pathol* 78(4): 259–266, 1997.
162. Freedman JE, et al. Alpha-tocopherol inhibits aggregation of human platelets by a protein kinase C-dependent mechanism. *Circulation* 94(10): 2434–2440, 1996.

163. Nakano Y, et al. Effect of 17-beta-estradiol on inhibition of platelet aggregation in vitro is mediated by an increase in NO synthesis. *Arterioscler Thromb Vasc Biol* 18(6): 961–967, 1998.

164. Berge LN, et al. Female sex hormones and platelet/endothelial cell interactions. *Haemostasis* 20(6): 313–320, 1990.

165. Ciavatti M, et al. Vitamin E prevents the platelet abnormalities induced by estrogen in rat. *Contraception* .30(3): 279–287, 1984.

166. Renaud S, et al. Influence of vitamin E administration on platelet functions in hormonal contraceptive users. *Contraception* .36(3): 347–358, 1987.

167. Qiu J, et al. Experimental study on antiatherosclerotic treatment by PGE2 combined with vitamin E and estradiol. *Chin Med J (Engl)* 108(1): 33–36, 1995.

168. Robinson JN, et al. Coagulopathy secondary to vitamin K deficiency in hyperemesis gravidarum. *Obstet Gynecol* 92(4 Pt 2): 673–675, 1998.

169. Ekenstam E, et al. The acute effect of high dose corticosteroid treatment on serum osteocalcin. *Metabolism* 37(2): 141–144, 1988.

170. Szulc P, et al. Serum undercarboxylated osteocalcin is a marker of the risk of hip fracture: a three year follow-up study. *Bone* 18(5): 487–488, 1996.

171. Szulc P, et al. Serum undercarboxylated osteocalcin is a marker of the risk of hip fracture in elderly women. *J Clin Invest* 91(4): 1769–1774, 1993.

172. Sharaev PN, et al. [Collagen metabolism in the skin with different vitamin K regimens]. [Article in Russian] *Biull Eksp Biol Med* 81(6): 665–666, 1976.

173. Pushina NG. [Relation between ascorbic acid metabolism and the body's supply of vitamin K]. [Article in Russian] *Vopr Pitan* 3: 36–42, 1982.

174. Willard ST, Frawley LS. Phytoestrogens have agonistic and combinatorial effects on estrogen-responsive gene expression in MCF-7 human breast cancer cells. *Endocrine* 8(2): 117–121, 1998.

175. Charland SL, et al. The effects of a soybean extract on tumor growth and metastasis. *Int J Mol Med* 2(2): 225–228, 1998.

176. Bingham SA, et al. Phyto-oestrogens: where are we now? *Br J Nutr* 79(5): 393–406, 1998.

177. Shoff SM, et al. Usual consumption of plant foods containing phytoestrogens and sex hormone levels in postmenopausal women in Wisconsin. *Nutr Cancer* 30(3): 207–212, 1998.

178. Same as 181.

179. Reinli K, Block G. Phytoestrogen content of foods—a compendium of literature values. *Nutr Cancer* 26(2): 123–148, 1996.

180. Hutchins AM, et al. Vegetables, fruits, and legumes: effect on urinary isoflavonoid phytoestrogen and lignan excretion. *J Am Diet Assoc* 95(7): 769–774, 1995.

181. Obermeyer WR, et al. Chemical studies of phytoestrogens and related compounds in dietary supplements: flax and chaparral. *Proc Soc Exp Biol Med* 208(1): 6–12, 1995.

182. Thompson LU. Antioxidants and hormone-mediated health benefits of whole grains. *Crit Rev Food Sci Nutr* 34(5–6): 473–497, 1994.

183. Slavin JL. Epidemiological evidence for the impact of whole grains on health. *Crit Rev Food Sci Nutr* 34(5–6): 427–434, 1994.

184. Mayr U, et al. Validation of two in vitro test systems for estrogenic activities with zearalenone, phytoestrogens and cereal extracts. *Toxicology* 74(2–3): 135–149, 1992.

185. Seely S. The possible connection between phytoestrogens, milk and coronary heart disease. *Med Hypotheses* 8(4): 349–354, 1982.

186. Goodman MT, et al. Association of soy and fiber consumption with the risk of endometrial cancer. *Am J Epidemiol* 146(4): 294–306, 1997.

187. Lewis RD, Modlesky CM. Nutrition, physical activity, and bone health in women. *Int J Sport Nutr* 8(3): 250–284, 1998.
188. Fanti P, et al. The phytoestrogen genistein reduces bone loss in short-term ovariectomized rats. *Osteoporos Int* 8(3): 274–281, 1998.
189. Murkies AL, et al. Clinical review 92: Phytoestrogens. *J Clin Endocrinol Metab* 83(2): 297–303, 1998.
190. Knight DC, Eden JA. A review of the clinical effects of phytoestrogens. *Obstet Gynecol* 87(5 Pt 2): 897–904, 1996.
191. Barnes S. Evolution of the health benefits of soy isoflavones. *Proc Soc Exp Biol Med* 217(3): 386–392, 1998.
192. Same as 181.
193. Brandi ML. Natural and synthetic isoflavones in the prevention and treatment of chronic diseases. *Calcif Tissue Int* 61(suppl 1): S5–S8, 1997.
194. Tansey G, et al. Effects of dietary soybean estrogens on the reproductive tract in female rats. *Proc Soc Exp Biol Med* 217(3): 340–344, 1998.
195. Same as 191.
196. Murkies AL, et al. Dietary flour supplementation decreases post-menopausal hot flushes: effect of soy and wheat. *Maturitas* 21(3): 189–195, 1995.

Chapter 12

1. Sherman JA. *The Complete Botanical Prescriber.* Portland OR: John Sherman, 1993.
2. Duke JA. *CRC Handbook of Medicinal Herbs.* Boca Raton, FL: CRC Press, 1985.
3. Same as 2.
4. Singh HK, Dhawan BN. Effect of *Bacopa monniera* Linn. (*brahmi*) extract on avoidance responses in rat. *J Ethnopharmacol* 5(2): 205–214, 1982.
5. Bone, K, et al. *How to Prescribe Herbal Medicines.* Australia: Mediherb Pty Ltd, 1992.
6. Same as 5.
7. Bensky D, et al. *Chinese Herbal Medicine Materia Medica,* Seattle, WA: Eastland Press, 1986.
8. Jain SK. Ethnobotany and research on medicinal plants in India. *Ciba Found Symp* 185: 153–164; discussion 164–8, 1994.
9. Tripathi YB, et al. *Bacopa monniera* Linn. as an antioxidant: mechanism of action. *Indian J Exp Biol* 34(6): 523–526, 1996.
10. Same as 4.
11. Same as 5.
12. Same as 11.
13. Same as 9.
14. Same as 9.
15. Same as 10.
16. Brücker A. Essay on the phytotherapy of hormonal disorders in women. *Med. Welt.*; 44: 2331–2333, 1960.
17. Einer-Jensen N, et al. Cimicifuga and Melbrosia lack oestrogenic effects in mice and rats. *Maturitas* 25(2): 149–153, 1996.
18. Mills SY. *The Dictionary of Modern Herbalism.* Wellingborough, NY: Thorsons Publishing Group, 1985.
19. Same as 16.
20. Weiss RF. *Herbal Medicine.* Beaconsfield, England: Beaconsfield Publishers Ltd., 1988.
21. Lieberman S. A review of the effectiveness of *Cimicifuga racemosa* (black cohosh) for the symptoms of menopause. *J Women's Health.* 7(5): 525–529, 1998.
22. Same as 1.

23. Same as 18.
24. Priest AW, Priest, LR. *Herbal Medication: A Clinical and Dispensary Handbook.* Romford, Essex: L.N. Fowler & Co., Ltd., 1982.
25. Same as 2.
26. Chang HM et al. *Advances in Chinese Medicinal Materials Research.* Singapore: World Sci. Publ., 1985.
27. Chang H, But P. *Pharmacology and Application of Chinese Materia Medica,* Chinese University of Hong Kong, Singapore: World Scientific, 1987.
28. Hikino H, Kiso Y. Natural products for liver diseases. IN: Wagner H, et al., eds. *Economic and Medicinal Plant Research,* Vol 2. Orlando, FL: Academic Press, 1988.
29. Same as 11.
30. Same as 1.
31. Tyler VE, et al. *Pharmacognosy,* 9th Ed. Philadelphia: Lea & Febiger, 1988.
32. Felter JW, Lloyd JV. *Kings American Dispensatory.* Portland, OR: Eclectic Medical Publications, Republished 1983.
33. Same as 1.
34. Same as 32.
35. Grieve M. *A Modern Herbal.* New York, NY: Dover Publications, 1984.
36. Same as 1.
37. Same as 5.
38. Nicholson JA, et al. Viopudial, a hypotensive and smooth muscle antispasmodic from Viburnum opulus. *Proc Soc Exp Biol Med* 140(2): 457–461, 1972.
39. Same as 24.
40. *British Herbal Pharmacopoeia.* West Yorks, England: British Herbal Medicine Association, 1983.
41. Same as 35.
42. Alarcon-Aguilara FJ, et al. Study of the anti-hyperglycemic effect of plants used as antidiabetics. *J Ethnopharmacol* 61(2): 101–110, 1998.
43. Chang HM et al. *Pharmacology and Applications of Chinese Materia Medica,* Vol 1. Singapore: World Scientific Publ, 1986.
44. Hirata JD, et al. Does dong quai have estrogenic effects in postmenopausal women? A double-blind, placebo-controlled tiral. *Fertil Steril* 68(6): 981–986, 1997.
45. Wu H, et al. [Effects of different processed products of radix *Angelica sinensis* on clearing out oxygen free radicals and anti-lipid peroxidation]. [Article in Chinese] *Chung Kuo Chung Yao Tsa Chih* 21(10): 599–601, 639, 1996.
46. Choy YM, et al. Immunopharmacological studies of low molecular weight polysaccharide from *Angelica sinensis. Am J Chin Med* 22(2): 137–145, 1994.
47. Wang Y, Zhu B. [The effect of angelica polysaccharide on proliferation and differentiation of hematopoietic progenitor cell]. [Article in Chinese] *Chung Hua I Hsueh Tsa Chih* 76(5): 363–366, 1996.
48. Same as 1.
49. Ozaki Y. Antiinflammatory effect of tetramethylpyrazine and ferulic acid. *Chem Pharm Bull* 40(4): 954–956, 1992.
50. Same as 7.
51. Same as 1.
52. Same as 49.
53. Dai L, et al. [Using ligustrazini and *Angelica sinensis* to treat bleomycin-induced pulmonary fibrosis in rats]. [Article in Chinese] *Chung Hua Chieh Ho Ho Hu Hsi Tsa Chih* 19(1): 26–28, 1996.
54. Chen SG, et al. [Protective effects of *Angelica sinensis* injection on myocardial ischemia/reperfusion injury in rabbits]. [Article in Chinese] *Chung Kuo Chung Hsi I Chieh Ho Tsa Chih* 15(8) 486–488, 1995.
55. Same as 50.
56. Same as 55.

57. Same as 1.
58. Zhu DPQ. *American Journal of Chinese Medicine* 15(Nos. 3–4) 1987: 117–125, 1987.
59. Same as 35.
60. Same as 18.
61. Same as 59.
62. Same as 32.
63. Kuroda K, Takagi K. Physiologically active substance in Capsella bursa-pastoris. *Nature* 220(168): 707–708, 1968.
64. Hoffman D. *The Holistic Herbal.* Scotland, UK: Findhorn Press, 1983.
65. Same as 62.
66. Same as 62.
67. Same as 1.
68. Same as 42.
69. Shanmugasundaram KR, et al. The insulinotropic activity of Gymnema sylvestre, R. Br. An Indian medical herb used in controlling diabetes mellitus. *Pharmacol Res Commun* 13(5): 475–486.
70. Ajabnoor MA, Tilmisany AK. Effect of Trigonella foenum graceum on blood glucose levels in normal and alloxan-diabetic mice. *J. Ethnopharmacol* 22(1): 45–49, 1988.
71. Same as 11.
72. Same as 2.
73. Same as 7.
74. Same as 20.
75. Wong AH, et al. Herbal remedies in psychiatric practice. *Arch Gen Psychiatry* 55(11): 1033–1044, 1998.
76. Eckmann F. [Cerebral insufficiency—treatment with *ginkgo biloba* extract. Time of onset of effect in a double-blind study with 60 inpatients]. [Article in German.] *Fortschr Med* 108(29): 557–560, 1990.
77. Warburton DM. [Clinical psychopharmacology of *ginkgo biloba* extract]. Article in French. *Nouv Presse Med* 15(31): 1595–1604, 1986.
78. Weiss RF. *Herbal Medicine.* Beaconsfield, England: Beaconsfield Publishers Ltd. 1988.
79. Same as 78.
80. Milligan SR, et al. Identification of a potent phytoestrogen in hops (*Humulus lupulus* L.) and beer. *J Clin Endocrinol Metab* 84(6): 249–252, 1999.
81. Miranda CL, et al. Antiproliferative and cytotoxic effects of prenylated flavonoids from hops (*Humulus lupulus*) in human cancer cell lines. *Food Chem Toxicol* 37(4): 71–285, 1999.
82. Same as 18.
83. Same as 7.
84. Same as 1.
85. Same as 11.
86. Same as 11.
87. Same as 7.
88. Same as 1.
89. Same as 11.
90. Same as 7.
91. Same as 1.
92. Same as 11.
93. Tamaya T, et al. Inhibition by plant herb extracts of steroid bindings in uterus, liver and serum of the rabbit. *Acta Obstet Gynecol Scand* 65(8): 839–842, 1986.
94. Mooreville M, et al. Enhancement of the bladder defense mechanism by an exogenous agent. *J Urol* 130(3): 607–609, 1983.

95. Pantazopoulos, D. et al. The effect of pentosanpolysulphate and carbenox-olone on bacterial adherence to the injured urothelium. *Br J Urol* 59(5): 423–426, 1987.
96. Same as 7.
97. Goto H, et al., Effect of extract prepared from the roots of Paeonia lactiflora on endothelium-dependent relaxation and antioxidant enzyme activity in rats administered a high-fat diet. *Phytother Res* 13(6): 526–528, 1999.
98. Same as 1.
99. Same as 20.
100. Same as 18.
101. Same as 40.
102. Same as 24.
103. Same as 1.
104. Same as 11.
105. Kim H, et al. Effect of Rehmannia glutinosa on immediate type allergic re-action. *Int J Immunopharmacol* 1998 Apr–May; 20 (4–5): 231–240.
106. Kubo M, et al. Studies on rehmanniae radix. I. Effect of 50% ethanolic ex-tract from steamed and dried rehmanniae radix on hemorheology in arthritic and thrombosic rats. *Biol Pharm Bull* 17(9):1282–1286, 1994.
107. Miura T, et al. Antidiabetic effect of seishin-kanro-to in KK-Ay mice. *Planta Med* 63(4): 320–322, 1997.
108. Same as 7.
109. Same as 7.
110. Same as 2.
111. Same as 18.
112. Same as 18.
113. Schauenberg P, Paris F. *Guide to Medicinal Plants*. Cambridge, England: Lutterworth Press, 1977.
114. Same as 1.
115. Same as 18.
116. Same as 20.
117. Same as 1.
118. Lung A, Foster S. *Encyclopedia of Common Natural Ingredients*. New York: John Wiley & Sons, Inc., 1996.
119. Mowrey, DB. *Herbal Tonic Therapies*. New Canaan, CT: Keats Publishing, Inc., 1993.
120. Balch JF, Balch PA. *Prescription for Nutritional Healing*. Garden City Park, NY: Avery Publishing Group, 1990.
121. Same as 24.
122. Di Silverio F, et al. Effects of long-term treatment with *Serenoa repens* (Per-mixon) on the concentrations and regional distribution of androgens and epidermal growth factor in benign prostatic hyperplasia. *Prostate* 37(2): 77–83, 1998.
123. Di Silverio F, et al. Evidence that *Serenoa repens* extract displays an antiestro-genic activity in prostatic tissue of benign prostatic hypertrophy patients. *Eur Urol* 21(4): 309–314, 1992.
124. Same as 7.
125. Same as 27.
126. Same as 20.
127. Same as 35.
128. Same as 63.
129. Kuroda K, Takagi K. Studies on capsella bursa pastoris. II. Diuretic, anti-in-flammatory and anti-ulcer action of ethanol extracts of the herb. *Arch Int Pharmacodyn Ther* 178(2): 392–399, 1969.

130. Same as 63.
131. Shipochliev T. [Uterotonic action of extracts from a group of medicinal plants]. [Article in Bulgarian] *Vet Med Nauki* 18(4): 94–98, 1981.
132. Same as 11.
133. Same as 20.
134. Same as 11.
135. Farnsworth NR, et al. *Economic and Medicinal Plant Research*. Vol 1. London: Academic Press, 1985.
136. Fulder S. *The Root of Being*. London: Hutchinson and Co., 1980.
137. Same as 18.
138. Same as 1.
139. Same as 2.
140. Same as 24.
141. Same as 1.
142. Same as 2.
143. Houghton, P. J. The scientific basis for the reputed activity of valerian. *J Pharm Pharmacol* 51(5): 505–512, 1988.
144. Wagner H. et al. [Comparative studies on the sedative action of Valerian extracts, valepotriates and their degradation products.] [Article in German] *Planta Med* 39(4):, 358–365, 1980.
145. Same as 20.
146. Same as 20.
147. Same as 18.
148. Same as 35.
149. Same as 20.
150. Same as 18.
151. Same as 40.
152. Same as 40.
153. Trease GE, Evans WC. *Pharmacognosy*, 12th Ed., Kent, UK: Bailliere Tindall, 1983.
154. Same as 20.
155. Same as 153.
156. Same as 18.
157. Same as 2.
158. Same as 2.
159. Same as 20.
160. Same as 18.
161. Talalaj S, Czechowicz AS. *Herbal Remedies Harmful and Beneficial Effects*. Cincinnati, OH: Seven Hills Book Distributors, 1989.
162. Same as 24.
163. Same as 64.

Chapter 13

1. [Federal Register: September 23, 1997 (Volume 62, Number 184)] [Rules and Regulations] [Pages 49859–49868] From the Federal Register Online via GPO Access [wais.access.gpo.gov] [DOCID: fr23se97-16].
2. *Nobel Lectures, Physiology or Medicine 1922–1941*. Amsterdam: Elsevier Publishing Company, 1970.
3. Harrower HR. *An Endocrine Handbook*. Glendale, CA: The Harrower Laboratory, Inc., 1939.
4. Same as 3.
5. Gardner MLG. Intestinal assimilation of intact peptides and proteins from the diet—a neglected field? Cambridge Philosophical Society, *Biol Rev* 59: 289–331, 1984.

6. Low TLK, Goldstein AI. The thymic hormones; an overview. *Methods Enzymol* 16: 213–219, 1985.
7. Jankovick BD, Koroliyam P. et al. Immunorestorative effects in elderly humans of lipid and protein fractions from calf thymus: a double blind study. *Ann NY Acad Sci* 521: 247–257, 1988.
8. Simonet H, et al. Therapeutic use of enzymes as anti-inflammatory agents. *Ed Med Hyg* 1: 108, 1961.
9. Gardner ML. Gastrointestinal absorption of intact proteins. *Annu Rev Nutr* 8: 329–350, 1988.
10. Gall DG. Gastrointestinal uptake of macromolecules. *Chung Hua Min Kuo Hsiao Erh Ko I Hsueh Hui Tsa Chih* 39(1): 9–11, 1998.
11. Same as 9.
12. Same as 10.
13. Roberts PR, Zaloga GP. Dietary bioactive peptides. *New Horiz* 2(2): 237–243, 1994.
14. Schlimme E, Meisel H. Bioactive peptides derived from milk proteins. Structural, physiological and analytical aspects. *Nahrung* 39(1): 1–20, 1995.
15. Same as 9.
16. Brinson RR, et al. A reappraisal of the peptide-based enteral formulas: clinical applications. *Nutr Clin Pract* 4(6): 211–217,1989.
17. Webb KE Jr. Intestinal absorption of protein hydrolysis products: a review. *J Anim Sci* 68(9): 3011–3022, 1990.
18. Same as 3.
19. Harrower HR. Endocrine Diagnostic Charts. Glendale, CA: The Harrower Laboratory, Inc., 1929.
20. Harrower HR. Endocrine Pointers. Glendale, CA: The Harrower Laboratory, Inc., 1933.
21. Murray MT. *Glandular Extracts, What You Must Know.* New Canaan, CT: Keats Publishing, 1994.
22. Same as 3.

Chapter 14

1. Tyler VE, et al. *Pharmacognosy,* 9th Ed. Philadelphia: Lea & Febiger, 1988.
2. Minshall RD, et al. Ovarian steroid protection against coronary artery hyperreactivity in rhesus monkeys. *J Clin Endocrinol Metab* 83(2): 649–659, 1998.
3. Sandow N. Rxlist—The Internet Drug Index. Hyperlink: "www.rxlist.com", 1995.
4. Becker, KL, ed. *Principles and Practice of Endocrinology and Metabolism.* Philadelphia: JB Lippincott, 1995.
5. Goji K. Twenty-four-hour concentration profiles of gonadotropin and estradiol (E2) in prepubertal and early pubertal girls: the diurnal rise of E2 is opposite the nocturnal rise of gonadotropin. *J Clin Endocrinol Metab* 77(6): 1629–1635, 1993.
6. Lonning PE, et al. Lack of diurnal variation in plasma levels of androstenedione, testosterone, estrone and estradiol in postmenopausal women. *J Steroid Biochem* 34(1–6): 551–553, 1989.
7. Lobo RA, Cassidenti DL. Pharmacokinetics of oral 17-beta-estradiol. *J Reprod Med* 37(1): 77–84, 1992.
8. Scott RT Jr, et al. Pharmacokinetics of percutaneous estradiol: a crossover study using a gel and a transdermal system in comparison with oral micronized estradiol. *Obstet Gynecol* 77(5): 758–764, 1991.

9. Townsend PT, et al. The absorption and metabolism of oral oestradiol, oestrone and oestriol. *Br J Obstet Gynaecol* 88(8): 846–852, 1981.
10. Levrant SG, Barnes RB. Pharmacology of estrogens. IN: Lobo RA. *Treatment of the Postmenopausal Woman, Basic and Clinical Aspects*. Philadelphia: Lippincott-Raven Publishers, 1996: 59.
11. Same as 8.
12. Szymczak J, et al. Concentration of sex steroids in adipose tissue after menopause. *Steroids* 63(5–6): 319–321, 1998.
13. Deslypere JP, et al. Fat tissue: a steroid reservoir and site of steroid metabolism. *J Clin Endocrinol Metab* 61(3): 564–570, 1985.
14. Riad-Fahmy D, et al. Steroids in saliva for assessing endocrine function. *Endocr Rev*. 3(No. 4) 1982.
15. Same as 14.
16. Cauter EV. Endocrine rhythms. IN: Becker KL, ed. *Principles and Practice of Endocrinology and Metabolism*. Philadelphia: JB Lippincott, 1995.
17. Collins JJ. Circadian Activity of Progesterone. Unpublished research, 1999.
18. Hanggi W, et al. Comparison of transvaginal ultrasonography and endometrial biopsy in endometrial surveillance in postmenopausal HRT users. *Maturitas* 27(2): 133–143, 1997.
19. Yen SS, et al. Circulating estradiol, estrone and gonadotropin levels following the administration of orally active 17-beta-estradiol in postmenopausal women. *J Clin Endocrinol Metab* 40(3): 518–521, 1975.
20. Same as 7.
21. Schubert W, et al. Pharmacokinetic evaluation of oral 17-beta-oestradiol and two different fat soluble analogues in ovariectomized women. *Eur J Clin Pharmacol* 44(6): 563–568, 1993.
22. Mijatovic V, et al. Postmenopausal oral 17-beta-estradiol continuously combined with dydrogesterone reduces fasting serum homocysteine levels. *Fertil Steril* 69(5): 876–882, 1998.
23. Belfort MA, et al. Hormonal status affects the reactivity of the cerebral vasculature. *Am J Obstet Gynecol* 172(4 Pt 1): 1273–1278, 1995.
24. Hartmann BW, et al. Absorption of orally supplied natural estrogens correlated with age and somatometric parameters. *Gynecol Endocrinol* 8(2): 101–107, 1994.
25. Callantine MR, et al. Micronized 17-beta-estradiol for oral estrogen therapy in menopausal women. *Obstet Gynecol* 46(1): 37–41, 1975.
26. Alfie J, et al. Hemodynamic effects of transdermal estradiol alone and combined with norethisterone acetate. *Maturitas* 27(2): 163–169, 1997.
27. Oosterbaan HP, et al. The effects of continuous combined transdermal oestrogen-progestogen treatment on bleeding patterns and the endometrium in postmenopausal women. *Maturitas* 21(3): 211–219, 1995.
28. Wiklund I, et al. Long-term effect of transdermal hormonal therapy on aspects of quality of life in postmenopausal women. *Maturitas* 14(3): 225–236, 1992.
29. Gabrielsson J, et al. Pharmacokinetic data on estradiol in light of the estring concept. Estradiol and estring pharmacokinetics. *Acta Obstet Gynecol Scand Suppl* 163: 26–31; discussion 32–34, 1996.
30. Johnston A. Estrogens—pharmacokinetics and pharmacodynamics with special reference to vaginal administration and the new estradiol formulation—Estring. *Acta Obstet Gynecol Scand Suppl* 163: 16–25, 1996.
31. Barentsen R, et al. Continuous low dose estradiol released from a vaginal ring versus estriol vaginal cream for urogenital atrophy. *Eur J Obstet Gynecol Reprod Biol* 71(1): 73–80, 1997.
32. Henriksson L, et al. A one-year multicenter study of efficacy and safety of a continuous, low-dose, estradiol-releasing vaginal ring (Estring) in post-

menopausal women with symptoms and signs of urogenital aging. *Am J Obstet Gynecol* 174(1 Pt 1): 85–92, 1996.

33. Same as 32.
34. Same as 29.
35. Same as 32.
36. Schmidt G, et al. Release of 17-beta-oestradiol from a vaginal ring in postmenopausal women: pharmacokinetic evaluation. *Gynecol Obstet Invest* 38(4): 253–260, 1994.
37. Snow JM, *The Natural Pharmacist: Natural Treatments for Menopause.* Rocklin, CA: Prima Publishing, 1999.
38. Chang M, et al. Inhibition of glutathione S-transferase activity by the quinoid metabolites of equine estrogens. *Chem Res Toxicol* 11(7): 758–765, 1998.
39. Bhavnani BR. Pharmacokinetics and pharmacodynamics of conjugated equine estrogens: chemistry and metabolism. *Proc Soc Exp Biol Med* 217(1): 6–16, 1998.
40. Genant HK, et al. Low-dose esterified estrogen therapy: effects on bone, plasma estradiol concentrations, endometrium, and lipid levels. Estratab/Osteoporosis Study Group. *Arch Intern Med* 157(22): 2609–2615, 1997.
41. van Haaften M, et al. Biochemical and histological effects of vaginal estriol and estradiol applications on the endometrium, myometrium and vagina of postmenopausal women. *Gynecol Endocrinol* 11(3): 175–185, 1997.
42. Hustin J, Van den Eynde JP. Cytologic evaluation of the effect of various estrogens given in postmenopause. *Acta Cytol* 21(2): 225–228, 1977.
43. Melis GB, et al. Salmon calcitonin plus intravaginal estriol: an effective treatment for the menopause. *Maturitas* 24(1–2): 83–90, 1996.
44. van der Linden MC, et al. The effect of estriol on the cytology of urethra and vagina in postmenopausal women with genito-urinary symptoms. *Eur J Obstet Gynecol Reprod Biol* 51(1): 29–33, 1993.
45. Arteaga E, et al. [Comparison of the antioxidant effect of estriol and estradiol on low density lipoproteins in post-menopausal women]. [Article in Spanish] *Rev Med Chil* 126(5): 481–487, 1998.
46. Nishibe A, et al. [Effect of estriol and bone mineral density of lumbar vertebrae in elderly and postmenopausal women]. [Article in Japanese] *Nippon Ronen Igakkai Zasshi* 33(5): 353–359, 1996.
47. Devogelaer JP, et al. Long-term effects of percutaneous estradiol on bone loss and bone metabolism in postmenopausal hysterectomized women. *Maturitas* 28(3): 243–249, 1998.
48. Barentsen R, et al. Continuous low dose estradiol released from a vaginal ring versus estriol vaginal cream for urogenital atrophy. *Eur J Obstet Gynecol Reprod Biol* 71(1): 73–80, 1997.
49. Vooijs GP, Geurts TB. Review of the endometrial safety during intravaginal treatment with estriol. *Eur J Obstet Gynecol Reprod Biol* 62(1): 101–106, 1995.
50. Di Stefano L, et al. [Transvaginal administration of estriol in postmenopausal urogynecological disorders]. [Article in Italian] *Minerva Ginecol* 45(11): 551–556, 1993.
51. Stapleton A, Stamm WE. Prevention of urinary tract infection. *Infect Dis Clin North Am* 11(3): 719–733, 1997.
52. Koloszar S, Kovacs L. [Treatment of climacteric urogenital disorders with an estriol-containing ointment]. [Article in Hungarian] *Orv Hetil* 136(7): 343–345, 1995.
53. Schar G, et al. [Effect of vaginal estrogen therapy on urinary incontinence in postmenopause]. [Article in German] *Zentralbl Gynakol* 117(2): 77–80, 1995.
54. Same as 52.
55. Kanne B, Jenny J. [Local administration of low-dose estriol and vital *Lactobacillus acidophilus* in postmenopause]. [Article in German] *Gynakol Rundsch* 31(1): 7–13, 1991.

56. Vasquez JM, et al. Endocrine studies in postmenopausal women during oral replacement therapy with unconjugated oestrogens. *Reproduction* 6(2): 49–59, 1982.

57. Townsend PT, et al. The absorption and metabolism of oral oestradiol, oestrone and oestriol. *Br J Obstet Gynaecol* 88(8): 846–852, 1981.

58. Habiba M, et al. Effect of a new cyclical sequential postmenopausal HRT on lipoprotein, apoprotein and thrombophilia profile. *Eur J Obstet Gynecol Reprod Biol* 62(1): 89–94, 1995.

59. Akkad A, et al. Carotid plaque regression on oestrogen replacement: a pilot study. *Eur J Vasc Endovasc Surg* 11(3): 347–348, 1996.

60. Johnson SR. Menopause and hormone replacement therapy. *Med Clin North Am* 82(2): 297–320, 1998.

61. Kenya PR. Effects of steroidal contraceptives on gallbladder: a review. *East Afr Med J* 67(9): 661–666, 1990.

62. Hulley S, et al. Randomized trial of estrogen plus progestin for secondary prevention of coronary heart disease in postmenopausal women. Heart and Estrogen/Progestin Replacement Study (HERS) Research Group. *JAMA* 280(7): 605–613, 1998.

63. Barrett-Connor E, Grady D. Hormone replacement therapy, heart disease, and other considerations. *Annu Rev Public Health* 19: 55–72, 1998.

64. Saleh AA, et al. Thrombosis and hormone replacement therapy in postmenopausal women. *Am J Obstet Gynecol* 169(6): 1554–1557, 1993.

65. Seelig MS. Increased need for magnesium with the use of combined oestrogen and calcium for osteoporosis treatment. *Magnes Res* 3(3):197–215, 1990.

66. Heckers H, Platt D. [Lipoprotein metabolism in menopause. Effect of hormonal substitution therapy]. [Article in German] *Fortschr Med* 109(18): 379–382, 1991.

67. Chang AY. Megestrol acetate as a biomodulator. *Semin Oncol* 25(2 suppl 6): 58–61, 1998.

68. Gutierrez M, et al. Cyproterone acetate displaces opiate binding in mouse brain. *Eur J Pharmacol* 328(1): 99–102, 1997.

69. Sandow N. Rxlist—The Internet Drug Index. Hyperlink: "www.rxlist.com", 1995.

70. Wolfe BM, et al. Effects of adding C-19 versus C-21 progestin to conjugated estrogen in moderately hypercholesterolemic postmenopausal women. *Am J Obstet Gynecol* 178(4): 787–792, 1998.

71. Same as 66.

72. Wilde MI, Balfour JA. Gestodene. A review of its pharmacology, efficacy and tolerability in combined contraceptive preparations. *Drugs* 50(2): 364–395, 1995.

73. Same as 69.

74. Simon JA, et al. The absorption of oral micronized progesterone: the effect of food, dose proportionality, and comparison with intramuscular progesterone. *Fertil Steril* 60(1): 26–33, 1993.

75. McAuley JW, et al. Oral administration of micronized progesterone: a review and more experience. *Pharmacotherapy* 16(3): 453–457, 1996.

76. Arafat ES, et al. Sedative and hypnotic effects of oral administration of micronized progesterone may be mediated through its metabolites. *Am J Obstet Gynecol* 159(5): 1203–1209, 1988.

77. Maxson WS, Hargrove JT. Bioavailability of oral micronized progesterone. *Fertil Steril* 44(5): 622–626, 1985.

78. Freeman EW, et al. A placebo-controlled study of effects of oral progesterone on performance and mood. *Br J Clin Pharmacol* 33(3): 293–298, 1992.

79. Same as 75.

80. Same as 77.

81. Sitruk-Ware R, et al. Oral micronized progesterone. Bioavailability pharma-cokinetics, pharmacological and therapeutic implications—a review. *Contra-ception* 36(4): 373–402, 1987.

82. Same as 74.

83. Jasionowski EA, Jasionowski PA. Further observations on the effect of topical progesterone on vulvar disease. *Am J Obstet Gynecol* 134(5): 565–567, 1979.

84. Jasionowski EA, Jasionowski P. Topical progesterone in treatment of vulvar dystrophy: preliminary report of five cases. *Am J Obstet Gynecol* 127(6): 667–670, 1977.

85. Simpson NB, et al. The effect of topically applied progesterone on sebum excretion rate. *Br J Dermatol* 100(6): 687–692, 1979.

86. Mauvais-Jarvis P, et al. [Progesterone administered by percutaneous route: an an-tiandrogen locally useful]. [Article in French] *Ann Endocrinol* 36(2): 55–62, 1975.

87. Sitruk-Ware R. Transdermal delivery of steroids. *Contraception* 39(1): 1–20, 1989.

88. Krause W, et al. [Resorption of progesterone through the intact skin of the breast in comparison with other body regions]. [Article in German] *Geburtshilfe Frauenheilkd* 47(8): 562–564, 1987.

89. Cataldi U, et al. [Authors' experience with transvaginal administration of progestagens]. [Article in Italian] *Clin Ter* 148(4): 165–172, 1997.

90. Pouly JL, et al. [Luteal phase support after vaginal progesterone: compara-tive study with micronized oral progesterone]. [Article in French] *Contracept Fertil Sex* 25(7–8): 596–601, 1997.

91. Pouly JL, et al. Luteal support after in-vitro fertilization: Crinone 8%, a sus-tained release vaginal progesterone gel, versus Utrogestan, an oral mi-cronized progesterone. *Hum Reprod* 11(10): 2085–2089, 1996.

92. Casanas-Roux F, et al. Morphometric, immunohistological and three-dimensional evaluation of the endometrium of menopausal women treated by oestrogen and Crinone, a new slow-release vaginal progesterone. *Hum Reprod* 11(2): 357–363, 1996.

93. Balasch J, et al. Further data favoring the hypothesis of the uterine first-pass effect of vaginally administered micronized progesterone. *Gynecol Endocrinol* 10(6): 421–426, 1996.

94. Kimble-Haas SL. The intrauterine device: dispelling the myths. *Nurse Pract* 23(11): 58, 63–69, 73, 1998.

95. Kaunitz AM. Reappearance of the intrauterine device: a 'user-friendly' con-traceptive. *Int J Fertil Womens Med* 42(2): 120–127, 1997.

96. Same as 94.

97. Soderstrom RM. Will progesterone save the IUD? *J Reprod Med* 28(5): 305–308, 1983.

98. Sievers S, Dallenbach-Hellweg G. [Clinical and morphological studies in patients with a progesterone-releasing intrauterine contraceptive device (Progestasert-System)]. [Article in German] *Geburtshilfe Frauenheilkd* 36(4): 334–340, 1976.

99. Sheppard BL. Endometrial morphological changes in IUD users: a review. *Contraception* 36(1): 1–10, 1987.

100. Ermini M, et al. Distribution and effect on the endometrium of proges-terone released from a progestasert device. *Hum Reprod* 4(3): 221–228, 1989.

101. Bergqvist A, Rybo G. Treatment of menorrhagia with intrauterine release of progesterone. *Br J Obstet Gynaecol* 90(3): 255–258, 1983.

102. Scholten PC, et al. Intrauterine steroid contraceptives. *Wien Med Wochenschr* 137(20–21): 479–483, 1987.

103. Sievers S. [The progestasert system—a 24-month-long active spiral. Clinical experiences with an intrauterine progesterone-releasing system]. [Article in German] *Fortschr Med* 102(39): 982–984, 1984.

104. Speroff L, et al. The comparative effect on bone density, endometrium, and lipids of continuous hormones as replacement therapy (CHART study). A randomized controlled trial. *JAMA* 276(17): 1397–1403, 1996.

105. Gambrell RD Jr. Strategies to reduce the incidence of endometrial cancer in postmenopausal women. *Am J Obstet Gynecol* 177(5): 1196–1204; discussion 1204–1207, 1997.

106. Same as 104.

107. Taskinen MR, et al. Hormone replacement therapy lowers plasma Lp(a) concentrations. Comparison of cyclic transdermal and continuous estrogen-progestin regimens. *Arterioscler Thromb Vasc Biol* 16(10): 1215–1221, 1996.

108. Warenik-Szymankiewicz A, et al. [Effect of Kliogest therapy on serum blood lipids in postmenopausal women]. [Article in Polish] *Ginekol Pol* 66(9): 541–546, 1995.

109. Same as 104.

110. Farish E, et al. Effects of postmenopausal hormone replacement therapy on lipoproteins including lipoprotein(a) and LDL subfractions. *Atherosclerosis* 126(1): 77–84, 1996.

111. Hellberg D, Nilsson S. Pilot study to evaluate a new regimen to treat climacteric complaints with cyclic combined oestradiol valerate/medroxyprogesterone acetate. *Maturitas* 9(1): 103–107, 1987.

112. Gibbons WE, et al. Biochemical and histologic effects of sequential estrogen/progestin therapy on the endometrium of postmenopausal women. *Am J Obstet Gynecol* 154(2): 456–461, 1986.

113. Schiff I, et al. Oral medroxyprogesterone in the treatment of postmenopausal symptoms. *JAMA* 244(13): 1443–1445, 1980.

114. Bullock JL, et al. Use of medroxyprogesterone acetate to prevent menopausal symptoms. *Obstet Gynecol* 46(2): 165–168, 1975.

115. Yen SS. Estrogen and the menopause. *Am Fam Physician* 16(1): 87–91, 1977.

116. Lobo RA, et al. Depo-medroxyprogesterone acetate compared with conjugated estrogens for the treatment of postmenopausal women. *Obstet Gynecol* 63(1):1–5, 1984.

117. Same as 116.

118. Snow GR, Anderson C. The effects of continuous progestogen treatment on cortical bone remodeling activity in beagles. *Calcif Tissue Int* 37(3): 282–286, 1985.

119. Haller DG, Glick JH. Progestational agents in advanced breast cancer: an overview. *Semin Oncol* 13(4 Suppl 4): 2–8, 1986.

120. van Veelen H, et al. Adrenal suppression by oral high-dose medroxyprogesterone acetate in breast cancer patients. *Cancer Chemother Pharmacol* 12(2): 83–86, 1984.

121. Izuo M, et al. A phase III trial of oral high-dose medroxyprogesterone acetate (MPA) versus mepitiostane in advanced postmenopausal breast cancer. *Cancer* 56(11): 2576–2579, 1985.

122. Hirvonen E, et al. Clinical and lipid metabolic effects of unopposed oestrogen and two oestrogen–progestogen regimens in post-menopausal women. *Maturitas* 9(1): 69–79, 1987.

123. Hirvonen E, et al. Effects of different progestogens on lipoproteins during postmenopausal replacement therapy. *N Engl J Med* 304(10): 560–563, 1981.

124. Notelovitz M, et al. Oestrogen–progestin therapy and the lipid balance of post-menopausal women. *Maturitas* 4(4): 301–308, 1982.

125. Miodrag A, et al. Sex hormones and the female urinary tract. *Drugs* 36(4): 491–504, 1988.

126. Warnock JK, et al. Female hypoactive sexual desire disorder due to androgen deficiency: clinical and psychometric issues. *Psychopharmacol Bull* 33(4): 761–766, 1997.

127. Sherwin BB. Use of combined estrogen–androgen preparations in the post-menopause: evidence from clinical studies. *Int J Fertil Womens Med* 43(2): 98–103, 1998.
128. Davis SR, Burger HG. Use of androgens in postmenopausal women. *Curr Opin Obstet Gynecol* 9(3): 177–180, 1997.
129. Sands R, Studd J. Exogenous androgens in postmenopausal women. *Am J Med* 98(1A): 76S–79S, 1995.
130. Coope J. Hormonal and non-hormonal interventions for menopausal symptoms. *Maturitas* 23(2): 159–168, 1996.
131. Same as 126.
132. Same as 128.
133. Kennedy RG, et al. Sexual interest in postmenopausal women is related to 5alpha-reductase activity. *Hum Reprod* 12(2): 209–213, 1997.
134. Same as 130.
135. Same as 129.
136. Persky H, et al. Plasma testosterone level and sexual behavior of couples. *Arch Sex Behav* 7(3): 157–173, 1978.
137. Hickok LR, et al. A comparison of esterified estrogens with and without methyltestosterone: effects on endometrial histology and serum lipoproteins in postmenopausal women. *Obstet Gynecol* 82(6): 919–924, 1993.
138. Sarrel PM. Cardiovascular aspects of androgens in women. *Semin Reprod Endocrinol* 16(2): 121–128, 1998.
139. Same as 138.
140. Sarrel PM, Wiita B. Vasodilator effects of estrogen are not diminished by androgen in postmenopausal women. *Fertil Steril* 68(6): 1125–1127, 1997.
141. Murphy S, et al. Endogenous sex hormones and bone mineral density among community-based postmenopausal women. *Postgrad Med J* 68(805): 908–913, 1992.
142. Same as 128.
143. Gitlin N, et al. Liver function in postmenopausal women on estrogen-androgen hormone replacement therapy: a meta-analysis of eight clinical trials. *Menopause* 6(3): 216–224, 1999.
144. Paradinas FJ, et al. Hyperplasia and prolapse of hepatocytes into hepatic veins during long-term methyltestosterone therapy: possible relationships of these changes to the development of peliosis hepatitis and liver tumours. *Histopathology* 1(4): 225–246, 1977.
145. Westaby D, et al. Liver damage from long-term methyltestosterone. *Lancet* 2(8032): 262–263, 1977.
146. Bird D, et al. Spontaneous rupture of a liver cell adenoma after long-term methyltestosterone: report of a case successfully treated by emergency right hepatic lobectomy. *Br J Surg* 66(3): 212–213, 1979.

Chapter 15

1. Morse CA, et al. Relationships between premenstrual complaints and peri-menopausal experiences. *J Psychosom Obstet Gynaecol* 19(4): 182–191, 1998.
2. Burg MA, et al. Lifetime use of alternative therapy: a study of Florida residents. *South Med J* 91(12): 1126–1131, 1998.
3. Gordon NP, et al. Use of and interest in alternative therapies among adult primary care clinicians and adult members in a large health maintenance organization. *West J Med* 169(3): 153–161, 1998.
4. Damkier A, et al. Nurses' attitudes to the use of alternative medicine in cancer patients. *Scand J Caring Sci* 12(2): 119–126, 1998.
5. Willhite L. Osteoporosis in women: prevention and treatment. *J Am Pharm Assoc* 38(5): 614-623; quiz 623–624, 1998.

Appendix A

1. Erickson GF, Schreiber JR. Morphology and physiology of the ovary. IN: Becker KL, ed. *Principles and Practice of Endocrinology and Metabolism.* Philadelphia: JB Lippincott, 1995: 864–865.
2. Same as 1.
3. Levrant SG, Barnes RB. Pharmacology of estrogens. IN: Lobo RA, ed. *Treatment of the Postmenopausal Woman, Basic and Clinical Aspects.* Philadelphia: Lippincott-Raven Publishers, 1996: 58.
4. Liehr JG, et al. 4-Hydroxylation of estradiol by human uterine myometrium and myoma microsomes: implications for the mechanism of uterine tumorigenesis. *Proc Natl Acad Sci USA* 92(20): 9220–9224, 1995.
5. Liehr JG, Ricci MJ. 4-Hydroxylation of estrogens as marker of human mammary tumors. *Proc Natl Acad Sci USA* 93(8): 3294–3296, 1996.
6. Bradlow HL, et al. 2-hydroxyestrone: the 'good' estrogen. *J Endocrinol* 150 (suppl): S259–S265, 1996.
7. Guyton AC, *Textbook of Medical Physiology.* Philadelphia: WB Saunders, 1986: 972.
8. Schiff I, Walsh B. Menopause. IN: Becker KL, ed. *Principles and Practice of Endocrinology and Metabolism.* Philadelphia: JB Lippincott, 1995: 916.
9. Levrant SG, Barnes RB. Pharmacology of estrogens. IN: Lobo RA. *Treatment of the Postmenopausal Woman, Basic and Clinical Aspects.* Philadelphia: Lippincott-Raven Publishers, 1996: 64.
10. Schiff I, Walsh B. Menopause. IN: Becker KL, ed. *Principles and Practice of Endocrinology and Metabolism.* Philadelphia: JB Lippincott, 1995: 922.
11. Walsh BW, et al. Effects of postmenopausal estrogen replacement on the concentrations and metabolism of plasma lipoproteins. *N Engl J Med* 325(17): 1196–1204, 1991.
12. Same as 10.
13. Levrant SG, Barnes RB. Pharmacology of estrogens. IN: Lobo RA. *Treatment of the Postmenopausal Woman, Basic and Clinical Aspects.* Philadelphia: Lippincott-Raven Publishers, 1996: 60.
14. Same as 11.
15. Levrant SG, Barnes RB. Pharmacology of estrogens. IN: Lobo RA. *Treatment of the Postmenopausal Woman, Basic and Clinical Aspects.* Philadelphia: Lippincott-Raven Publishers, 1996: 64.
16. Schiff I, Walsh B. Menopause. IN: Becker KL, ed. *Principles and Practice of Endocrinology and Metabolism.* Philadelphia: JB Lippincott, 1995, 922.
17. Levrant SG, Barnes RB. Pharmacology of estrogens. IN: Lobo RA. *Treatment of the Postmenopausal Woman, Basic and Clinical Aspects.* Philadelphia: Lippincott-Raven Publishers, 1996: 65.
18. Mashchak CA, Lobo RA. Estrogen replacement therapy and hypertension. *J Reprod Med* 30(10 suppl): 805–810, 1985.
19. Same as 17.
20. Levrant SG, Barnes RB. Pharmacology of estrogens. IN: Lobo RA. *Treatment of the Postmenopausal Woman, Basic and Clinical Aspects.* Philadelphia: Lippincott-Raven Publishers, 1996: 57.
21. Same as 20.
22. Levrant SG, Barnes RB. Pharmacology of estrogens. IN: Lobo RA. *Treatment of the Postmenopausal Woman, Basic and Clinical Aspects.* Philadelphia: Lippincott-Raven Publishers, 1996: 59.
23. Lemon HM, et al. Reduced estriol excretion in patients with breast cancer prior to endocrine therapy. *JAMA* 196(No. 3), 1966.
24. Same as 23.
25. Follingstad AH. Estriol, the forgotten estrogen? *JAMA* 239(No. 1), 1978.

26. Gronroos M, et al. Ovarian production of estrogens in postmenopausal women. *Int J Gynaecol Obstet* 18(2): 93–98, 1980.
27. Same as 23.
28. Same as 25.
29. Same as 26.
30. Wright JV, Morgenthaler J. *Natural Hormone Replacement*. Petaluma, CA: Smart Publications, 1997.
31. Martin L, et al. Oestriol, oestradiol-17-beta and the proliferation and death of uterine cells. *J Endocrinol* 69(1): 103–115, 1976.
32. Lemon HM. Clinical and experimental aspects of the anti-mammary carinogenic activity of estriol. *Front Horm Res* 5: 155–173, 1977.
33. van Haaften M, et al. Identification of 16 alpha-hydroxy-estrone as a metabolite of estriol. *Gynecol Endocrinol* 2(3): 215–221, 1988.
34. Same as 33.
35. Newfield L, et al. Estrogen metabolism and the malignant potential of human papillomavirus immortalized keratinocytes. *Proc Soc Exp Biol Med* 217(3): 322–326, 1998.
36. Ursin G, et al. A pilot study of urinary estrogen metabolites (16alpha-OHE1 and 2-OHE1) in postmenopausal women with and without breast cancer. *Environ Health Perspect* 105(suppl 3): 601–605, 1997.
37. Same as 35.
38. Zhu BT, Conney AH. Functional role of estrogen metabolism in target cells: review and perspectives. *Carcinogenesis* 19(1): 1–27, 1998.
39. Alanko J, et al. Catechol estrogens as inhibitors of leukotriene synthesis. *Biochem Pharmacol* 55(1): 101–104, 1998.
40. Same as 6.
41. Dubey RK, et al. 17-Beta-estradiol, its metabolites, and progesterone inhibit cardiac fibroblast growth. *Hypertension* 31(1 Pt 2): 522–528, 1998.
42. Same as 41.
43. Seeger H, et al. Effect of estradiol metabolites on the susceptibility of low density lipoprotein to oxidation. *Life Sci* 61(9): 865–868, 1997.
44. Same as 43.
45. Miura T, et al. Inhibition of lipid peroxidation by estradiol and 2-hydroxyestradiol. *Steroids* 61(6): 379–383, 1996.
46. Same as 43.
47. Yagi K. Female hormones act as natural antioxidants—a survey of our research. *Acta Biochim Pol* 44(4): 701–709, 1997.
48. Liehr JG, et al. 4-Hydroxylation of estradiol by human uterine myometrium and myoma microsomes: implications for the mechanism of uterine tumorigenesis. *Proc Natl Acad Sci USA* 92(20): 9220–9224, 1995.
49. Liehr JG, Ricci MJ. 4-Hydroxylation of estrogens as marker of human mammary tumors. *Proc Natl Acad Sci USA* 93(8): 3294–3296, 1996.
50. Tabakovic K, et al. Oxidative transformation of 2-hydroxyestrone. Stability and reactivity of 2,3-estrone quinone and its relationship to estrogen carcinogenicity. *Chem Res Toxicol* 9(5): 860–865, 1996.
51. Newfield L, et al. Estrogen metabolism and the malignant potential of human papillomavirus immortalized keratinocytes. *Proc Soc Exp Biol Med* 217(3): 322–326, 1998.
52. Pizzorno J. *Total Wellness, Improve Your Health by Understanding the Body's Healing Systems*. Rocklin, CA: Prima Publishing, 1996.
53. Sasson S. Equilibrium binding analysis of estrogen agonists and antagonists: relation to the activation of the estrogen receptor. *Pathol Biol* 39(1): 59–69, 1991.
54. Same as 22.
55. Martin L, et al. Oestriol, oestradiol-17-beta and the proliferation and death of uterine cells. *J Endocrinol* 69(1): 103–115, 1976.

56. Same as 55.
57. Guyton AC, *Textbook of Medical Physiology.* Philadelphia: WB Saunders, 1986: 972.
58. Levrant SG, Barnes RB. Pharmacology of estrogens. IN: Lobo RA. *Treatment of the Postmenopausal Woman, Basic and Clinical Aspects.* Philadelphia: Lippincott-Raven Publishers, 1996: 61.
59. Same as 6.
60. Kall MA, et al. Effects of dietary broccoli on human in vivo drug metabolizing enzymes: evaluation of caffeine, oestrone and chlorzoxazone metabolism. *Carcinogenesis* 17(4): 793–799, 1996.
61. Same as 6.
62. Michnovicz JJ, et al. Changes in levels of urinary estrogen metabolites after oral indole-3-carbinol treatment in humans. *J Natl Cancer Inst* 89(10): 718–723, 1997.
63. Same as 35.
64. Same as 62.
65. Michnovicz JJ. Increased estrogen 2-hydroxylation in obese women using oral indole-3-carbinol. *Int J Obes Relat Metab Disord* 22(3):227–229, 1998.
66. Same as 60.

Appendix B

1. Stancyz FZ. Structure–function relationships, potency, and pharmacokinetics or progestogens. IN: Lobo RA. *Treatment of the Postmenopausal Woman, Basic and Clinical Aspects.* Philadelphia: Lippincott-Raven Publishers, 1996: 96.
2. Same as 1.
3. Same as 1.
4. Boonkasemsanti W, et al. Relative binding affinity of various progestins and antiprogestins to a rabbit myometrium receptor. *Arzneim-Forsch* 39(2): 195–199, 1989.
5. Radwanska E. The role of reproductive hormones in vascular disease and hypertension. *Steroids* 58(12): 605–610, 1993.
6. Ottosson UB, et al. Subfractions of high-density lipoprotein cholesterol during estrogen replacement therapy: a comparison between progestogens and natural progesterone. *Am J Obstet Gynecol* 151(6): 746–750, 1985.

Appendix C

1. Nakano Y, et al. The receptor, metabolism and effects of androgen in osteoblastic MC3T3-E1 cells. *Bone Miner* 26(3): 245–259, 1994.
2. Takeuchi M, et al. Androgens directly stimulate mineralization and increase androgen receptors in human osteoblast-like osteosarcoma cells. *Biochem Biophys Res Commun* 204(2): 905–911, 1994.

Appendix D

1. Fitzgerald PA. Adrenal cortex physiology. In: Tierney LM Jr, McPhee J, Papadakis MA, eds. *Current Medical Diagnosis and Treatment.* Los Altos, CA: MA Lange Publishers, 1995: 982.
2. Berdanier CD, et al. Is dehydroepiandrosterone an antiobesity agent? *FASEB J* 7(5): 414–419, 1993.
3. Rosenfeld RS, et al. 24-hour secretory pattern of dehydroisoandrosterone and dehydroisoandrosterone sulfate. *J Clin Endocrin Metab* 40: 850–855, 1975.

4. Rosenfeld RS, et al. Metabolism and interconversion of dehydroepiandrosterone and dehydroepiandrosterone sulfate. *J Clin Endocrinol Metab* 35: 187–193, 1972.

5. Same as 3.

6. Singh VB, et al. Intracranial dehydroepiandrosterone blocks the activation of tryptophan hydroxylase in response to acute sound stress. *Mol Cell Neurosci* 5: 176–181, 1994.

7. Namiki, M. Aged people and stress. *Jpn J Geriatr* 31: 85–95, 1994.

8. Freiss E, et al. DHEA administration increases rapid eye movement sleep and EEG power in the sigma frequency range. *Am J Physiol* 268(31): E107–E113, 1995.

9. Bologa L, et al. Dehydroepiandrosterone and its sulfated derivative reduce neuronal death and enhance astrocytic differentiation in brain cell cultures. *J Neurosci Res* 17: 225–234, 1987.

10. Maes M, et al. Protection from glucocorticoid induced thymic involution by dehydroepiandrosterone. *Life Sci* 46: 1627–1631, 1990.

11. Meikle AW, et al. The presence of a dehydroepiandrosterone-specific receptor binding complex in murine T cells. *Am J Med Sci* 303: 366–371, 1992.

12. Gordon GB, et al. Modulation of growth, differentiation and carcinogenesis by dehydroepiandrosterone. *Adv Enzymol Regul* 26: 255–282, 1987.

13. Hedman M, et al. Low blood and synovial fluid levels of sulpho-conjugated steroids in rheumatoid arthritis. *Clin Exp Rheumatol* 10: 25–30, 1992.

14. Cutolo M, et al. Androgen replacement therapy in male patients with rheumatoid arthritis. *Arthritis Rheum* 34: 1–5, 1991.

15. Hedman M, et al. Low sulpho-conjugated steroid hormone levels in systemic lupus erythematosus. *Clin Exp Rheumatol* 7: 583–588, 1989.

16. Hall GM, et al. Depressed levels of dehydroepiandrosterone sulfate in postmenstrual women with rheumatoid arthritis but no relation with axial bone density. *Ann Rheum* 52:211–214, 1993.

17. Cleary MP, Zisk JF. Anti-obesity effect of two different levels of dehydroepiandrosterone in lean and obese middle-aged female zucker rats. *Int J Obes* 10: 193–204, 1986.

18. Usiskin KS, et al. Lack of effect of dehydroepiandrosterone in obese men. *Int J Obes* 14: 457–453, 1990.

19. Welle S, et al. Failure of dehydroepiandrosterone to influence energy and protein metabolism in humans. *J Endocrinol Metab* 21: 1197–1207, 1990.

20. Nowaczynski WF, et al. Further evidence of altered adrenocortical functions in hypertension: dehydroepiandrosterone secretion rate. *Can J Biochem* 46: 1031–1038, 1968.

21. Herrington DM, et al. Plasma dehydroepiandrosterone and dehydroepiandrosterone sulfate in patients undergoing diagnostic coronary angiography. *J Am Coll Cardiol* 16(4): 862–870, 1990.

22. Nestler JE, et al. Dehydroepiandrosterone reduces serum low density lipoprotein levels and body fat but does not alter insulin sensitivity in normal men. *J Endocrinol Metab* 66: 57–61, 1988.

23. Falcone T, et al. Effect of hyperprolactinemia on the androgen response to an oral glucose load. *Fertil Steril* 58(6): 1119–1122, 1992.

24. Nestler JE, et al. Dehydroepiandrosterone: the "missing link" between hyperinsulinemia and atherosclerosis? *FASEB J* 6(12): 3073–3075, 1992.

25. Ebeling P, et al. Androgens and insulin resistance in type 1 diabetic men. *Clin Endocrinol* 43(5): 601–607, 1995.

26. Han DH, et al. DHEA treatment reduces fat accumulation and protects against insulin resistance in male rats. *J Gerontol A Biol Med Sci* 53(1): B19–B24, 1998.

27. Paolisso G, et al. Insulin resistance and advancing age: what role for dehydroepiandrosterone sulfate? *Metabolism* 46(11): 1281–1286, 1997.
28. Yamauchi A, et al. Hyperglycemia decreases dehyroepiandrosterone in Japanese male with impaired glucose tolerance and low insulin response. *Endocr J* 43(3): 285–290, 1996.
29. Same as 24.
30. Buffington CK, et al. Case report: amelioration of insulin resistance in diabetes with dehydroepiandrosterone. *Am J Med Sci* 306(5): 320–324, 1993.
31. Haffner SM, et al. Decreased testosterone and dehydroepiandrosterone sulfate concentrations are associated with increased insulin and glucose concentrations in nondiabetic men. *Metabolism* 43(5): 599–603, 1994.
32. Buffington CK, et al. Enhanced adrenocortical activity as a contributing factor to diabetes in hyperandrogenic women. *Metabolism* 43(5): 584–590, 1994.
33. Foldes JL, et al. Dehydroepiandrosterone sulfate (DS), dehydroepiandrosterone (D) and "free" dehydroepiandrosterone (FD) in the plasma with thyroid diseases. *Horm Metab Res* 15: 623–624, 1983.
34. Fitzgerald PA. Adrenal cortex physiology. In: Tierney LM Jr, McPhee J, Papadakis MA, eds. *Current Medical Diagnosis and Treatment.* Los Altos, CA: MA Lange Publishers, 1995: 982.
35. Sunderland T, et al. Reduced plasma dehydroepiandrosterone concentrations in Alzheimer's disease. *Lancet* 2: 570, 1989.
36. Gordon GB, et al. Serum levels of dehydroepiandrosterone and its sulfate and the risk of developing bladder cancer. *Cancer Res* 51(5): 1366–1369, 1991.
37. Gordon GB, et al. Serum levels of dehydroepiandrosterone and dehydroepiandrosterone sulfate and the risk of developing gastric cancer. *Cancer Epidemiol Biomarkers Prev* 2(1): 33–35, 1993.
38. Stahl H, et al. Dehydro-epiandrosterone (DHEA) levels in patients with prostatic cancer, heart diseases and under surgery stress. *Exp Clin Endocrinol* 99: 68–70, 1992.
39. Bhatavdekar JM, et al. Levels of circulating peptide and steroid hormones in men with lung cancer. *Neoplasma* 41(2): 101–103, 1994.
40. Gordon GB, et al. Relationship of serum levels of dehydroepiandrosterone and dehydroepiandrosterone sulfate to the risk of developing postmenopausal breast cancer. *Cancer Res* 50(13): 3859–3862, 1990.
41. Vermeulen A. Adrenal androgens and aging. In: Genazzani AR, Thijssen JH, Siiteri PK, eds. *Adrenal Androgens.* New York: Raven Press, 1980: 27–42.
42. Bonney RC, et al. The interrelationship between plasma 5-ene adrenal androgens in normal women. *J Steroid Biochem* 20: 1353–1355, 1984.
43. Wong L, et al. A genetic component to the variation of dehydroepiandrosterone. *Metab Clin Exp* 34: 731–736, 1985.
44. Born J, et al. Night-time plasma cortisol secretion is associated with specific sleep stages. *Biol Psychiatry* 21: 1415–1424, 1986.
45. Born J, et al. Gluco- and antimineralocorticoid effects on human sleep: a role of central corticosteroid receptors. *Am J Physiol* 260(2 Pt 1): E183–E188, 1991.
46. Guechot J, et al. Simple laboratory test of neuroendocrine disturbance in depression: 11 p.m. saliva cortisol. *Biol Psychiatry* 18: 1–4, 1987.
47. Guechot J, et al. Physiological and pathological variations in saliva cortisol. *Horm Res* 16: 357–364, 1982.
48. Galard R, et al. Salivary cortisol levels and their correlation with plasma ACTH levels in depressed patients before and after DST. *Am J Psychiatry* 148: 505–508, 1991.
49. Goodyer I, et al. Cortisol hypersecretion in depressed school-aged children and adolescents. *Psychiat Res* 37: 237–244, 1991.

50. von Zerssen D, et al. Diurnal variation of mood and the cortisol rhythm in depression and normal states of mind. *Eur Arch Psychiat Neurol Sci* 237: 36–45, 1987.

51. Opstad K. Circadian rhythm of hormones is extinguished during prolonged physical stress, sleep and energy deficiency in young men. *Eur J Endocrinol* 131: 56–66, 1994.

52. Blood GW, et al. Subjective anxiety measurements and cortisol responses in adults who stutter. *J Speech Hear Res* 37: 760–768, 1994.

53. Demitrack MA. Chronic fatigue syndrome: a disease of the hypothalamic–pituitary–adrenal axis? [editorial] *Ann Med* 26(1): 1–5, 1994.

54. Demitrack MA, et al. Evidence for impaired activation of the hypothalamic–pituitary–adrenal axis in patients with chronic fatigue syndrome. *J Clin Endocrinol Metab* 73: 1224–1234, 1991.

55. Jeffries WM. Mild adrenocorticol deficiency, chronic allergies, autoimmune disorders and the chronic fatigue syndrome: a continuation of the cortisone story. *Med Hypotheses* 42(3): 183–189, 1994.

56. Araneo B, Daynes R. Dehydroepiandrosterone functions as more than an antiglucocorticoid in preserving immunocompetence after thermal injury. *Endocrinology* 136: 393–401, 1995.

57. Goulding NS, Guyre PM. Glucocorticoids, lipocortins and the immune response. *Curr Opin Immunol* 5: 108–113, 1993.

58. Filipovsky J, et al. The relationship of blood pressure with glucose, insulin, heart rate, free fatty acids and plasma cortisol levels according to degree of obesity in middle-aged men. *J Hypertens* 14(2): 229–235, 1996.

59. Schnorr D, et al. Dehydroepiandrosterone (DHEA) levels in patients with prostatic cancer, heart diseases and under surgery stress. *Exp Clin Endocrinol* 99: 68–70, 1992.

60. Tsuda K, et al. Electrocardiographic abnormalities in patients with Cushing's syndrome. *Jpn Heart J* 36(3): 333–339, 1995.

61. Walker BR. Abnormal glucocorticoid activity in subjects with risk factors for cardiovascular disease. *Endocr Res* 22(4): 710–708, 1996.

62. Pasquali R, et al. Hypothalamic–pituitary–adrenal axis activity and its relationship to the autonomic nervous system in women with visceral and subcutaneous obesity: effects of the corticotropin-releasing factor/arginine-vasopressin test and of stress. *Metabolism* 45(3): 351–356, 1996.

63. Ljung T, et al. Inhibition of cortisol secretion by dexamethasone in relation to body fat distribution: a dose-response study. *Obese Res* 4(3): 277–282, 1996.

64. McErin P, et al. Cortisol secretion in relation to body fat distribution in obese premenopausal women. *Metabolism* 41: 882–886, 1992.

65. Champe PC, Harvey RA, eds. Lippincott Illustrated Reviews. Biochemistry. New York: JB Lippincott, 1992.

66. De Feo P, et al. Contribution of cortisol to glucose counterregulation in humans. *Am J Physiol* 257: E35–E42, 1989.

67. Barnes BO, Galton L. *Hypothyroidism: The Unsuspected Illness*. New York: Harper and Row, 1976: 206–207.

68. Bockman RS, Weinerman SA. Steroid-induced osteoporosis. *Orthop Clin North Am* 21(1): 97–107, 1990.

69. Catargi B, et al. Development of bone mineral density after cure of Cushing's syndrome. *Ann Endocrinol* 57(3): 203–208, 1996.

70. Manolagas SC, et al. Adrenal steroids and the development of osteoporosis in oophorectomized women. *Lancet* 2: 597, 1979.

71. George MS, et al. CSF neuroactive steroids in affective disorders: pregnenolone, progesterone, and DBI. *Biol Psychiatry* 35(10): 775–780, 1994.

72. Holsboer F, et al. Steroid effects on central neurons and implications for psychiatric and neurological disorders. *Ann N Y Acad Sci* 746: 345–359; discussion 359–61, 1994.

73. Pallares M, et al. The neurosteroid pregnenolone sulfate infused into the nucleus basalis increases both acetylcholine release in the frontal cortex or amygdala and spatial memory. *Neuroscience* 87(3): 551–558, 1998.

74. Rupprecht R. The neuropsychopharmacological potential of neuroactive steroids. *J Psychiatr Res* 31(3): 297–314, 1997.

75. Same as 73.

76. Same as 72.

77. Vallee M, et al. Neurosteroids: deficient cognitive performance in aged rats depends on low pregnenolone sulfate levels in the hippocampus. *Proc Natl Acad Sci USA* 94(26): 14865–14870, 1997.

78. Khalsa DS. Integrated medicine and the prevention and reversal of memory loss. *Altern Ther Health Med* 4(6): 38–43, 1998.

79. Sahelian, R. *Pregnenolone: Nature's Feel Good Hormone*. Garden City Park, NY: Avery Publishing Group, 1997: 28–29.

80. Hedman M, Nilsson E, de la Torre B. Low blood and synovial fluid levels of sulpho-conjugated steroids in rheumatoid arthritis. *Clin Exp Rheumatol* 10(1): 25–30, 1992.

81. Sahelian, R. *Pregnenolone: Nature's Feel Good Hormone*. Garden City Park, NY: Avery Publishing Group, 1997: 57–64.

82. Dollins AB, et al. Effect of inducing nocturnal serum melatonin concentrations in daytime on sleep, mood, body temperature, and performance. *Proc Natl Acad Sci USA* 91: 1824–1828, 1994.

83. Wehr TA. The durations of human melatonin secretion and sleep respond to changes in daylength (photoperiod). *J Clin Endocrinol Metab* 73: 1276–1280, 1991.

84. Campbell SS, Broughton RJ. Rapid decline in body temperature before sleep. *Chronobiol Int* 11(2): 126–131, 1994.

85. Axelrod J. The pineal gland: a neurochemical transducer. *Science* 184: 1341–1348, 1974.

86. Pang SF, et al. Melatonin receptors in peripheral tissues: a new area of melatonin research. *Biol Signals* 2(4): 177–180, 1993.

87. Bojkowski C, Arendt J. Factors influencing urinary 6-sulphatoxymelatonin, a major melatonin metabolite, in normal human subjects. *Clin Endocrinol* 33: 435–444, 1990.

88. Wever RA. Characteristics of circadian rhythms in human functions; melatonin in humans. *J Neural Trans* (suppl 21): 323–374, 1986.

89. Reiter RJ. Neuroendocrine effects of light. *Int J Biometeorol* 35(3): 169–175, 1991.

90. Dahlitz M, et al. Delayed sleep phase syndrome response to melatonin. *Lancet* 337: 1121–1124, 1991.

91. Petrie K, et al. A double-blind trial of melatonin as a treatment for jet lag in international cabin crew. *Biol Psychiatry* 33: 526–530, 1993.

92. Reiter RJ, et al. Reduction of the nocturnal rise in pineal melatonin levels in rats exposed to 60-Hz electric fields in utero and for 23 days after birth. *Life Sci* 42: 2203–2206, 1988.

93. Wilson BW, et al. 60-Hz electric-field effects on pineal melatonin rhythms: time course for onset and recovery. *Bioelectromagnetics* 7: 239–242, 1986.

94. Wilson BW, et al. Chronic exposure to 60-Hz electric fields: effects on pineal function in the rat. *Bioelectromagnetics* 2: 371–380, 1981.

95. Welker HA, et al. Effects of an artificial magnetic field on serotonin N-acetyltransferase activity and melatonin content of the rat pineal gland. *Exp Brain Res* 50: 426–432, 1983.

96. Brugger P, et al. Impaired nocturnal secretion of melatonin in coronary heart disease. *Lancet* 345: 1408, 1995.
97. Chan TY, Tang PL. Effect of melatonin on the maintenance of cholesterol homeostasis in the rat. *Endocr Res* 21(3): 681–696, 1995.
98. Cardinali DP, et al. The effects of melatonin in human platelets. *Acta Physiol Pharmacol Ther Latinaom* 43: 1–13, 1993.
99. Cutando A, Silvestre FJ. Melatonin: implications at the oral level. *Bull Group Int Rech Sci Stomatol Odontol* 38: 81–86, 1995.
100. Maestroni GJ. The immunoneuroendocrine role of melatonin. *J Pineal Res* 14(1): 1–10, 1993.
101. Armstrong SM, Redman JR. Melatonin: a chronobiotic with anti-aging properties? *Med Hypotheses* 34(4): 300–309, 1991.
102. Poeggeler B, et al. Melatonin, hydroxyl radical-mediated oxidative damage, and aging: a hypothesis. *J Pineal Res* 14(4): 151–168, 1993.
103. Reiter RJ. The role of the neurohormone melatonin as a buffer against macromolecular oxidative damage. *Neurochem Int* 27(6): 453–460, 1995.
104. Reiter RJ. Interactions of the pineal hormone melatonin with oxygen-centered free radicals: a brief review. *Braz J Med Biol Res* 26(11): 1141–55, 1993.
105. Reiter RJ, et al. A review of the evidence supporting melatonin's role as an antioxidant. *J Pineal Res* 18: 1–11, 1995.
106. Vijayalaxmi BZ, et al. Melatonin protects human blood lymphocytes from radiation induced chromosomal damage. *Mutat Res* 346(1): 23–31, 1995.
107. Shida CS, et al. High melatonin solubility in aqueous medium. *J Pineal Res* 16: 198–201, 1994.
108. Ram PT, et al. Estrogen receptor transactivation in MCF-7 breast cancer cells by melatonin and growth factors. *Mol Cell Endocrinol* 141(1–2): 53–64, 1998.
109. Cos S, et al. Influence of melatonin on invasive and metastatic properties of MCF-7 human breast cancer cells. *Cancer Res* 58(19): 4383–4390, 1998.
110. Cos S, Blask DE. Melatonin modulates growth factor activity in MCF-7 human breast cancer cells. *J Pineal Res* 17(1): 25–32, 1994.
111. Okatani Y, et al. Nocturnal changes in pineal melatonin synthesis during puberty: relation to estrogen and progesterone levels in female rats. *J Pineal Res* 22(1): 33–41, 1997.
112. Okatani Y, et al. Effect of estrogen on melatonin synthesis in female peripubertal rats. *J Pineal Res* 24(2): 67–72, 1998.
113. Danforth DN, Jr, et al. Melatonin increases oestrogen receptor binding activity of human breast cancer cells. *Nature* 305(5932): 323–325, 1983.
114. Murphy DL, et al. Effects of antidepressants and other psychotropic drugs on melatonin release and pineal gland function. *J Neural Transm Suppl* 21: 2291–2309, 1986.
115. Murphy DL, et al. Human plasma melatonin is elevated during treatment with the monoamine oxidase inhibitors clorgyline and tranylcypromine but not deprenyl. *Psychiatry Res* 17(2): 119–127, 1986.
116. Murphy DL, et al. Marked enhancement by clorgyline of nocturnal and daytime melatonin release in rhesus monkeys. *Psychopharmacology* 92(3): 382–387, 1987.
117. Golden RN, et al. Antidepressants reduce whole-body norepinephrine turnover whle enhancing 6-hydroxymelatonin output. *Arch Gen Psychiatry* 45(2): 150–154, 1988.
118. Childs PA, et al. Effect of fluoxetine on melatonin inpatients with seasonal affective disorder and matched controls. *Br J Psychiatry* 166(2): 196–198, 1995.
119. Murphy PJ, et al. Nonsteroidal anti-inflammatory drugs alter body temperature and suppress melatonin in humans. *Physiol Behav* 59(1): 133–139, 1996.

120. Surrall K, et al. Effect of ibuprofen and indomethacin on human plasma melatonin. *J Pharm. Pharmacol* 39(10): 840–843, 1987.
121. Ritta MN, Cardinali DP. Prostaglandin E2 increases adenosine 3', 5'-monophosphate concentration and binding-site occupancy, and stimulates serotonin-N-acetyltransferase activity in rat pineal glands in vitro. *Mol Cell Endocrinol* 23(2): 151–159, 1981.
122. Rommel T, Demisch L. Influence of chronic beta-adrenoreceptor blocker treatment on melatonin secretion and sleep quality in patients with essential hypertension. *J Neural Transm Gen Sect* 95(1): 39–48, 1994.
123. Hanssen T, et al. Propranolol in schizophrenia. Clinical, metabolic, and pharmacological findings. *Arch Gen Psychiatry* 37(6): 685–690, 1980.
124. Ekman AC, et al. Ethanol inhibits melatonin secretion in healthy volunteers in a dose-dependent randomized double blind cross-over study. *J Clin Endocrinol Metab* 77(3): 780–783, 1993.
125. Wright KP Jr, et al. Caffeine and light effects on nighttime melatonin and temperature levels in sleep-deprived humans. *Brain Res* 30; 747(1): 78–84, 1997.
126. Monteleone P, et al. Preliminary observations on the suppression of nocturnal plasma melatonin levels by short-term administration of diazepam in humans. *J Pineal Res* 6(3): 253–258, 1989.
127. Touitou Y, et al. Age- and sex-associated modification of plasma melatonin concentrations in man. Relationship to pathology, malignant or not, and autopsy findings. *Acta Endocrinol* 108(1): 135–144, 1985.
128. Ronkainen H, et al. Effects of physical exercise on the serum concentration of melatonin in female runners. *Acta Obstet Gynecol Scand* 65(8): 827–829, 1986.
129. Theron JJ, et al. Effect of physical exercise on plasma melatonin levels in normal volunteers. *S Afr Med J* 66(22): 838–841, 1984.
130. Bullen BA, et al. Exercise effect upon plasma melatonin levels in women: possible physiological significance. *Can J Appl Sport Sci* 7(2): 90–97, 1982.
131. Monteleone P, et al. The human pineal gland responds to stress-induced sympathetic activation in the second half of the dark phase: preliminary evidence. *J Neural Transm Gen Sect* 92(1): 25–32, 1993.
132. Monteleone P, et al. Physical exercise at night blunts the nocturnal increase of plasma melatonin levels in healthy humans. *Life Sci* 47(22): 1989–1995, 1990.
133. Guardiola-Lemaitre B. Toxicology of melatonin. *J Biol Rhythms* 12(6): 697–706, 1997.
134. Weaver DR. Reproductive safety of melatonin: a "wonder drug" to wonder about. *J Biol Rhythms* 12(6): 682–689, 1997.
135. Affinito P, et al. Effects of thyroxine therapy on bone metabolism in postmenopausal women with hypothyroidism. *Acta Obstet Gynecol Scand* 75(9): 843–848, 1996.
136. Guo CY, et al. Longitudinal changes of bone mineral density and bone turnover in postmenopausal women on thyroxine. *Clin Endocrinol* 46(3): 301–307
137. Williams JB. Adverse effects of thyroid hormones. *Drugs Aging* 11(6): 460–469, 1997.
138. Lecomte P, et al. Effects of suppressive doses of levothyroxine treatment on sex-hormone-binding globulin and bone metabolism. *Thyroid* 5(1): 19–23, 1995.
139. Same as 137.
140. De Rosa G, et al. Prospective study of bone loss in pre- and postmenopausal women on L-thyroxine therapy for non-toxic goitre. *Clin Endocrinol* 47(5): 529–535, 1997.

141. Schneider DL, et al. Thyroid hormone use and bone mineral density in elderly women. Effects of estrogen. *JAMA* 271(16): 1245–1249, 1994.
142. Franklyn JA, et al. Effect of estrogen replacement therapy upon bone mineral density in thyroxine-treated postmenopausal women with a past history of thyrotoxicosis. *Thyroid* 5(5): 359–363, 1995.
143. Benencia H, et al. Thyroid profile modifications during oral hormone replacement therapy in postmenopausal women. *Gynecol Endocrinol* 12(3): 179–184, 1998.
144. Benencia H, et al. Thyroid profile modifications during oral hormone replacement therapy in postmenopausal women. *Gynecol Endocrinol* 12(3): 179–184, 1998.
145. National Physicians Group Debunks Human Growth Hormone "Fountain Of Youth" And "Super Athlete" Claims. Press Release. For Immediate Release—September 16, 1998. Contact: Stephanie Barker. American Association of Clinical Endocrinologists, 1000 Riverside Ave. Suite 205, Jacksonville, FL 32204.

Glossary

In most cases, new words and concepts are defined or described briefly the first time that they appear in this book. This glossary provides an easy review of these terms as well as other terms related to menopause.

Adaptogen: A substance that helps the body adapt to stress. Adaptogens appear to have their most specific effects on the adrenal glands, nervous system, and immune system, but may affect other tissues as well. Adaptogens may be able to decrease deterioration, slow aging of tissues, and revitalize the body.

Adrenal glands: These two endocrine glands secrete important steroid hormones and catecholamines. Located above each kidney, each adrenal gland is composed of two sections: an outer part, called the adrenal cortex; and an inner part, called the adrenal medulla. The adrenal cortex creates androgens, estrogens, glucocorticoids, and mineralocorticoids. The adrenal medulla produces catecholamines.

Adrenal recruitment: The process by which the adrenal glands are "recruited" to help make up for the decreased production of steroid hormones that occurs when a woman goes through menopause. Some of the production is transferred to the adrenal glands. This adrenal recruitment should result in increased production of androstenedione and other steroid hormones.

Agonist: A substance that stimulates the response at cell receptors by acting in the same way as a substance occurring naturally in the body. In the context of this book, the term usually refers to a hormone agonist, which behaves like a hormone such as estrogen when it binds to the receptor, and thereby affects similar changes in cells or tissues in a woman's body.

Aldosterone: Produced by the adrenal glands, aldosterone is a mineralocorticoid hormone that regulates the body's balance of water and electrolytes such as potassium and sodium. Aldosterone stimulates the kidney to eliminate potassium from the body and retain sodium and water.

Anabolic: The anabolic process (anabolism) is the part of the body's metabolic process that involves tissue or protein building and thus uses energy. Androgens such as testosterone have anabolic activity, which results in increased production of muscle, bone, and other structures. Estrogens such as estradiol also have anabolic activity, which increases production of blood proteins such as sex-hormone-binding globulin from the liver. Estrogens also exert some anabolic influence on bone and other tissues. Together, anabolic and catabolic hormones affect both aspects of the metabolic process.

Androgens: A group of hormones traditionally associated with the masculine traits of males (*andro* means "male"). Science now recognizes androgens as vital for both genders. In women, the ovaries and the cortex of the adrenal glands produce these hormones, which include testosterone, DHEA, androstenedione, and androstenediol, as well as their metabolites. Androgens promote protein building in every tissue of the body, and develop and maintain bone growth and health.

Androstenedione/Androstenediol: These are androgens that have their own actions, but are usually converted into testosterone or estrogens. In women, these androgens are produced predominantly by the adrenal glands, though the ovaries manufacture a portion.

Antagonist: A substance that negates the action of another substance. In the context of this book, the term usually refers to a hormone antagonist. These substances work against or compete with hormones, generally by blocking the ability of hormones to bind to receptors and thereby affect changes in cells or tissues.

Antiandrogens: Drugs, herbs, or other substances that decrease the production or actions of testosterone or other androgens are known as antiandrogens. An antiandrogen can decrease the actions of an androgen by binding to androgen receptors and blocking the action of the hormone, or it may both decrease production and block the receptor.

Antiestrogens: Drugs, herbs, or other substances that decrease the production or actions of estradiol or other estrogens are termed antiestrogens. An antiestrogen can decrease the actions of an estrogen by binding to estrogen receptors and blocking the action of the hormone, or it may both decrease production and block the receptor.

Antihormones: Drugs, herbs, or other substances that decrease the production or actions of a hormone are called antihormones. An antihormone can decrease the actions of a hormone by binding to the hormone receptors and blocking the action of the hormone, or it may both decrease production and block the receptor. Though the antihormones discussed in this book are those working against androgens, estrogens, and progestogens, other hormones have antihormone counterparts.

Antioxidant: A substance that prevents or counteracts the damaging effects of oxidation (oxygen reactions), an antioxidant helps decrease the formation of and damage caused by free radicals.

Antiprogestogens: Drugs, herbs, or other substances that decrease the production or actions of progesterone or other progestogens are called antiprogestogens. An antiprogestogen can decrease the actions of a progestogen by binding to progestogen receptors and blocking the action of the hormone, or it may both decrease production and block the receptor.

Bio-compatible: A bio-compatible substance is one that is similar enough to be used as a substitute for a naturally occurring substance. For example, a hormone that is bio-compatible reacts similarly to the body's natural hormone and is able to elicit a response even though it is not bio-identical.

Bio-identical: A substance that is biologically identical to the substance occurring naturally in an organism is termed bio-identical. For instance, the estradiol that is manufactured from soy or wild yam is bio-identical to estradiol occurring in women.

Blood lipids: A generic term for all the lipids or "fats" in the blood, blood lipids include total cholesterol, HDL ("good") cholesterol, LDL ("bad") cholesterol, VLDL (a precursor to LDL), and triglycerides.

Catabolic: The catabolic process (catabolism) is the part of metabolism that involves protein or tissue breakdown and creates energy, often in the form of glucose. Glucocorticoids such as cortisol are involved in catabolic activity, though progesterone also has some catabolic activity, especially in high doses. Together, catabolic and anabolic hormones affect both aspects of the metabolic processes that take place in the body.

Catecholamines: Hormones manufactured and released by the adrenal medulla or the nervous system. Catecholamines, which include adrenaline, noradrenaline, and dopamine, act as neurotransmitters, having a direct effect on the brain and nerves.

Cholesterol side chain cleavage system: This system is comprised of enzymes required for the first step of steroidogenesis. This group, or system, of enzymes in the adrenal glands is needed to convert cholesterol to pregnenolone. This is often called the rate-limiting step because all other reactions in steroidogenesis depend upon this first step. As with most enzyme reactions, this process requires a number of different vitamins in order to occur properly.

Circadian rhythm: A pattern that repeats itself daily. Most steroid hormones have a circadian rhythm in which levels are highest in the morning or the first half of the day and lowest at midnight.

Collagen: A fibrous protein that makes up a major part of connective tissue in bones, tendons, skin, and other tissues. Collagen provides a structured framework that holds cells and tissues together.

Cortisol: Also known as hydrocortisone, cortisol is a steroid hormone secreted by the adrenal cortex. In the sub-group of steroid hormones called glucocorticos-teroids, cortisol is both the most potent and most abundantly produced.

Dehydroepiandrosterone (DHEA): An androgen produced by the adrenal glands, DHEA has actions of its own, but can also be converted into androgens and estrogens. DHEA-S is the most abundant form of DHEA in the body and the form used as a precursor for androgens and estrogens.

Delivery system: See drug delivery system.

DHEA/DHEA-S: See dehydroepiandrosterone.

Diosgenin: A substance isolated from wild yam and other plants that can be converted in a laboratory into pregnenolone, progesterone, estradiol, and other hormones.

Dopamine: A neurotransmitter that affects mood and mental function, dopamine is also a precursor of adrenaline and noradrenaline.

Drug delivery system: This term refers to the way in which hormones and drugs are delivered to the body. Drug delivery systems for hormones include oral (by mouth), topical (skin cream or gel), injection (intramuscular or subcutaneous), transvaginal (vaginal suppository or cream), sublingual (under the tongue), or transbuccal (held inside the mouth against the cheek and absorbed through the mouth's lining).

Endocrine: This word literally means "secreting internally." The endocrine system is a group of glands producing secretions (hormones) that are distributed throughout the body via the bloodstream.

Endometrial hyperplasia: Abnormal thickening of the endometrium (see next page). Endometrial hyperplasia can cause abnormal bleeding in postmenopausal women, and is associated with an increased risk of endometrial cancer. Unopposed estrogen can result in endometrial hyperplasia.

Endometrium: The mucous membrane lining the uterus. It is sloughed off during menstruation and grows back after a period, slowly getting thicker until the next menstrual period.

Enzymes: Special proteins in the body that act as catalysts which speed up chemical or metabolic reactions but are not used up or changed in the process.

Equilibrium: A state of balance in which no change occurs. For example, after starting on any hormone, it is best to wait at least one month before testing to allow time for the hormones to reach equilibrium in the blood.

Estradiol (E_2): The most potent of the naturally occurring estrogens, estradiol is formed primarily by the ovaries, but also by the adrenal cortex, placenta, and testes to a lesser degree. Its chemical name is 17-beta-estradiol, or estra-1,3,5(10)-triene-3,17beta-diol.

Estriol (E_3): As an end product of estrogen metabolism, estriol is usually the major metabolite found in urine, especially during pregnancy. Estriol is currently used in some hormone replacement protocols.

Estrogen: This is actually a generic term for any substance, whether natural or synthetic, that has the same biological effect as the hormone estradiol. Estrogens are predominantly made by the ovaries, but also by the adrenal cortex, placenta, and testes to a lesser degree. Estradiol is the most potent estrogen that occurs naturally in the human body. Other estrogens include estrone and metabolites such as estriol.

Estrogen mimetics: Substances, such as herbs or foods, that mimic the effects of estrogen, though the effects are weaker than those of the hormone.

Estrone (E_1): An estrogen produced by the adrenal glands and ovaries. It is also a metabolite of estradiol that is less potent than estradiol and more potent than estriol. Estrone is commonly found in the ovaries, placenta, and urine. It has much less biological activity than estradiol.

FAD/FMN (Flavin Adenine Dinucleotide/Flavin Mononucleotide): Molecules that contain riboflavin (vitamin B_2) and work with enzymes in various metabolic processes requiring energy.

Free radicals: Overactive chemicals caused by oxidation (oxygen reactions) are known as free radicals. The strong reactions of free radicals harm molecules by changing their structure. This molecular change can affect the function of cells and tissues.

GABA/GABAA (Gamma-amino-butyric acid): A neurotransmitter that helps keep the nerve cells from being too reactive, so the nervous system does not overload. Actions of GABA type A (GABAA) include calming and sedating the nervous system. GABA agonists are also calming and sedating to the nervous system and include progesterone and progesterone metabolites, as well as benzodiazepine drugs such as Valium.

Glandular extracts: Extracts of specific animal tissues or glands are used to restore the health and function of the corresponding tissue or gland in humans. Usually taken orally, glandular extracts can help rejuvenate, strengthen, tonify, and nourish the target tissues.

Glucocorticosteroid/glucocorticoid: Manufactured by the adrenal cortex, these hormones mainly affect the metabolism of carbohydrates such as blood glucose. Cortisol is the major natural glucocorticoid.

Growth hormone: A hormone produced by the pituitary gland, which, in turn, stimulates the liver to produce a number of different insulin-like-growth-factors (IGFs). These IGF hormones promote growth and maintain function of tissues.

Homeostasis: A state of balance, or equilibrium, between different (and often opposing) functions, chemicals, or actions in the body.

Hormone: A chemical substance formed in one part of the body and carried in the blood to another part where it exerts its effects. Hormones may affect more than one part of the body. Glands that do not have ducts form most hormones, so the hormone is secreted directly into the bloodstream.

Hormone receptors: See receptor.

Insulin-like-growth-factor: See growth hormone.

Liver first pass: This term refers to the effect of the liver on hormones taken by mouth in which approximately 90% of them are broken down or metabolized as they pass through the liver before going into general circulation in the body.

Menopause Type Questionnaire (MTQ): A questionnaire designed to determine what type of menopause a women is experiencing.

Menorrhagia: Excessive uterine bleeding occurring at the regular intervals of menstruation.

Metabolism/metabolic process: Refers to the chemical changes taking place in cells, and includes all anabolic and catabolic processes; that is, energy being created by catabolic activity, and energy being used by anabolic activity. The chemical processes of metabolism allow various functions to occur, including both the production and destruction of molecules, cells, and tissues.

Metabolite: A substance, such as a specific hormone, produced as part of a metabolic process. For example, estriol is a metabolite resulting from the metabolism of estradiol.

Metalloenzymes: Enzymes that contain metals as part of their structure.

Micronized: Reduced particle size of a substance, such as progesterone or estradiol, which enables the substance to be absorbed through the lymphatic system and slow its degradation by the liver.

Mineralocorticoid: A group of hormones produced by the adrenal cortex, mineralocorticoids regulate the body's balance of water and electrolytes such as potassium and sodium. Aldosterone is the most potent mineralocorticoid.

NADH/NADPH [Nicotinamide adenine dinucleotide(H)/Nicotinamide adenine dinucleotide phosphate(H)]: Molecules that contain niacin (vitamin B3) and work with enzymes in various metabolic processes requiring energy.

Natural hormone: For the purpose of this book, the phrase "natural hormone" means a hormone that is exactly the same as, or bio-identical to, the hormone that occurs naturally in the human body.

Neurotransmitter: Molecules that affect the brain and nerves due to their action on nerve cells. Neurotransmitters, which include adrenaline, noradrenaline, and dopamine, influence mood, memory, and other mental functions.

Ovaries: Two small, oval glands located on either side of the uterus, ovaries function as endocrine glands by releasing estradiol, progesterone, testosterone, and other hormones into the blood. In reproductive terms, the ovaries are where the ova (eggs) are developed, to be released during ovulation.

Oxidation: The chemical process that takes place when oxygen reacts with another substance. Rusting iron is oxidation, as is the browning of a sliced apple left exposed to air. Oxidation changes the very structure and nature of a substance, therefore substances do not function in exactly the same way after undergoing oxidation. When oxidation is controlled, it is a vital part of metabolism. When oxidation is not controlled, it can result in the production of harmful free radicals.

Phytoestrogens: Plant substances that have an estrogenlike activity or, more specifically, bind to estrogen receptor sites in cells.

Precursor: A substance that is transformed into another substance which is usually more active. For instance, androstenedione is a precursor for testosterone, a more potent hormone.

Pregnenolone: The first steroid hormone made in the steroidogenic pathway, pregnenolone acts as a precursor for all other hormones.

Progesterone: A steroid hormone in the progestogen family, progesterone has antiestrogen actions and is manufactured by the corpus luteum (a yellow mass of cells in the ovary formed after the egg has been released) during the second half of the menstrual cycle. It is made in increased quantities by the placenta during pregnancy. Classically referred to as the pregnancy hormone, since it is required for pregnancy, progesterone can even be used to prevent some forms of miscarriage.

Progestogens: A generic term for any substance, natural or synthetic, that affects some or all of the biological changes produced by progesterone.

Quartile: One-fourth of a reference range.

Receptor: A certain structured molecule, either on the surface of a cell or within a cell, to which a certain substance such as a hormone binds, allowing the hormone to affect the cell.

Reference Range: The normal range of a lab result.

Steroid hormones/steroids: A generic term for a class of hormones and drugs that are closely related and based on the cholesterol molecule, which is the precursor for all steroid hormones. Steroid hormones control sex characteristics and the growth and maintenance of many tissues. The receptors for steroid hormones are inside the cell on the nucleus instead of on the cell membrane.

Steroidogenesis/steroidogenic pathway: This process and pathway refers to the biological formation of steroid hormones, such as estrogens, progesterone, testosterone, DHEA, and cortisol.

Subclinical: This term refers to the early stage of a condition before major signs or symptoms become apparent, or such a mild form of the condition that it is not apparent.

Testosterone: The most potent of the naturally occurring androgens. In women, the ovaries and adrenal cortex manufacture testosterone.

Transvaginal: A drug delivery system using vaginal suppositories or creams.

Unopposed estrogen: Estrogen that is not balanced or opposed by progesterone is known as unopposed estrogen.

Uterus: The hollow muscular organ in women in which a fertilized ovum (egg) becomes implanted and the developing embryo and fetus is nourished. The lining of the uterus is the endometrium.

Resources

For more information about treatment of menopause and other health-related issues, e-mail the author directly at Dr.Collins@yourmenopausetype.com or visit *www.yourmenopausetype.com*, a Web site that currently features the following sections:

- Your Menopause Type
- Ask Dr. Collins
- Find a Physician
- Choose a Pharmacist
- Resources for Women
- Nutritional Supplements
- Health Spas and Resorts
- Fitness Centers & Gyms
- Resources for Physicians
- Resources for Pharmacists
- Lab Tests

This site will continue to grow and change based upon reader feedback and current information.

SALIVA HORMONE TESTS

Many physicians, pharmacists, and other health-care professionals are currently using the professional saliva hormone tests that measure each hormone three times. You can order your test directly through many of these professionals by phone, mail, or the Internet. Many of them are also available to assist with interpretation and consultation. See an example of a saliva testing report below.

Your Menopause Type

An analysis of salivary estradiol, progesterone and testosterone levels. Based on *Discover Your Menopause Type* by Joseph Collins, N.D.

Test ID#: 040200-0143
Patient: Sample Patient
Address: 82953 Anystreet Ave.
Anytown, ST 26643
Date: January 6, 2000

Ordered by:
John Q. Smith, M.D.
5432 Physician Lane
Anytown, ST 26643
(123) 456-7980

Your Saliva Test Hormone Levels

	Specimen 1	Specimen 2	Specimen 3	Average levels*	Result
Estradiol	4.1	3.4	4.3	3.9 pmol/L	Low
Progesterone	38	62	58	53 pmol/L	Low
Testosterone	216	168	189	191 pmol/L	High

*Each hormone was measured three times. The ideal reference range for estradiol is 4.4–17.3 pmol/L, for progesterone it is 64–300 pmol/L, and for testosterone it is 64–164 pmol/L.

Commentary:

This report is designed to reveal risks associated with the specific menopause type.

The tests reveal: Estradiol and Progesterone Deficiency with High Testosterone Menopause Type.

With this menopause type there is increased risk of oily skin, acne, hirsutism (facial hair) and deepening of the voice due to the high testosterone.

Hyperinsulinemia and insulin resistance risk is also high, due to the elevated testosterone levels with low estradiol.

The elevated testosterone and increased risk for hyperinsulinemia result in a higher risk for endometrial cancer, breast cancer, non-insulin–dependent diabetes, and heart disease.

Vaginal dryness due to the low estradiol is likely in this menopause type.

The low estradiol may result in difficulty in remembering name- and word-related things, while new learning will become a struggle.

Shrinking of the breasts may occur due to estradiol deficiency with a testosterone excess.

The progesterone-to-estradiol ratio (P:E) of 13:1 is below ideal P:E ratio ranges. This increases risk for irritability, inflammation, abnormal uterine bleeding, and cancer risks.

To learn more about the Estradiol and Progesterone Deficiency with High Testosterone Menopause Type, talk to your health-care provider, and review the book *Discover Your Menopause Type* by Joseph Collins, N.D.

PHYSICIANS AND OTHER HEALTH-CARE PROFESSIONAL ORGANIZATIONS

The following organizations are very useful resources for finding a practitioner in your area that can assist you in the following areas:

The American Association
of Naturopathic Physicians
8201 Greensboro Drive, Suite 300
McLean, VA 22102
Phone: (703) 610-9037
Fax: (703) 610-9005
www.naturopathic.org
Licensed Naturopathic
Physician (N.D. or N.M.D.)

American Holistic Medical
Association
6728 McLean Village Drive
McLean, VA 22101-8729
www.holisticmedicine.org
Medical doctors (M.D.) and
doctors of osteopathic medicine (D.O.)

American College for
Advancement in Medicine
23121 Verdugo Drive, Suite 204
Laguna Hills, CA 92653
e-mail: acam@acam.org
www.acam.org
Physicians with various degrees.

American Osteopathic Association
142 E. Ontario Street
Chicago, IL 60611
Phone: (312) 202-8000
Fax: (312) 202-8200
www.aoa-net.org
Doctors of osteopathic
medicine (D.O.).

The American Chiropractic
Association
1701 Clarendon Boulevard
Arlington, VA 22209
Fax: (703) 243-2593
www.amerchiro.org
Doctors of chiropractic (D.C.).

American Association
of Oriental Medicine
433 Front Street
Catasauqua, PA 18032
Phone: (610) 266-1433
Fax: (610) 264-2768
www.aaom.org
Licensed Acupuncturist
(L.Ac.) and Doctor of
Oriental Medicine (D.O.M.).

Homeopathic Academy
of Naturopathic Physicians
12132 S.E. Foster Place
Portland, OR 97266
Phone: (503) 761-3298
Fax: (503) 762-1929
Email: hanp@igc.apc.org
www.healthy.net/Pan/pa
/Homeopathic/hanp/
Licensed naturopathic physicians
board certified as diplomates
of the Homeopathic Academy
of Naturopathic Physicians
(DHANP).

The National Center
for Homeopathy
801 North Fairfax Street,
Suite 306
Alexandria, VA 22314
www.healthy.net/Pan/pa
/Homeopathic/Natcenhom/
Homeopathic practitioners
with various degrees.

International Academy of
Compounding Pharmacists
(IACP)
P.O. Box 1365
Sugar Land, TX 77487
Phone: (800) 927-4227
Fax: (281) 495-0602
www.iacprx.org
Pharmacists who compound
custom medications to meet
unique patient needs.

Professional Compounding
Centers of America
9901 S. Wilcrest
Houston, TX 77099
Phone: (800) 331-2498
Fax: (800) 874-5760
www.pccarx.com
Compounding pharmacists.

The North American
Menopause Society
P.O. Box 94527
Cleveland, OH 44101-4527
Phone: (440) 442-7550
www.menopause.org
The leading nonprofit scientific
organization devoted to promoting
understanding of menopause.

The American Academy
of Anti-Aging Medicine
2415 N. Greenview
Chicago, IL 60614
Phone: (773) 528-4333
Fax: (773) 528-5390
www.worldhealth.net
Physicians and scientists dedicated
to improve the quality of life while
extending the quantity of life.

The Institute for Functional Medicine
P.O. Box 1729
Gig Harbor, WA 98335
Phone: (800) 228-0622; (253) 858-4724
www.fxmed.com
A provider of educational activities
and materials on functional medicine.

Index